Contributions to Nephrology

Vol. 88

Series Editors
G. M. Berlyne, Brooklyn, N.Y.
S. Giovannetti, Pisa

Editorial Board
J. Churg, New York, N.Y.; *K. D. G. Edwards,* New York, N.Y.;
E. A. Friedman, Brooklyn, N.Y.; *S. G. Massry,* Los Angeles, Calif.;
R. E. Rieselbach, Milwaukee, Wisc.; *J. Traeger,* Lyon

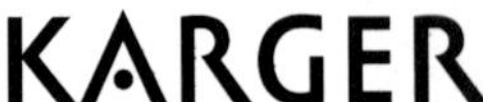

Basel · München · Paris · London · New York · New Delhi · Bangkok · Singapore · Tokyo · Sydney

Erythropoietin in Renal and Non-Renal Anemias

Update on Basic Research and Clinical Applications

Volume Editors

H. J. Gurland, Munich; *J. Moran,* Melbourne; *W. Samtleben,* Munich;
P. Scigalla, L. Wieczorek, Mannheim

101 figures and 77 tables, 1991

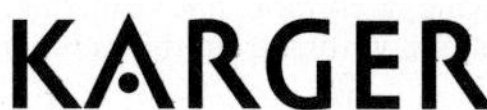

Basel · München · Paris · London · New York · New Delhi · Bangkok · Singapore · Tokyo · Sydney

Contributions to Nephrology

Library of Congress Cataloging-in-Publication Data
International Workshop on Treatment of Anemia with Recombinant Human Erythropoietin
(3rd: 1990: Telfs-Buchen, Austria)
Erythropoietin in renal and non-renal anemias: update on basic research and clinical applications /
3rd International Workshop on Treatment of Anemia with Recombinant Human Erythropoietin,
Telfs-Buchen, June 7–10, 1990; volume editors, H.J. Gurland... [et al.].
(Contributions to nephrology; vol. 88)
Includes bibliographical references.
Includes index.
1. Recombinant erythropoietin – Therapeutic use – Congresses.   2. Anemia – Hormone therapy –
Congresses.   3. Renal anemia – Hormone therapy – Congresses.   I. Gurland, H.J. (Hans Jürgen),
1930–.   II. Title.   III. Series: Contributions to nephrology; v. 88.
[DNLM: 1. Anemia – drug therapy – congresses.   2. Erythropoietin – genetics – congresses.
3. Erythropoietin – therapeutic use – congresses.   4. Recombinant Proteins – congresses.
W1 CO778UN v. 88 / WH 150 I618e 1991]
RC641.7.R44I57   1991
616.1'5206–dc20
ISBN 3-8055-5272-6

Bibliographic Indices
This publication is listed in bibliographic services, including Current Contents® and Index Medicus.

Contents

Treatment of Renal Anemia with Recombinant Human Erythropoietin

Safety Profile of Intravenous Treatment with Recombinant Human Erythropoietin in ESRD Patients

Experience with Subcutaneous Recombinant Human Erythropoietin in ESRD Patients

Experience with Recombinant Human Erythropoietin in Predialytic Renal Failure

Experience with Recombinant Human Erythropoietin in Children with Renal Anemia

Panel Discussion

Use of Recombinant Human Erythropoietin in Non-Renal Anemia and Surgery

Hematology and Oncology

Contents VIII

Infectious and Inflammatory Diseases

Neonatology

Surgery

Preface

The 3rd International Workshop on Treatment of Anemia with Recombinant Human Erythropoietin, following the 1st in Wolfenbüttel with 80 and the 2nd in Cologne with 120 participants, was held in Telfs-Buchen in the Austrian Alps, and was attended by 160 participants. The increase in the number of participants reflects the increasing use of erythropoietin and the importance of exchanging research and clinical experience with such a novel agent. Thirty-eight international experts participated as speakers or chairmen and made the workshop a significant and timely scientific event. At this meeting, indications other than the anemia of end-stage renal disease were discussed comprehensively for the first time. Important examples include the anemias of pre-end-stage renal disease, of cancer and of AIDS.

On behalf of all the participants we would like to express our gratitude to Boehringer Mannheim GmbH for enabling us to hold the meeting in such pleasant surroundings, with special thanks to Mr. Rühl for the faultless organization of the workshop. The efforts of Dr. Schöpe of Boehringer Mannheim GmbH and especially those of the staff of S. Karger AG, Basel, made a rapid publication of the proceedings possible.

In their concluding remarks Drs. Goldwasser and Eschbach evince the wide scope of erythropoietin research in both the basic and clinical areas presented at this meeting, and suggest future research directions. It is clear that more such workshops will be necessary!

The Editors

Advances in Basic Erythropoietin Research

Gurland HJ, Moran J, Samtleben W, Scigalla P, Wieczorek L (eds): Erythropoietin in
Renal and Non-Renal Anemias. Contrib Nephrol. Basel, Karger, 1991, vol 88, pp 2–7

The Regulation of Erythropoietin Gene Expression[1]

Eugene Goldwasser[a], *Nega Beru*[b]

[a]Department of Biochemistry and Molecular Biology, and [b]Department of Medicine,
Section of Hematology/Oncology, The University of Chicago, Chicago, Ill., USA

Regulation of the circulating erythropoietin (EPO) level in mammals is
most probably very complex, involving many factors that can operate to keep
the supply of oxygen to the tissues adequate for metabolic purposes. Some of
the regulatory mechanisms operate at the level of the expression of the EPO
gene [1, 2]. In adults, the major source of EPO is the kidney [3] but in fetal life
it is the liver [4], which is also an erythroid organ, and control of erythropoiesis
in the fetal liver may be a paracrine process. Adult liver also produces a small,
but finite amount of circulating EPO [5]. Nothing is yet known concerning the
fascinating problem of the mechanism of the switch from hepatic to renal EPO
formation that occurs about the time of birth.

The site of EPO formation in the kidney has been determined variously to
be either a small subset of endothelial, peritubular cells [6, 7], or epithelial,
tubular cells [8, 9]. Kidney tumors of tubular origin also have been shown to
produce EPO [10]. Additionally, it has been demonstrated by in situ hybridization studies that the response to increasing degree of anemic stress in mice
involves recruiting an increased number of cells expressing EPO mRNA
rather than by increasing the intensity of the signal per cell [11]. There is clearly
much more work needed to clarify the exact nature of the renal cells that can
sense an oxygen deficit and respond by increasing EPO secretion.

Some important progress has been made in the study of the mechanism by
which cells (in this case a human hepatocarcinoma cell line) can detect a
change in oxygen availability. As will be discussed in detail later in this

[1] The work described was done with funding from the National Heart, Lung and Blood
Institute, National Institutes of Health (grants HL30121 and HL21676) to E.G. and the
American Cancer Society, Illinois Division, Inc. (grant 90–16) to N.B.

5′<u>CCCCCACCCCCACCCGC</u>GCACGCACACATGC3′

−61   −31

Fig. 1. Upstream sequence identical in mouse and human EPO genes. Numbering starts at the start site of transcription of the mouse gene. The 17 mer (EP17) used for the mobility shift assays is underlined.

symposium, this process appears to involve a membrane bound heme protein [12]. The linkage between sensing an oxygen deficit at the cell surface and communicating that to the cell nucleus to activate the EPO gene is still not at all understood, although it does not appear to involve any of the usual second messengers.

At the level of nuclear function we have been studying the possible role of trans-acting factors in the regulation of EPO gene expression [13]. These experiments were initiated when we found a region of the near upstream sequences of the human and mouse EPO gene to be identical for the two species (fig. 1). We used a synthetic oligodeoxynucleotide (31 mer) end-labeled with ^{32}P to search, by the mobility shift assay, for factors that might bind to this sequence. In extracts of mouse kidney nuclei we found clear evidence for such binding factors; the binding was competed for by unlabeled homologous oligonucleotide but not by irrelevant oligonucleotides. Further study by this method showed that only the 17 base sequence at the 5′ end of the 31 mer was involved in the binding and that 17 mer (EP17) was used for subsequent experiments. The 3′ portion (EP14) was used as a control in some experiments.

To summarize our findings: (a) binding of material contained in extracts of kidney cell nuclei to the 17 base oligonucleotide is specific for that sequence (fig. 2); (b) cross-linking experiments show that there is a protein of mass about 47,000 that binds to the 17 mer and is present in kidney nuclei from normal and stimulated mice (fig. 3a); (c) in normal kidney nuclei there are, at least, four ribonucleoproteins present that can bind to the specific 17 mer (fig. 3b), and (d) at least one of the ribonucleoproteins in kidney cell nuclei (fig. 3a, I) decreases very significantly upon stimulation with cobalt chloride and hypoxia (fig. 4). The amount of this RNA-containing binding factor in kidney extracts from animals stimulated by hypoxia was decreased severalfold relative to unstimulated controls, but not decreased to the same extent as in cobalt-treated animals. This may be due to the type and time of stimulation used. We have found that cobalt causes increased EPO gene expression in

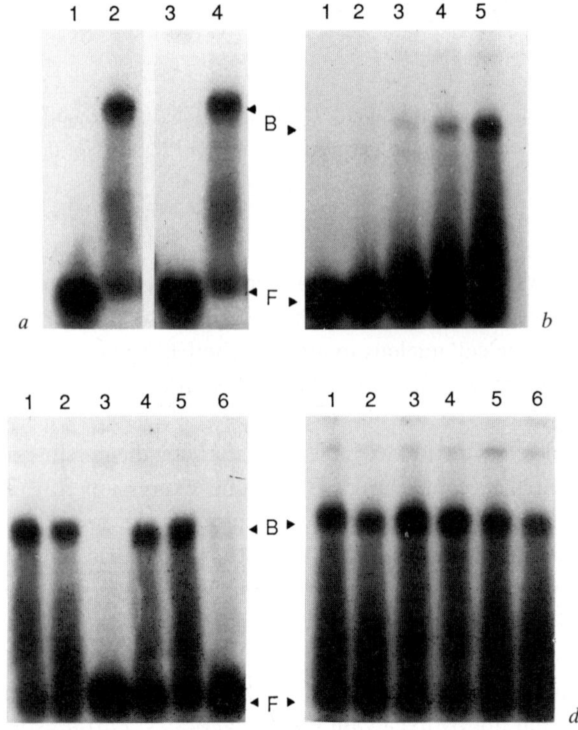

Fig. 2. Presence of trans-acting factors binding to EP17. *a* Mobility shift assay using ^{32}P-EP17 or ^{32}P-14 and about 7 µg of nuclear extract either from the kidneys of control animals (1,2) or those injected with cobalt (3,4). 1, 3 binding using ^{32}P-EP14; 2, 4, binding using ^{32}P-EP17. *b* Mobility shift assay using ^{32}P-EP17 and 0.5 (lane 1), 1 (lane 2), 2 (lane 3), 4 (lane 4) and 6 µg (lane 5) of extract. *c* Mobility shift assay using ^{32}P-EP17 and 9 µg of kidney nuclear extract in the absence of competitor (lane 1) and presence of 500-fold molar excess of EP14 (lane 2), EP17 (lane 3), EP19 (lane 4), EP22 (lane 5) and EP31 (lane 6). *d* Mobility shift assay using ^{32}P-EP17 and 9 µg of kidney nuclear extract using 3 types of bulk nonspecific competitor DNA. 1 and 4 µg of poly(dA-dT) · poly(dA-dT), lanes 1 and 2; 1 and 4 µg of poly(dG-dC) · poly(dG-dC), lanes 3 and 4; 1 and 4 µg of poly(dI-dC) · poly(dI-dC), lanes 5 and 6. B = Bound ^{32}P-EP17; F = free ^{32}P-EP17. From 13, with permission.

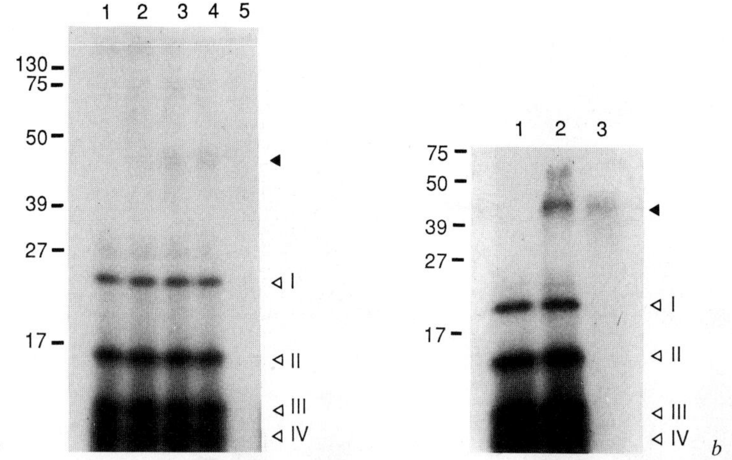

Fig. 3. Analysis of EP17-bound factors by SDS-PAGE. *a* Binding assay using ^{32}P-EP17 and 7 µg of extract from the kidney of control animals was set up and exposed to UV light for 0 (lane 1), 5 (lane 2), 15 (lane 3) and 30 min (lanes 4 and 5). Lanes 1–4 were in the absence of excess unlabeled EP17 while lane 5 was in the presence of 500-fold molar excess of unlabeled EP17. The positions of the protein molecular weight standards are indicated. *b* The 47-kd factor (indicated by a closed arrow) is protease-sensitive while the low molecular weight factors (indicated by open arrows) are RNase-sensitive but protease-resistant. Binding assays were set up as above and exposed to UV light for 30 min followed by treatment with 20 µg of proteinase K in the presence of 0.5% SDS for 1 h at 50°C (lane 1); 0.5% SDS for 1 h at 50°C (lane 2); 10 µg of RNase A for 1 h at 37°C (lane 3). From 13, with permission.

mice sometime between 7 and 10 h following injection, as determined by Northern blotting [1]. In the present experiment the interval was 6 h because we were interested in the early events during EPO gene activation. Under these conditions the serum EPO level was 47 mU/ml (contrasted to 5 mU/ml in controls); hypoxia on the other hand causes an earlier switch-on of the EPO gene [14] and at 5 h, the time at which we harvested the kidneys for this experiment, the serum EPO level was 485 mU/ml. The smaller decrease in amount of RNA-containing, trans-acting factor using hypoxic vs. cobalt stimuli could well have been due to the response to hypoxia being more rapid and past its maximal effect by the time we extracted the kidneys.

We propose the following: the EPO gene is under dual control by trans-acting factors; the 47-kd protein may be a positive acting factor formed constitutively. It does not activate the EPO gene until one or more of the ribonucleoproteins that bind to the same sequence has been dissociated from

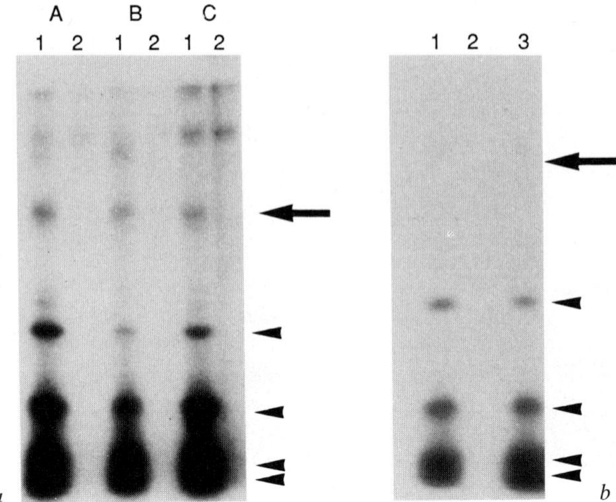

Fig. 4. Comparison of the levels of various factors that bind to EP17 in extracts of kidneys from control animals as well as animals subjected to hypoxic stimulation. *a* Binding assays were carried out using ^{32}P-EP17 and kidney nuclear extracts from control mice (A: 7 µg extract), mice injected with cobalt (B: 5 µg extract) and mice subjected to hypoxia (C: 12 µg extract) in the absence of competitor (lane 1) or 500-fold molar excess of the unlabeled EP17 (lane 2). Following exposure to UV light for 30 min, EP17-bound factors were resolved by SDS-PAGE on 12% polyacrylamide gels. The four RNA species that bind to EP17 as well as the 47-kd protein are indicated by triangles, the 47-kd protein is indicated by arrows. The high molecular weight RNA species is greatly reduced in the extracts derived from the animals stimulated by cobalt or hypoxia while the 47-kd protein is relatively unaffected. *b* The same experiment as above showing that binding of the factors to EP17 is specific. The binding assays were carried out in the absence of competitor (lane 1), presence of 500-fold molar excess EP17 (lane 2) or 500-fold molar excess of EP22 (lane 3). From 13, with permission.

the chromosome or until the synthesis of that ribonucleoprotein has been arrested. Activation of the EPO gene then, at a minimum, would involve loss of the negative trans-acting factor (ribonucleoprotein) upon cobalt or hypoxic stimulation and positive, stimulatory interaction of the 47-kd protein with the same site on the chromosome, resulting in transcription of the EPO gene.

The molecular nature of these trans-acting factors, the details of their interaction with the EPO gene and the regulation of the expression of the genes for these factors need to be understood before a complete analysis of the regulation of EPO secretion can be presented. These topics are currently under intensive study.

References

1 Beru N, McDonald J, Lacombe C, Goldwasser E: Expression of the erythropoietin gene. Mol Cell Biol 1986;6:2571–2575.
2 Schuster SJ, Badiavas EV, Costa-Giomi P, Weinman R, Erslev AJ, Caro J: Stimulation of erythropoietin gene transcription during hypoxia and cobalt exposure. Blood 1989;73:13–16.
3 Jacobson LO, Goldwasser E, Fried W, Plzak LF: Role of the kidney in erythropoiesis. Nature 1957;179:633–634.
4 Zanjani ED, Foster I, Burlington H, Wasserman LR: Liver as the primary site of erythropoietin formation in the fetus. J Lab Clin Med 1977;89:640–644.
5 Fried W: The liver as a source of extrarenal erythropoietin production. Blood 1972;40:671–677.
6 Lacombe C, DaSilva JL, Bruneval P, Fournier J-G, Wendling F, Casadevall N, Camilleri J-P, Bariety J, Varet B, Tambourin P: Peritubular cells are the site of erythropoietin synthesis in the murine hypoxic kidney. J Clin Invest 1987;81:620–623.
7 Koury ST, Bondurant MC, Koury MJ: Localization of erythropoietin synthesizing cells in murine kidneys by in situ hybridization. Blood 1987;71:524–527.
8 Maxwell AP, Lappin TRJ, Johnston CF, Bridges JM, McGeown MG: Erythropoietin gene expression in kidney tissue detected by in situ hybridization. Br J Haematol 1990;74:535–539.
9 Maples PB, Smith DH, Beru N, Goldwasser E: Identification of EPO-producing cells in mammalian tissue by in situ hybridization. Blood 1986;68:170A.
10 Da Silva JL, Lacombe C, Bruneval P, Casadevall N, Leporrier M, Camilleri J-P, Bariety J, Tambourin P, Varet B: Tumor cells are the site of erythropoietin synthesis in human renal cancers associated with polycythemia. Blood 1990;75:577–582.
11 Koury ST, Koury M, Bondurant MC, Caro J, Graber S: Quantitation of erythropoietin-producing cells in kidneys of mice by in situ hybridization: Correlation with hematocrit, renal erythropoietin mRNA and serum erythropoietin concentration. Blood 1989;74:645–651.
12 Goldberg MA, Dunning SP, Bunn HF: Regulation of the erythropoietin gene: Evidence that the oxygen sensor is a heme protein. Science 1988;242:1412–1415.
13 Beru N, Smith D, Goldwasser E: Evidence suggesting negative regulation of the erythropoietin gene by ribonucleoprotein. J Biol Chem, in press.
14 Nishida J, Hirai H, Kubota M, Lin F-K, Okabe T, Urabe A, Takaku F: Detection of erythropoietin message in hypoxic mouse kidney. Jpn J Exp Med 1986;56:321–323.

Eugene Goldwasser, PhD, Department of Biochemistry and Molecular Biology, The University of Chicago, 920 East 58th Street, Chicago, IL 60637 (USA)

Gurland HJ, Moran J, Samtleben W, Scigalla P, Wieczorek L (eds): Erythropoietin in Renal and Non-Renal Anemias. Contrib Nephrol. Basel, Karger, 1991, vol 88, pp 8–9

Discussion

to the Paper by E. Goldwasser and N. Beru

Kurtz (Zurich): You suggest from your data that the regulation of hypoxia-induced EPO production includes a region of the EPO gene very close to the starting point of transcription. On the other hand, there are the data from Semenza in the transgenic mouse. They suggested that, at least in the kidney, hypoxia-induced regulation of EPO formation occurs far more distant from the transcription initiation site.

Goldwasser: Their interpretation does not concern negative regulation but what they are saying, if I remember the paper correctly, is that positive regulation does not occur nearby. Therefore, it must occur some distance away, beyond the scope of the constructs they have used. I hope I did not get too enthusiastic about the close-in control; I think the control is multifactorial. What we are describing may be necessary but not sufficient. I think the experiments with the transgenic mice may not be suitable for addressing negative controls, which is what we have been finding. They were looking for positive control elements.

Rich (Ulm): You postulated an on/off mechanism for EPO. As you know, EPO is really modulated, so how do you explain this modulation with respect to the model you have postulated here?

Goldwasser: The modulation of EPO expression was shown fairly clearly by Mark Koury's experiments, which demonstrate that hypoxia causes recruitment of cells rather than increased activity per cell. I think that is a very important result. What we may be seeing, although we don't understand all the details, is how cells become recruited. I think our model, crude as it is, is compatible with an all-or-none mechanism of the cell being recruited. In view of Mark Koury's data, I might suggest that there are regional differences in the kidney, and that the cells which are on all the time and produce the steady state level of 20 mU/ml in man are in at a site where the kidney is hypoxic enough so that they are turned on by the same mechanism. And as hypoxia becomes more extensive, more cells are recruited, using the same mechanism of removing the negative suppressor and permitting the positive trans-acting factor to operate. That is a crude answer to an elegant question.

Cotes (Harrow): Has the glycosylation of the IW32 EPO been studied? Is glycosylation of the abnormal gene EPO identical with that of normal mouse EPO?

Goldwasser: That is one of the hard problems. The mouse EPO that is formed in IW32, Dr. Lacombe can bear me out, appears to be similar in all respects to serum EPO from anemic mice. The exact carbohydrate structure of neither is known. In order to do that, someone is going to have to express the mouse gene and get a very large quantity of pure mouse EPO to do the rather difficult job of looking at the structure of the carbohydrate. I'd love to know the answer but I wouldn't like to do the experiment.

Erslev (Philadelphia): You have on occasion proposed the existence of a number of different erythropoietins. What is the data right now on the difference, if any, between the hepatic EPO, the renal EPO, the cobalt-induced EPO and the hypoxia-induced EPO?

Goldwasser: I don't think I ever proposed any different erythropoietins. I think the evidence right now is virtually iron-clad: there is one EPO gene, it's a single-copy gene, therefore, whatever is made in whatever tissue is making it, under whatever stimulus you propose, is going to be the same material. I don't think we can find a way out of that, it has to be the same. There may be slight differences in glycosylation pattern depending on the cell, although I wouldn't be too sure about that, because Chinese hamster ovary cells seem to make the same carbohydrate structure as the human kidney. So I don't think, and I hope that I never said publicly, that there is anything but a single EPO.

Goldberg (Boston): I found your model very interesting. You described oxygen binding to the receptor on the cell surface. You don't necessarily have to have the receptor on the cell surface since oxygen can diffuse into the cell. I was wondering, is it possible, for example, that your 47-kD protein might contain a heme moiety, or might change conformation with hypoxia. Although it's difficult to do DNA band-shifts in hypoxia, is it possible that you might see different binding or an increase in binding if you ran your gels hypoxically versus non-hypoxically?

Goldwasser: That's a very good idea. I put the hypoxic sensor at the cell membrane in honour of a very important paper by Goldberg and Bunn. And because esthetically it seems rather pleasing to have it there. The data, as you know, are not yet definitive. I like the idea of the 47-kD protein being a hypoxic sensor or an oxygen binder. We don't have enough of it yet to do even the most rudimentary kind of study of its properties, but we're in the process of cloning it. The recent method of Singh makes cloning such a protein relatively simple, because we have the probe in hand. If we can clone it and express it in a mammalian cell, we can ask the question very easily whether it does have heme in it, and that's obviously one of the things we will do and let you know by phone.

Gurland HJ, Moran J, Samtleben W, Scigalla P, Wieczorek L (eds): Erythropoietin in
Renal and Non-Renal Anemias. Contrib Nephrol. Basel, Karger, 1991, vol 88, pp 10–16

Transcriptional Regulation of the Erythropoietin Gene

J. Caro, P. Costa-Giomi, I. Beck, S. Ramirez, S.J. Schuster

Cardeza Foundation for Hematologic Research, Thomas Jefferson Medical College,
Philadelphia, Pa., USA

Erythropoietin is the glycoprotein growth factor that regulates red cell
production by stimulating proliferation and differentiation of erythroid precursor cells. Originally purified in small quantities from human urine [1] it is
now massively produced by recombinant DNA techniques and used for the
treatment of various anemias. Since the early work by Jacobson et al. [2] the
kidney has been known to be the main source of erythropoietin production.
While extrarenal sources also exist, they probably do not account for more
than 10–15% of total [3] erythropoietin production in adult individuals.

Erythropoietin synthesis and secretion is greatly stimulated by anemic or
hypoxic hypoxia and also by pharmacological exposure to cobalt chloride. In
patients with various types of anemias, plasma erythropoietin levels increase
exponentially and levels as high as 1,000 times normal and found in cases of
severe anemias [4]. In patients with renal diseases, however, the erythropoietin response to anemia is markedly blunted [5].

The recent cloning of the human [6, 7] and mouse [8, 9] erythropoietin
genes has increased enormously our understanding of the mechanism that
regulate erythropoietin production. There appears to be only one gene for
erythropoietin in the human genome, localized in chromosome 7. The erythropoietin gene is composed by five exons which encode for a 27 amino acids
leader sequence followed by a 166 amino acids mature protein. Comparison of
coding sequences between the mouse and human genes reveals about 80%
homology between both species. However, the most highly conserved sequence of the gene with more than 90% homology is located within about 150
bp 5' upstream of the transcription start site. This high degree of homology
between different species suggests that important regulatory sequences are
probably contained in this region.

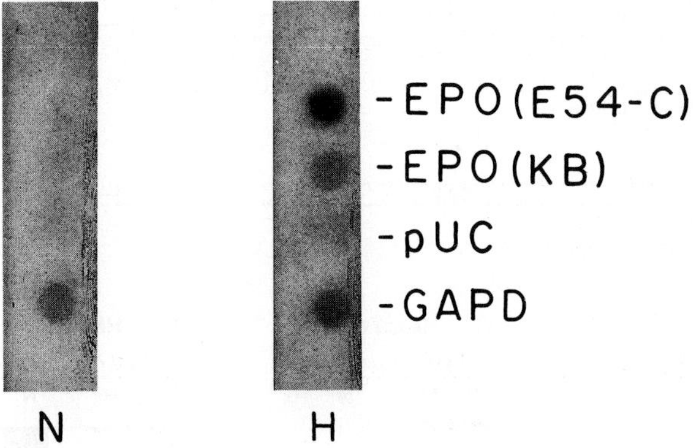

Fig. 1. Effect of hypoxia on erythropoietin gene transcription in Hep 3B cells. Nuclei were isolated from normal (N) or hypoxic (H) cells and incubated in vitro with ^{32}P UTP. Labelled RNA transcripts were hybridized against human erythropoietin cDNA (E54-C and KB) and against glyceraldehyde phosphate dehydrogenase (GAPD) cDNA.

Studies in experimental animals have shown that exposure to anemia, hypoxia or cobalt result in a rapid accumulation of erythropoietin mRNA in the kidney that precedes the appearance of the hormone in the plasma [10–12]. Discontinuation of the stimulus results in a rapid disappearance of the erythropoietin messenger [12]. It thus appears that erythropoietin synthesis is regulated at the level of its specific mRNA and that these levels follow very closely the degree of tissue oxygenation. Regulated expression of the erythropoietin gene has also been recently described in human hepatoma cell lines [13]. These cell lines respond to hypoxia or cobalt in vitro with accumulation of erythropoietin mRNA and secretion of the hormone to the culture medium.

Transcriptional activation of the erythropoietin gene appears to play a primary role in regulation of erythropoietin mRNA levels in the response to hypoxia or stimulation by cobalt. Run-on assays utilizing isolated nuclei from normal or hypoxic rat kidneys have shown a significant increase in transcription rate of the erythropoietin gene in stimulated animals [14]. A similar effect on transcription has been observed in the hepatoma cell line Hep 3B when exposed to 1% oxygen. Figure 1 shows a run-on assay using isolated nuclei from normal and hypoxic stimulated Hep 3B cells. As shown, the transcription rate of the erythropoietin gene is greatly increased in the hypoxic as compared

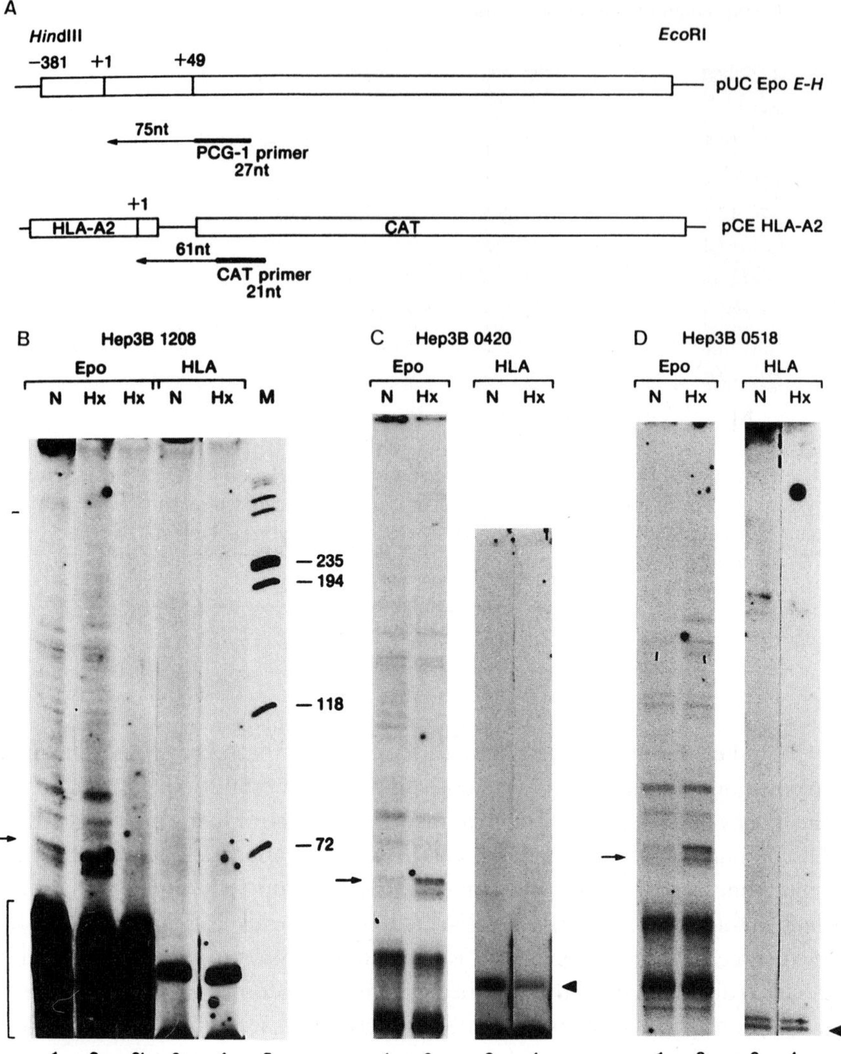

Fig. 2. In vitro transcription of the human erythropoietin gene by nuclear extracts of normal (N) or hypoxic (H) Hep 3B cells. *A* Diagram of the erythropoietin (pUC Epo E-H) and HLA (pCE HLA-A2) templates utilized for in vitro transcription analysis. Primers for erythropoietin (PCG-1) and HLA (CAT) are indicated. The diagram indicates also the predicted length of the primer extension products corresponding to in vitro synthesized RNA from erythropoietin promoter (75 nucleotides) and HLA promoter (61 nucleotides). *B – D* Results of primer extension analysis of in vitro transcription from three different nuclear extract preparations. Lanes 1 and 2 correspond to the erythropoietin gene and lanes 3 and 4 to the HLA gene (transcript products are indicated by arrows). Lane 2' in *A* corresponds to a reaction performed in the presence of α-amanitin (1 mg/ml).

with normal nuclei. In order to study further the mechanisms that regulate transcription of the erythropoietin gene, we have prepared nuclear extracts from Hep 3B cells which accurately transcribe the erythropoietin gene and reproduce in vitro the response to hypoxia. Nuclei were isolated from suspensions of normal or hypoxic Hep 3B cells and extracts were prepared after precipitation of DNA essentially as described [15]. These nuclear extracts were utilized for in vitro transcription reactions using as DNA template an erythropoietin genomic fragment containing 380 bp of 5′ flanking region. An unrelated DNA template, the major histocompatibility gene (HLA), was used as control for transcription. In vitro transcription reactions were carried out as already described [15] and the RNAs transcribed in vitro were analyzed by 5′ extension reactions. Figure 2A depicts the templates and primers utilized and figure 2B shows results of in vitro transcription reactions from three independent, normal and hypoxic nuclear extract preparations. As seen, the erythropoietin gene is expressed more intensively in the hypoxic than in the normal extracts. No differences in expression were observed with the HLA gene suggesting that the hypoxia-induced enhanced transcription is specific for the erythropoietin gene. Moreover, nuclear extracts prepared from HeLa cells, a non-erythropoietin producing cell line, failed to show differences in erythropoietin gene transcription between normal or hypoxic extracts (not shown). This data suggests that nuclear extracts obtained from hypoxic Hep 3B cells contain functional factors that can specifically stimulate transcription of the erythropoietin gene. These factors appear not to be present in HeLa cells. Furthermore, it indicates that DNA sequences contained in the erythropoietin genomic fragment utilized (which included 380 bp 5′ and about 600 bp 3′ flanking regions) were sufficient to confer regulated hypoxia responsiveness in Hep 3B cells. These results agree with results published recently by Semenza et al. [16] in transgenic mice, where a similar genomic fragment was sufficient to confer hypoxia responsiveness and expression in the liver but not in the kidney of transgenic animals.

Information regarding regulatory elements necessary for regulated expression of the erythropoietin gene was also obtained by the use of transient transfection assays in Hep 3B cells. Erythropoietin mini-genes were constructed by deletion of internal sequences of the human erythropoietin gene and utilized for transient transfections. As shown in figure 3 deletions of Kpn-Hinc II or Kpn-Acc fragments result in two mini-genes whose mRNA would be 201 and 384 nt respectively shorter than the normal RNA transcript. Northern blot analysis of RNA from normal and hypoxic cells transfected with erythropoietin mini-genes are shown in figure 4. The mini-genes were introduced by

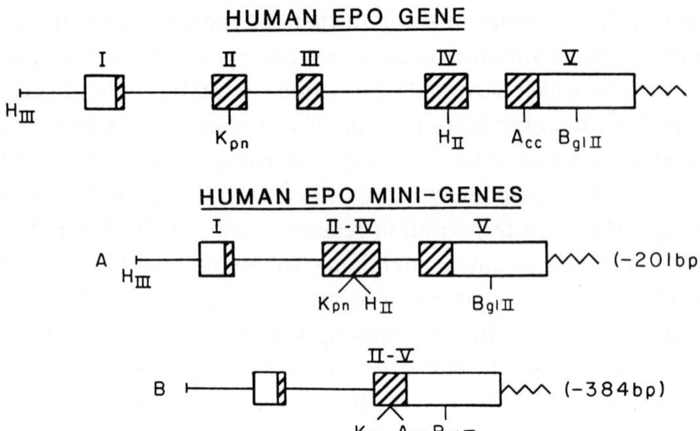

Fig. 3. Diagram represents the structure of the human erythropoietin gene and mini-gene constructs. Mini-gene A results from deletion of a Kpn-Hinc II fragment (201 bp) and mini-gene B is the result of a Kpn-Acc (384 bp) deletion.

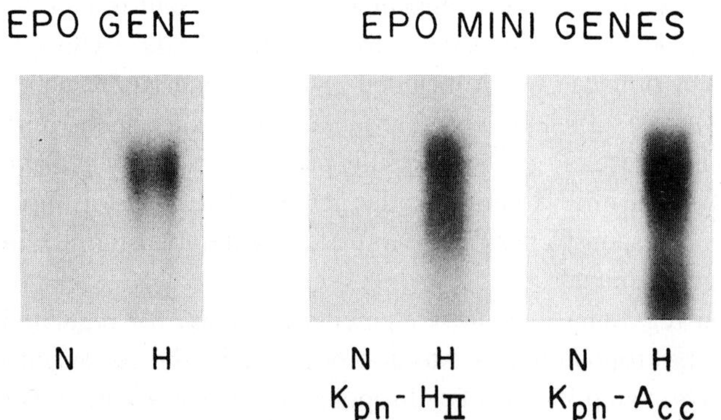

Fig. 4. Expression of mini-genes in transfected Hep 3B cells. Mini-genes containing 380 bp of 5' upstream region were transfected by electroporation Hep 3B cells. Forty-eight hours later the cells were either maintained at normoxic conditions (N) or stimulated with hypoxia (H) for 16 h. Northern blot analysis utilizing a human erythropoietin cDNA are shown. Left panel shows nontransfected cells, middle and right panels are cells transfected with the Kpn-Hinc II and Kpn-Acc mini-genes respectively.

electroporation into Hep 3B cells, RNA extracted and analyzed using a human erythropoietin cDNA probe. As shown, both mini-genes are expressed in Hep 3B cells after exposure to hypoxia, paralleling the expression of the erythropoietin endogenous gene. These results confirm the results of in vitro transcription suggesting that genomic sequences comprised between -380 5' and $+600$ 3' of the erythropoietin gene are sufficient to confer regulated expression in Hep 3B cells. Unfortunately, it is not yet clear whether the same sequences would be sufficient for regulated expression of the erythropoietin gene in kidney cells.

References

1 Miyake, T.; Kung, C. K. H.; Goldwasser, E.: Purification of human erythropoietin. J. Biol. Chem. *252:* 5558–5564 (1977).
2 Jacobson, L. O.; Goldwasser, E.; Fried, W.; Plzak, L.: Role of the kidney in erythropoiesis. Nature *179:* 633–634 (1957).
3 Erslev, A. J.; Caro, J.; Kansu, E.; Silver, R.: Renal and extrarenal erythropoietin production in anaemic rats. Br. J. Haematol. *45:* 65–72 (1980).
4 Erslev, A. J.; Wilson, J.; Caro, J.: Erythropoietin titers in anemic, nonuremic patients. J. Lab. Clin. Med. *109:* 429–433 (1987).
5 Caro, J.; Brown, S.; Miller, O. P.; Murray, T.; Erslev, A. J.: Erythropoietin levels in uremic nephric and anephric patients. J. Lab. Clin. Med. *93:* 449–458 (1979).
6 Lin, F.-K.; Suggs, S.; Lin, C.-H.; Browne, J. K.; Smalling, R.; Egrie, J. C.; Chen, K. K.; Fox, G. M.; Martin, F.; Stabinsky, Z.; Badrawi, S. M.; Lai, P.-H.; Goldwasser, E.: Cloning and expression of the human erythropoietin gene. Proc. Natl. Acad. Sci. USA *82:* 7580–7584 (1985).
7 Jacobs, K.; Shoemaker, C.; Rudersdorf, R.; Neill, S. D.; Kaufman, R. J.; Mufson, A.; Seehra, J.; Jones, S. S.; Hewick, R.; Fritsch, E. F.; Kawakita, M.; Shimizu, T.; Miyake, T.: Isolation and characterization of genomic and cDNA clones of human EPO. Nature *313:* 806–810 (1985).
8 Shoemaker, C.; Mitsock, L. D.: Murine erythropoietin gene: cloning, expression and human gene homology. Mol. Cell. Biol. *6:* 849–858 (1986).
9 McDonald, J. D.; Lin, F.-K.; Goldwasser, E.: Cloning, sequencing, and evolutionary analysis of the mouse erythropoietin gene. Mol. Cell. Biol. *6:* 842–848 (1986).
10 Beru, W.; McDonald, J.; Lacombe, C.; Goldwasser, E.: Expression of the mouse erythropoietin gene. Mol. Cell. Biol. *6:* 2571–2575 (1986).
11 Bondurant, M. C.; Koury, M. J.: Anemia induces accumulation of erythropoietin mRNA in the kidney and liver. Mol. Cell. Biol. *6:* 2731–2733 (1986).
12 Schuster, S. J.; Wilson, J. H.; Erslev, A. J.; Caro, J.: Physiologic regulation and tissue localization of renal erythropoietin messenger RNA. Blood *70:* 316–318 (1987).
13 Goldberg, M. A.; Glass, G. A.; Cunningham, J. M.; Bunn, H. F.: The regulated expression of erythropoietin by two human hepatoma cell lines. Proc. Natl. Acad. Sci. USA *84:* 7972–7976 (1987).

14 Schuster, S. J.; Badiavas, E. V.; Costa-Giomi, P.; Weinmann, R.; Erslev, A. J.; Caro, J.: Stimulation of erythropoietin gene transcription during hypoxia and cobalt exposure. Blood *73:* 13–16 (1989).
15 Costa-Giomi, P.; Caro, J.; Weinmann, R.: Enhancement by hypoxia of human erythropoietin gene transcription in vitro. J. Biol. Chem. *265:* 10185–10188 (1990).
16 Semenza, G. L.; Dureza, R. C.; Traystman, M. D.; Gearhart, J. D.; Antonarakis, S. E.: Human erythropoietin gene expression in transgenic mice: multiple transcription initiation sites and *cis*-acting regulatory elements. Mol. Cell. Biol. *10:* 930–938 (1990).

J. Caro, MD, Cardeza Foundation for Hematologic Research, Thomas Jefferson Medical College, 1015 Walnut Street, Philadelphia, PA 19107 (USA)

Gurland HJ, Moran J, Samtleben W, Scigalla P, Wieczorek L (eds): Erythropoietin in
Renal and Non-Renal Anemias. Contrib Nephrol. Basel, Karger, 1991, vol 88, p 17

Discussion

to the Paper by J. Caro et al.

Lacombe (Paris): Did you try using antibodies such as Mac 1, F4/80, or anti-von Willebrand factor to characterise these small cells?

Caro: We are in the process of trying to characterize them. It has been more difficult than what we thought. We are using von Willebrand factor for the small cells, cytokeratins for the large cells, and we also have probes for both. I cannot tell you what they are yet.

Rich (Ulm): Perhaps I can get into the controversy of EPO localisation too. Using non-radioactive in situ hybridization we have obtained similar results to those of Maxwell, and have found gene expression in mouse tubular cells rather than in peritubular cells. We have recently extended those studies using human kidney. In this case we have used oligonucleotide 40mers and again found positive in situ hybridization in the human tubular cells. As you say, there are three groups for the peritubular cell and two against at the moment.

Goldberg (Boston): With your in vitro transcription assays that you did on the HEP3B cells – although you used hypoxic extracts – have you ever tried taking those extracts and doing the transcription hypoxically? I don't think you can assume that because you expose under hypoxia you made something that wasn't there before. It may well be a change in something that is already there, and you may need continued hypoxia to see an optimal effect. So whereas you saw a three-or fivefold effect, you might see a much greater one if you actually did it hypoxically.

Caro: That's right. First of all, it is very difficult to prepare the nuclear extract under completely hypoxic conditions. We have tried using xenon in our incubation mixtures, since it is heavier than oxygen and will displace oxygen from the reaction, but it has been very difficult to be sure that we have maintained hypoxic conditions all the way through. It is possible that we don't see a bigger difference between normal and hypoxic extracts because these factors may be very labile, and while we are doing the extractions these factors already may be deactivated. We have thought about that, but technically it is very, very difficult since we are dealing with a large volume of cells.

Gurland HJ, Moran J, Samtleben W, Scigalla P, Wieczorek L (eds): Erythropoietin in
Renal and Non-Renal Anemias. Contrib Nephrol. Basel, Karger, 1991, vol 88, pp 18–31

Unutilized Reserves: The Production Capacity for Erythropoietin Appears to Be Conserved in Chronic Renal Disease

Kai-Uwe Eckardt[a], *Tilman Drüeke*[b], *Michel Leski*[c], *Armin Kurtz*[a,1]

[a]Physiologisches Institut der Universität Zürich, Switzerland; [b]Département de
Néphrologie, INSERM U90, Hôpital Necker, Paris, France, and [c]Division de
Néphrologie, Hôpital Cantonal Universitaire, Genève, Switzerland

A relative deficiency of erythropoietin (EPO) has been recognized as the
major reason for the anemia accompanying chronic renal failure (CRF).
While in nonrenal anemias any reduction in hemoglobin results in an exponen-
tial rise in serum EPO, EPO levels in CRF remain within, only slightly above
or even below the normal range (fig. 1). There even appears to be a positive
correlation between EPO levels and hemoglobin, suggesting that hemoglobin
concentrations are determined by a given amount of EPO produced instead of
circulating EPO levels responding to a fall in red cell mass. The reason why the
adaptation of EPO levels to hemoglobin concentrations is lost during end-
stage renal disease has not been investigated systematically. Since the damage
to the kidneys in chronic renal disease is usually associated with a dramatic
decrease in renal cell mass it is generally assumed that destruction of renal
EPO producing cells is the reason for inappropriately low EPO production.
An alternative explanation that has so far not been sufficiently considered is
that it is not the capability to produce EPO but rather the adaptation of EPO
production to the hemoglobin concentration (commonly referred to as the
oxygen sensor function) that is disturbed during CRF.

In this paper we will summarize some evidence in favor of this second
possibility, that may arise in subgroups of renal patients or in certain clinical
settings. In particular, we will consider EPO production by renal patients in
response to acute hypoxia, and in situations where renal anemia is less severe

---

[1] We are grateful to Dr. U. Nattermann, Munich, for allowing us to present data from his
patients.

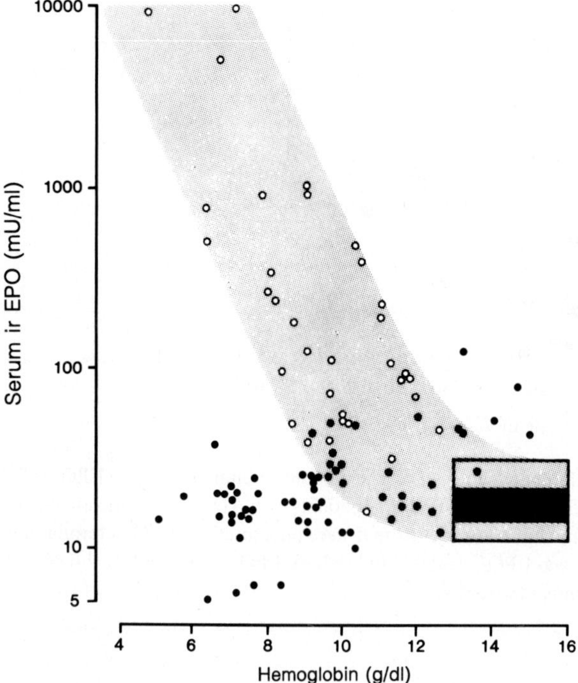

Fig. 1. Relationship between serum immunoreactive EPO (ir EPO) levels and hemoglobin concentrations in hypo- and hyperregenerative nonrenal anemias (○) and in patients with CRF (●) (excluding only patients with polycystic kidney disease). The rectangle depicts interquartile range (dark stippled) and 95% confidence range of EPO levels in nonanemic healthy adults. Values in renal failure patients were determined prior to kidney transplantation. [Reproduced with permission from 1.]

than usual, as in polycystic kidney disease, or improves during the course of renal failure, as may be observed after parathyroidectomy, or is even 'overcorrected' as in patients developing polycythemia after renal allotransplantation.

EPO Levels in Uremic Patients with Polycystic Kidney Disease

The assumption that severe kidney damage resulting in negligible excretory function does not necessarily extinguish the endocrine reserve for EPO production is clearly substantiated in patients with autosomal-dominant poly-

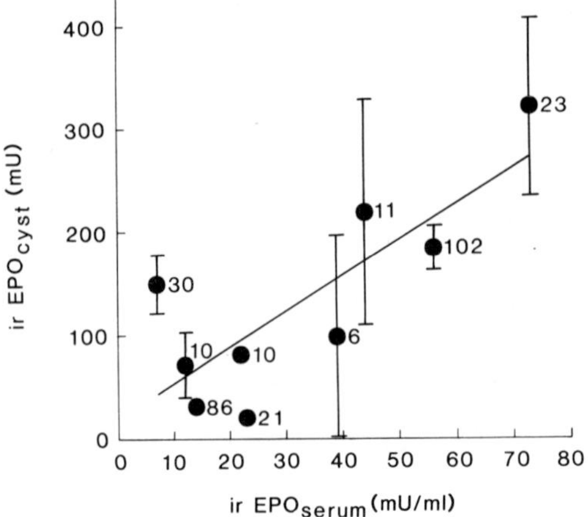

Fig. 2. Relationship between the average amount of immunoreactive EPO (ir EPO) in renal cysts and serum EPO concentrations in 9 patients with ADPKD. Values are mean ± SE; the numbers indicate the numbers of cysts that were punctured for EPO determination. The linear regression curve was EPO_{cyst} (mU) = 19.1 + 3.5 × EPO_{serum} (mU/ml) (r = 0.80; p<0.01). [Reproduced with permission from 4.]

cystic kidney disease (ADPKD). If it occurs at all, renal anemia is often strikingly mild in ADPKD. Plasma EPO levels in these patients have been found to be on average twofold higher than in patients with CRF of other etiologies [2, 3], suggesting that the better hematological situation in this particular renal disease is due to increased availability of EPO. In fact, we have recently obtained direct evidence for substantial EPO production by polycystic kidneys by measuring a significant difference in serum EPO levels between renal arteries and veins (23.8±8.2 vs. 35.4±10.1 mU/ml; mean ± SE; n = 5) and high EPO concentrations in cyst fluid, most likely resulting from intrarenal EPO formation [4]. The amount of EPO found in cysts appeared to reflect the production capacity for the hormone, since it was positively correlated with serum levels (fig. 2). Thus, polycystic kidneys without excretory function appear capable of producing sufficient EPO to maintain near normal erythropoiesis in a uremic individual. Interestingly however, EPO levels in ADPKD also fail to display the characteristic inverse relationship to the circulating hemoglobin concentration, but rather are positively correlated with hemoglobin levels [3], suggesting that the production capacity but not the 'physiological' regulation of EPO is retained.

The comparatively high EPO secretion rate in ADPKD appears not to be genetically linked to the underlying cystic disease since increased serum EPO levels were also found to accompany secondary cyst formation in long-term hemodialysis patients [5]. Furthermore, although in no subgroup of renal disease other than cystic kidneys has a sustained elevation of serum EPO so regularly been observed, quite significant temporary increases in EPO may also be seen in other renal failure patients, indicating that cyst formation in damaged kidneys is not a prerequisite for EPO formation, although it might promote it. Examples of increased EPO production independent of the etiology of renal disease include acute hypoxic episodes and, as recently observed, parathyroidectomy.

EPO Levels in Uremic Patients Experiencing Hypoxic Episodes

Despite their inability to respond to chronic anemia with a sustained increase in serum EPO, uremic patients have been reported to produce substantial amounts of EPO upon acute reductions of oxygen saturation. Blumberg et al. [6] exposed 6 anemic hemodialysis patients to an altitude of 3,450 m and observed a significant increase in Fe incorporation when testing their sera in the polycythemic mouse bioassay ($2.18 \pm 1.9\%$ vs. a baseline level of $0.39 \pm 0.34\%$; mean $\pm$ SD). More recently, Chandra et al. [7] reported the time course of serum immunoreactive EPO levels in uremic children during episodes of acute hypoxic stress, including pulmonary edema, acute hemolysis, heart failure and hypotension from sepsis. Serum EPO levels obtained during these episodes (273 ± 76 mU/ml; mean $\pm$ SE; n = 6) were tenfold higher than EPO levels during steady-state CRF (26 ± 6 mU/ml), even though EPO levels were inappropriately low for the degree of anemia in stable state (Hct $21.2 \pm 1.8\%$). Others have also demonstrated significant, albeit smaller, opposite changes of serum EPO in response to either a rise or a further decrease in hemoglobin concentrations in adult uremic patients experiencing blood loss or receiving transfusions [8].

Since these hypoxic episodes were terminated by therapeutic intervention, the short duration of elevation of EPO levels cannot be expected to result in increased erythropoiesis. However, increases in EPO have also been observed in situations where an improvement in renal anemia was the primary clinical observation which initiated further study of EPO production in order to elucidate the cause of this hematological improvement. Thus a marked increase in serum EPO has recently been observed in CRF patients who were parathyroidectomized for severe secondary hyperparathyroidism.

EPO Levels in Uremic Patients Undergoing Parathyroidectomy (PTx)

Secondary hyperparathyroidism has long been considered a contributory factor in the development of anemia during CRF. This view results from the observation that primary hyperparathyroidism may also be associated with anemia [9, 10], and that PTx has been shown to correct the anemia observed during primary hyperparathyroidism [9, 10] and to improve the anemia in some patients with CRF [11, 12]. The question of the role of EPO in this situation prompted us to determine the time course of EPO levels in uremic patients before and after PTx. As shown in figure 3, PTx in uremic patients resulted in a marked delayed but transient increase in their serum EPO levels. From a mean of 23.1 mU/ml before PTx, EPO levels rose to a peak of 245 mU/ml (n = 22) 2 weeks after PTx. When EPO levels were again measured after 1 year in a subgroup of 4 patients, their values had declined to 40.6 ± 8.4 mU/ml, while their hemoglobin concentration had slightly improved from 11 ± 0.9 to 12 ± 0.8 g/dl.

Although the mechanisms inducing this rise in EPO remain speculative, these observations further indicate that patients with CRF who display the characteristic inappropriately low EPO production of renal anemia can produce substantial amounts of EPO. This observation is important no matter where EPO is produced, but of course, for further understanding of the disturbance in EPO production in CRF, it is of great interest whether the increased amounts generated, for example, during hypoxia or after PTx are – as in ADPKD – secreted from the damaged kidneys or from the liver, an alternative production site for EPO. In another group of renal patients, those developing polycythemia after renal allotransplantation, significant EPO production by damaged kidneys can be clearly demonstrated.

EPO Production in Patients with Posttransplant Polycythemia

Some 10% of patients develop polycythemia after successful renal allotransplantation. Figure 4 shows the peripheral serum EPO values in polycythemic and nonpolycythemic kidney transplant patients. EPO values in both groups show a considerable variation, and on average serum EPO levels

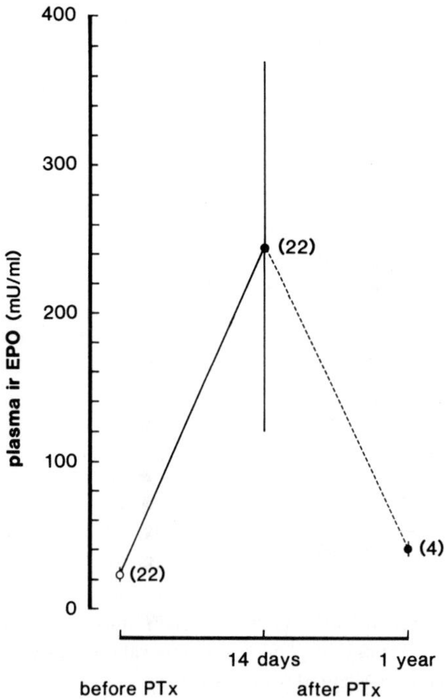

Fig. 3. Time course of plasma immunoreactive EPO (ir EPO) levels in hemodialysis patients undergoing PTx for severe secondary hyperparathyroidism. Values are mean ± SE. EPO levels 2 weeks after PTx were significantly elevated (p<0.001). In those 4 patients in whom EPO determinations could be performed 1 year after PTx, mean plasma EPO level 2 weeks after PTx was 382 ± 135 mU/ml (±SE). [Adapted from 13.]

in the polycythemic patients are not significantly elevated. However, in view of the normal inverse relationship between serum EPO levels and hemoglobin concentration, it is apparent that these patients have too high levels of EPO with respect to their hemoglobin concentration, suggesting that the feedback regulation of EPO production is somehow disturbed. The question of the source of EPO in this situation arises. Clinical experience that extirpation of the native kidneys usually cures posttransplant polycythemia suggests a role of the native diseased kidneys in this inappropriate (high) EPO formation. Dagher et al. [16] and Thevenod et al. [17] have further supported this assumption by measuring EPO levels in the veins draining the native kidneys. However, the low sensitivity of the bioassays available at that time precluded a

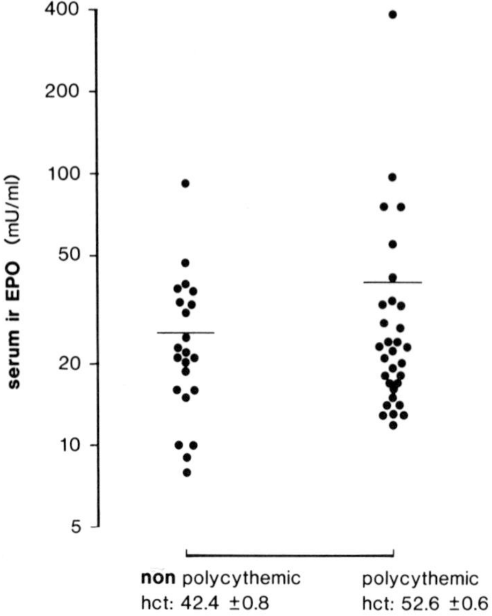

Fig. 4. Peripheral serum immunoreactive EPO (ir EPO) levels in renal transplant patients with and without polycythemia. Horizontal lines indicate mean values; EPO levels in both groups were not significantly different. [Adapted from 14 and 15.]

precise quantitation of the contribution of grafted and native kidneys to EPO production. Using a sensitive radioimmunoassay we have recently performed estimates of EPO concentrations in samples obtained by selective venous catheterization in polycythemic and nonpolycythemic posttransplant patients (table 1). In nonpolycythemic patients no concentration difference for EPO was found between femoral veins and the veins of either the native kidneys or grafts. However, in polycythemic patients, EPO levels in the veins draining the native kidneys were on average 15.6 mU/ml higher than in the femoral veins, while no difference was found between the values in the femoral and the graft veins. The difference between the renal veins and the femoral veins can be assumed to be identical with the arteriovenous (AV) concentration difference in the native kidneys. To assess the significance of such AV differences it is important to also consider renal plasma flow, since any reduction in plasma flow will automatically give rise to AV differences. In fact, due to the high plasma flow of normal kidneys, their AV concentration difference for EPO is

Table 1. Multiple-site estimates of immunoreactive EPO in polycythemic and nonpolycythemic kidney transplant patients

Sites	No.	Hct %	Vena cava (site 1)	Renal veins (endogenous kidneys) (site 2)	Graft vein (site 3)	Femoral vein (site 4)
Nonpolycythemic patients						
	1	41	10	13	11	10
	2	36	8	7	8	6
	3	46	9	10	9	10
	4	41	19	19	20	19
	x̄ ± SE		11.5 ± 2.6	11.9 ± 2.6	12.0 ± 2.8	11.3 ± 2.8
Polycythemic patients						
	1	46	24	36	22	21
	2	52	29	44	29	27
	3	51	17	32	19	15
	4	52	12	13	10	12
	5	54	13	22	14	13
	6	52	14	19	14	14
	7	50	41	95	37	35
	8	51	18	22	18	19
	x̄ ± SE		21.0 ± 3.5	35.1 ± 9.2	20.4 ± 3.1	19.5 ± 2.8

Blood samples at the locations indicated were obtained by selective venous catheterization. All patients received comparable immunosuppressive therapy with ciclosporin A. The 8 *polycythemic patients* were consecutive cases developing erythrocytosis after renal allotransplantation. Five were hypertensive, but none had diuretic treatment. Creatinine levels in all cases were below 140 µmol/l. The *nonpolycythemic controls* had severe hypertension, multiple-site estimates for renin being the indication for catheterization. From the renal veins of both native kidneys (site 2) up to three samples were obtained in different branches or at different distances from the vena cava. The values presented are the mean of the most proximal sample (generally the lowest value) obtained in the right and left renal vein, thus being characteristic for the effluent from the native kidneys. The mean difference between these values and the EPO concentration in femoral veins is 0.6 ± 0.8 mU/ml in nonpolycythemic and 15.6 ± 6.6 mU/ml (mean ± SE) in polycythemic patients. The difference between the right and left renal veins was 1.8 ± 0.8 mU/ml in nonpolythemic and 5.4 ± 1.7 mU/ml (mean ± SE) in polycythemic patients. In some branches of the renal veins, EPO levels up to 12 mU/ml higher than those presented were determined in the polycythemic patients. [Adapted from 15.]

normally too low to be detected with the assays presently available.[2] Although no direct measurements of plasma flow in the native kidneys and grafts of the above patients were performed, it can be calculated that the AV difference of 15.6 mU/ml EPO in the native kidneys would be sufficient to maintain the peripheral serum EPO concentration in these patients if the plasma flow through these kidneys is of the order of 12 ml/min.[3] This figure does not appear unrealistic, especially when one considers that EPO formation in the graft may not be completely suppressed. Thus, in conclusion, these data demonstrate that damaged kidneys without excretory function can produce EPO in amounts sufficient to maintain normal hemoglobin levels or even to induce erythrocytosis. Furthermore, these results indicate that in chronic renal disease not only the ability to increase EPO secretion in response to chronic anemia, but also the ability to down-regulate EPO formation under conditions of increased red cell mass may be disturbed. Again this supports the concept that a defect in the renal 'oxygen sensor' is a major cause for inappropriate EPO production in CRF.

Possible Reasons Why Damaged Kidneys Do Not Produce Sufficient Amounts of EPO in Spite of Their Ability to Do So

The above findings suggest that the diseased kidneys of patients with CRF retain the ability to produce substantial amounts of EPO in certain clinical situations, and therefore the question arises why this production capacity is not utilized when uremic patients develop chronic anemia, or in other words, why they become anemic at all.

In an attempt to give possible explanations to this question one should first consider the quantitative need for EPO. Relatively little is yet known

---

[2] A theoretical estimate of AV concentration differences for EPO in *normal* kidneys can be obtained on the basis of pharmacokinetic data for recombinant human EPO. Assuming a half-life time ($t_{1/2}$) of EPO in the order of 4.9 [18] to 9 h [19], a distribution volume (vol) of 0.073 l/kg [19], a body weight of 70 kg and an average serum EPO concentration ([EPO]) of 18 mU/ml, EPO production rate (PR_{EPO}) amounts to 7–13 U/h (PR_{EPO} = ln $2/t_{1/2}$ × [EPO] × vol). Assuming a normal renal plasma flow (RPF) of 700 ml/min, the AV concentration difference (Δ [EPO]$_{AV}$) would thus be about 0.2 mU/ml (PR_{EPO} = Δ [EPO]$_{AV}$ × RPF).

[3] According to the above equations, the average EPO production rate in the polycythemic patients is 8–14 U/h. At an average AV concentration difference of 15.6 mU/ml in the native kidneys, this production rate could be exclusively due to EPO formation in these kidneys if their plasma flow is 8 or 15 ml/min at a production rate of 8 or 14 U/h respectively.

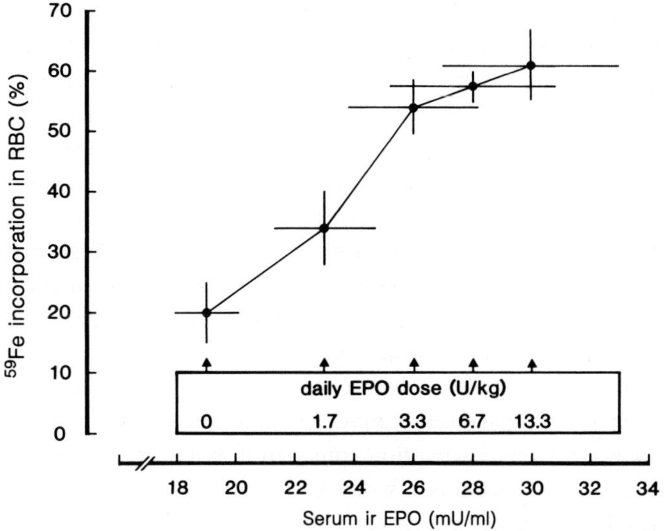

Fig. 5. Relationship between ^{59}Fe incorporation into red blood cells (RBC) and serum EPO concentrations in hypophysectomized rats receiving subcutaneous injections of EPO-enriched rat serum every 12 h for 4 days. EPO-enriched rat serum was prepared by exposing non-hypophysectomized donor animals to hypoxia. Values are mean ± SE of 5 animals each; EPO levels were determined 6 h after the last injection. [Adapted from 20.]

about the dose-response relationship of EPO, but a variety of observations indicate that slight increases in EPO levels are normally sufficient to enhance erythropoiesis. In hypophysectomized rats, for example, which show a significant reduction in red cell formation, due in part to diminished EPO formation, we observed a substantial increase of erythropoiesis when the serum EPO levels are raised by only 7 mU/ml with twice daily subcutaneous injections of the hormone (fig. 5). Furthermore, in humans the correction of renal anemia that follows renal allotransplantation is accompanied by only a two- to threefold elevation of serum EPO levels [21, 22]. In patients with secondary erythrocytosis, EPO determinations indicate that even slight increases in EPO are sufficient to maintain a red cell production rate above normal [23], a finding that is in accordance with our observations in polycythemic posttransplant patients. Although some uremic patients may show a resistance to EPO [24], for example due to aluminum intoxication [25], a recent comparison of the efficacy of EPO in uremic and nonuremic individuals provided no evidence for a generally diminished sensitivity to EPO in uremia

[26]. Growing experience with subcutaneous EPO administration in CRF patients confirms that in many patients only slight increases in EPO levels are required to correct renal anemia despite continued uremia [see chapters by Granolleras et al. and Slingeneyer et al., this volume]. It appears therefore that the increases in endogenous EPO described above, if persistent, would certainly be sufficient to correct the anemia of these patients. The main question therefore would seem to be, why the reduction in hemoglobin is no longer an efficient stimulus for EPO formation. Since the linkage of EPO formation to hemoglobin in healthy kidneys is only incompletely understood, the reasons for its disturbance during kidney disease remain speculative. At least three possibilities must be considered.

First it is possible that the *excretory renal function* that is decreased, or even entirely lacking in renal disease, plays an important role in the regulation of EPO. Evidence for this assumption comes from both clinical and experimental observations. For example, when EPO formation immediately after renal allotransplantation was investigated in patients with and without delayed excretory graft function, a 'physiological', oxygen-dependent regulation of EPO was only found in the presence of excretory function [22]. Since ongoing sodium reabsorption at the proximal tubular site appears necessary for the rise in EPO in response to hypoxia [27], it is possible that in the absence of tubular work in kidneys with negligible excretory function, as yet unidentified signals derived from tubular cells are missing, or renal oxygen consumption may be too low to achieve tissue oxygen tensions that normally induce enhanced EPO formation. Interestingly, parathyroid hormone is known to inhibit proximal tubular sodium reabsorption [28] and reducing this inhibition by PTx might partially account for the observed increased in EPO formation.

Second, it is possible that the oxygen-sensing function of the kidneys in CRF is at least partially intact, but that their *sensitivity towards changes in renal oxygen supply* is diminished. Uremic acidosis is one possible cause for such a desensitization of the renal oxygen sensor function. In animal experiments, metabolic acidosis inhibits those mechanisms that trigger EPO formation upon onset of hypoxic or anemic hypoxia [29] (table 2).

Finally, it is possible that adaptation occurs during chronic hypoxia. This would be compatible with the findings, mentioned above, that in uremic patients acute hypoxic episodes, but not chronic anemia, stimulate EPO formation. In fact, when humans or experimental animals with intact kidneys are exposed to high altitude, EPO levels soon increase but decline again after about 12 h despite continuing hypoxia, and adaptive processes are assumed to

Table 2. Effect of metabolic acidosis on immunoreactive EPO levels in mice exposed to normobaric hypoxia (8% O_2) or functional anemia (0.1% carbon monoxide) for 3 h

		Control	Acidosis
EPO, mU/ml	8% O_2	305 ± 20 (15)	197 ± 31 (15)
	0.1% CO	707 ± 56 (19)	440 ± 28 (20)
pH		7.34 ± 0.04 (8)	7.21 ± 0.03 (6)

Acidosis was induced by injection of ammonium chloride (10 mmol/kg) immediately prior to hypoxic exposure. pH values were determined in peripheral venous blood 1 h after injection of ammonium chloride. Values are mean ± SE. Numbers in parentheses are the numbers of animals. [Adapted from 29.]

account for this reduction [30, 31]. It is unknown why, in contrast, patients with chronic anemias of nonrenal origin seem to escape these adaptive processes and maintain elevated EPO levels.

In view of the broad spectrum of different etiologies and histomorphological as well as functional alterations in chronic kidneys disease, the cause for inappropriately low EPO formation may be quite different in individual patients and related to various combinations of the above mentioned and other, yet unconsidered factors. In any case, the oxygen sensor function of the kidney, that adapts EPO production to hemoglobin levels, appears much more sensitive towards an alteration of renal integrity than the production capacity itself.

References

1   Kurtz, A.; Eckardt, K.-U.: Erythropoietin production in chronic renal disease before and after transplantation. Contrib. Nephrol., in press.
2   Chandra, M; Miller, M. E.; Garcia, J. F.; Mossey, R. T.; McVicar, M.: Serum immunoreactive erythropoietin levels in patients with polycystic kidney disease as compared with other hemodialysis patients. Nephron *39:* 26–29 (1985).
3   Pavlovic-Kentera, V.; Clemons, G. K.; Djukanovic, L.; Biljanovic-Paunovic, L.: Erythropoietin and anemia in chronic renal failure. Exp. Hematol. *15:* 785–789 (1987).
4   Eckardt, K.-U.; Möllmann, M.; Neumann,R.; Brunkhorst, R.; Burger, H.-U.; Lonnemann, G.; Scholz, H.; Keusch, B.; Buchholz, B.; Frei, U.; Bauer, C.; Kurtz, A.: Erythropoietin in polycystic kidneys. J. Clin. Invest. *84:* 1160–1166 (1989).
5   Shaloub, R. J.; Rajan, U.; Kim, V.V.; Goldwasser, E.; Kark, J. A.; Antoniou, L. D.: Erythrocytosis in patients on long-term hemodialysis. Ann. Intern. Med. *97:* 686–690 (1982).

6 Blumberg, A.; Keller, H.; Marti, H. R.: Effect of altitude on erythropoiesis and oxygen affinity in anemic patients on maintenance hemodialysis. Eur. J. Clin. Invest. *3:* 93–97 (1973).

7 Chandra, M.; Clemons, G. K.; McVicar, M. I.: Relation of serum erythropoietin levels to renal excretory function: evidence for lowered set point for erythropoietin production in chronic renal failure. J. Pediatr. *113:* 1015–1021 (1988).

8 Walle, A. J.; Wong, G. Y.; Clemons, G. K.; Garcia, J. F.; Niedermayer, W.: Erythropoietin-hematocrit feedback circuit in the anemia of end-stage renal disease. Kidney Int. *31:* 1205–1209 (1987).

9 Falko, J. M.; Guy, J. T.; Smith, R. E.; Mazzaferri, E. L.: Primary hyperparathyroidism and anemia. Arch. Intern. Med. *136:* 887 (1976).

10 Boxer, M.; Ellmann, L.; Geller, R.; Wang, C.: Anemia in primary hyperparathyroidism. Arch. Intern. Med. *137:* 558 (1977).

11 Zingraff, J.; Drüeke, T.; Marie, P.; Man, N. K.; Jungers, P.; Bordier, P.: Anemia and secondary hyperparathyroidism. Arch. Intern. Med. *138:* 1650 (1978).

12 Barbour, G. L.: Effect of parathyroidectomy on anemia in chronic renal failure. Arch. Intern. Med. *139:* 889 (1979).

13 Ureña, P.; Eckardt, K.-U.; Zingraff, J.; Juquel, J. P.; Sarfati, E.; Kurtz, A.; Drüeke, T.: Blood reticulocytes, erythropoietin, and hemoglobin increase after parathyroidectomy in hemodialysis patients. Abstr. XXVIIth Congr. European Dialysis and Transplant Association, 1990.

14 Nattermann, U.; Hillebrand, G.; Kurtz, A.; Land, W.; Gurland, H. J.: Erythropoietinserumspiegel und Polyglobulie nach Nierentransplantation (Abstract). Nieren-Hochdruckkr. *9:* 392 (1988).

15 Aeberhard, J.-M.; Schneider, P.-A.; Vallotton, M. B.; Kurtz, A.; Leski, M.: Multiple-site estimates of erythropoietin and renin in polycythemic kidney transplant patients. Transplantation, in press.

16 Dagher, F. J.; Ramos, E.; Erslev, A. J.; Alongi, S. V.; Karmi, S. A.; Caro, J.: Are the native kidneys responsible for erythrocytosis in renal allorecipients? Transplantation *28:* 496–498 (1979).

17 Thevenod, F.; Radtke, H. W.; Grützmacher, P.; Vincent, E.; Koch, K. M.; Fassbinder, W.: Deficient feedback regulation of erythropoiesis in kidney transplant patients with polycythemia. Kidney Int. *24:* 227–232 (1983).

18 Cotes, P. M.; Pippard, M. J.; Reid, C. D. L.; Winearls, C. G.; Oliver, D. O.; Royston, J. P.: Characterization of the anemia of chronic renal failure and the mode of its correction by a preparation of human erythropoietin (rHuEPO). An investigation of the pharmacokinetics of intravenous erythropoietin and its effects on erythrokinetics. Q. J. Med. *70:* 113–137 (1989).

19 Kindler, J.; Eckardt, K.-U.; Ehmer, B.; Jandeleith, K.; Kurtz, A.; Schreiber A.; Scigalla, P.; Sieberth, H.-G.: Single dose pharmacokinetics of recombinant human erythropoietin (rHuEPO) in patients with various degrees of renal failure. Nephrol. Dial. Transplant. *4:* 345–349 (1989).

20 Kurtz, A.; Zapf, J.; Eckardt, K.-U.; Clemons, G.; Froesch, E. R.; Bauer, C.: Insulin-like growth factor I stimulates erythropoiesis in hypophysectomized rats. Proc. Natl. Acad. Sci. USA *85:* 7825–7829 (1988).

21 Besarab, A.; Caro, J.; Jarell, B. E.; Francos, G.; Erslev, A. J.: Dynamics of erythropoiesis following renal transplantation. Kidney Int. *32:* 526–536 (1987).

22 Eckhardt, K.-U.; Frei, U.; Kliem, V.; Bauer, C.; Koch, K. M.; Kurtz, A.: Role of excretory graft function for erythropoietin formation after renal transplantation. Eur. J. Clin. Invest., in press.

23 Cotes, P. M.; Dore, J. C.; Yin, J. A. L.; Lewis, S. M.; Messinezy, M.; Pearson, T. C.; Reid, C.: Determination of serum erythropoietin in the investigation of erythrocytosis. N. Engl. J. Med. *315:* 283–287 (1986).

24 Drüeke, T. B.: Resistance to recombinant human erythropoietin (rHuEPO) in hemodialysis (HD) patients (abstract). Eur. J. Clin. Invest. *20:* 56 (1990).

25 Losekann, A.; Ureña, P.; Khiraoui, F.; Casadevall; N.; Zins, B.; Bererhi, L.; Zingraff, J.; Bourdon, R.; Drüeke, T.: Aluminium intoxication in the rat induces partial resistance to the effect of recombinant human erythropoietin. Nephrol. Dial. Transplant *5:* 258–263 (1990).

26 Haley, N. R.; Eschbach, J. W.; Adamson, J. W.: Uremic inhibitors do not impair the response to erythropoietin (EPO) in chronic renal failure (CRF) (abstract). Blood *74:* suppl. 1, p. 15 (1989).

27 Eckardt, K.-U.; Kurtz, A.; Bauer, C.: Regulation of erythropoietin formation is related to proximal tubular function. Am. J. Physiol. *256:* F942–947 (1989).

28 Bank, N.; Aynedjian, H. S.: A micropuncture study of the effect of parathyroid hormone on renal bicarbonate reabsorption. J. Clin. Invest. *58:* 336 (1976).

29 Eckardt, K.-U.; Kurtz, A.; Bauer, C.: Triggering of erythropoietin production by hypoxia is inhibited by respiratory and metabolic acidosis. Am. J. Physiol. *258:* R678–683 (1990).

30 Abbrecht, P. H.; Littel, J. K.: Plasma erythropoietin in men and mice during acclimatization to different altitudes. J. Appl. Physiol. *32:* 54–58 (1972).

31 Eckardt, K.-U.; Dittmer, J.; Neumann, R.; Bauer, C.; Kurtz, A.: Decline of erythropoietin formation at continuous hypoxia is not due to feedback inhibition. Am. J. Physiol. *258:* F1432–1437 (1990).

Dr. Kai-Uwe Eckardt, Physiologisches Institut der Universität Zürich, Winterthurerstrasse 190, CH–8057 Zürich (Switzerland)

Gurland HJ, Moran J, Samtleben W, Scigalla P, Wieczorek L (eds): Erythropoietin in Renal and Non-Renal Anemias. Contrib Nephrol. Basel, Karger, 1991, vol 88, pp 32–34

Discussion

to the Paper by K.-U. Eckardt et al.

Cotes (Harrow): I enjoyed your talk and I think it may have therapeutic implications. I would like to draw attention to the fact that it is not only the secretion of EPO from diseased kidneys that can be increased, but also extrarenal EPO. In both cases the regulatory system is abnormal. Some time ago I saw an anephric patient under Dr. Shaldon's care. His anemia was worsened by an episode of hemolysis. This was followed by an enormous increase in endogenous EPO production. We have yet to learn appropriate pharmacological measures to increase endogenous production of EPO at times of physiological need in anephric patients and in nephric patients with renal disease.

Kurtz: Thank you very much for this comment, I can only agree. I have no doubts that extrarenal production occurs in these patients but we do not know the site. Probably it is the liver, but then again the question arises: the capability exists, but why do neither the liver nor the kidney produce sufficient EPO? We would only need an increase of serum levels by about 20 mU/ml to cure the anemia.

Shaldon (Montpellier): I'd like to follow-up your observation. 25 years ago we dialysed a Swiss patient. He went to live at an altitude of two thousand meters and his hematocrit spontaneously rose from 21 to 33%. How can you reconcile that with your proposed defect in oxygen regulation by the end-stage renal failure patient? This patient was an anuric non-polycystic end-stage renal patient.

Kurtz: I think there is no discrepancy between your finding and the data I have presented. I would say that the uremic patient has the capability to produce EPO and I think your observation supports the concept that there is a resetting of the oxygen sensor. Dr. Caro told me yesterday that patients who have hemoglobin concentrations of 5 g/dl have low EPO levels, but if they bleed and further lower their hemoglobin levels then their EPO levels increase. There is an oxygen-dependent regulation, but there is a resetting of this oxygen sensor to very low values. It is now the task of the physiologists to find out the reason for this resetting.

Goldwasser (Chicago): Your last comment implicates one of the factors that you listed on your slide but didn't really address very carefully and that is lack of adaptation. I would ask the physiologists among us to consider the fact that there are lots of other mechanisms that can operate to increase oxygenation in addition to simply the red cell level. That may be part of the operating difficulty that you are facing, trying to reconcile these various pathological phenomena.

Kurtz: Yes, I agree.

Cavill (Cardiff): Our unit is close to sea level so we have no confounding factors! These data are very interesting because it begins to explain to me some of the in vivo measurements of erythropoiesis using iron kinetics which we made some years ago in patients with end-stage renal failure. These were non-polycystic patients in whom we looked at the relationship between marrow iron turnover, which is an indicator of erythropoietic activity, and directly measured red cell life-span. In normal subjects there is an inverse, rather J-shaped relationship, such that any shortening of life-span is compensated by an increase in erythropoietic activity. That relationship was maintained in the patients with end-stage chronic renal failure, but was shifted to the left. It appeared to us that the fundamental mechanism remained intact but was attenuated and set at a lower level.

Eschbach (Seattle): I would like to suggest another interpretation of some of your data based upon Dr. Goldberg's theory. It has been known for years that dialysis patients can produce an EPO response to acute severe hypoxia, but they cannot produce any significant erythropoiesis unless the hypoxia is prolonged. We also know that the diseased kidney may be very damaged, including the EPO-producing cells. I suspect there are only some of these cells left which can respond to hypoxia. Dr. Goldberg has suggested that the cells don't make more EPO per cell but that more and more cells are brought into EPO production with greater degrees of hypoxia. Since there are less EPO-producing cells in kidney failure, you might consider that phenomenon to explain part of your data.

We have done ferrokinetic studies which indicate that patients with renal failure have an identical erythropoietic response to rhEPO to that of normal subjects. So I am not convinced that decreased excretory function, per se, explains why these patients do not respond to the EPO that they produce endogenously.

Kurtz: This is of course one possible reason among others. Acidosis perhaps could also play a role and there may be other factors. But I really want to stress the point that a uremic patient is capable of producing major amounts of EPO. For instance, in the study with the patients after parathyroidectomy we measured EPO values that were fully bioactive, as measured in the polycythemic mouse assay – levels as high as 2,000 mU/ml. And the patients were anemic and they had low EPO levels. If regulation of EPO production means the recruitment of EPO producers, there must be sufficient EPO producers in uremic patients but they don't get recruited.

Erslev (Philadelphia): Are you saying that there is an inhibitor?

Kurtz: No.

Shaldon: I would like to pick up that point. Lets talk about cytokine RIAs. It is very fashionable today to have circulating receptor antagonists which you cannot pick up by RIA, but which interfere with the biological activity by blocking the receptor. This is particularly so for Il-1, Can you be certain that your RIA is, in fact, measuring biologically active EPO?

Kurtz: I cannot say that the material that is measured by the RIA is really active in terms of bioactivity in vivo. I would say it is active in terms of in vitro bioactivity because I am fairly sure that the antibody we use for RIA also detects desialated EPO, i.e. EPO with free galactosyl residues which are then caught by the asialo receptor in the liver, resulting in a very short half-life. These molecules will not be very effective in vivo. I am pretty sure that the material we measure by RIA is active on the target cell, but we cannot say for certain that the material is really active in vivo.

Goldwasser: I want to respond somewhat differently to Dr. Shaldon's question. We have already reported that, with our RIA and our particular antibody, we can detect biologically inactive fragments, smaller than EPO. Therefore, there is the possibility of any RIA picking up materials which may have been derived from EPO, but no longer have any biological activity, whether it is in vitro or in vivo.

Rich (Ulm): I'd like to agree with Dr. Goldwasser: using our ELISA we see the same sort of thing. But I would like to come back to the oxygen sensor setpoints. As you know, we have published data showing that macrophages – in particular bone marrow macrophages – can express the EPO gene and produce the hormone and we have been thinking for a long time that the difference between the renal and the extrarenal production of EPO is basically due to a difference in oxygen sensor setpoints and the range at which those sensors can respond to oxygen.

Gurland HJ, Moran J, Samtleben W, Scigalla P, Wieczorek L (eds): Erythropoietin in Renal and Non-Renal Anemias. Contrib Nephrol. Basel, Karger, 1991, vol 88, pp 35–45

Erythropoietin Gene Regulation: From the Laboratory to the Bedside

Mark A. Goldberg[a], *Christopher C. Gaut*[a], *Lidia Schapira*[a], *Joseph H. Antin*[a], *Bernard J. Ransil*[c], *Karen H. Antman*[b,c], *J. Paul Eder*[b,c], *Carol J. McGarigle*[a], *H. Franklin Bunn*[a]

[a]Hematology Division, Department of Medicine, Brigham and Women's Hospital, [b]Department of Medicine, Dana-Farber Cancer Institute, and [c]Charles A. Dana Research Institute, Harvard-Thorndike Laboratory, Division of Medical Oncology, Department of Medicine, Beth Israel Hospital, Harvard Medical School, Boston, Mass., USA

We have previously demonstrated that the human hepatoma cell line, Hep 3B, synthesizes large quantities of erythropoietin (EPO) in a regulated manner in response to hypoxia and cobaltous chloride ($CoCl_2$) and that this regulation occurs at the EPO mRNA level [1, 2]. From Northern blot analyses of RNA from murine kidneys [3, 4] and Hep 3B [1, 2], it appears that EPO mRNA steady-state levels increase at least 50-fold with hypoxia. However, nuclear run-off experiments which we have performed on Hep 3B cells suggest that EPO gene transcription increases only 10-fold with hypoxia [5]. We have therefore begun to investigate posttranscriptional components to EPO gene regulation in Hep 3B cells. To do this in a cell culture system we have utilized inhibitors of gene transcription and protein synthesis, namely actinomycin D and cycloheximide. In addition, to study the clinical importance of the effects of inhibitors of DNA and protein synthesis in man, we have begun to investigate the effects of combination chemotherapy and radiation therapy on the ability of patients to make EPO in response to anemia.

Materials and Methods

Cell Culture. Hep 3B cells were obtained through American Type Culture Collection. They were cultured in MEM Alpha medium (Gibco) supplemented with penicillin (100 units/ml), streptomycin (100 µg/ml) and 10% defined supplemented bovine calf serum (Hyclone) and were maintained in a humidified 5% CO_2 incubator at 37°C. The cells were grown hypoxically either as described previously [1] or in a controlled atmosphere chamber (Plas Labs, Lansing, Mich.) supplied with a constant flow of a hydrated 1% O_2, 5% CO_2, balance N_2 gas mixture. All experiments were begun when the Hep 3B cells approached confluence.

EPO Radioimmunoassay (RIA). Serum immunoreactive EPO was measured by a method similar to that described by Egrie et al. [6]. The RIA for EPO was performed using a high titer polyclonal rabbit anti-rhEPO serum produced in our laboratory. ^{125}I rhEPO was obtained from Amersham, Inc. Standards were prepared using rhEPO from Amgen, Inc, diluted in MEM Alpha medium containing 0.5% bovine serum albumin and 0.05% sodium azide, pH 7.4. Aliquots of 0.2 ml of standard or sample were placed in 5 ml conical polypropylene tubes. To this was added 0.1 ml of rabbit antiserum diluted 1:15,000 in phosphate-buffered saline (PBS) containing 0.5% bovine serum albumin. The mixture was diluted to 0.7 ml using the same diluent used for the recombinant EPO standards and was incubated at room temperature for 2 h. 0.1 ml (approximately 15,000 cpm) of ^{125}I EPO prepared in the same diluent was then added, the mixture was briefly vortexed and incubated for 12–16 h at 4°C. 0.6 ml of Tachisorb® immunoabsorbent (goat anti-rabbit γ-globulin conjugated Pansorbin *Staphylococcus aureus* cells; Calbiochem) was then added to each tube and the tubes were placed at 4°C with constant shaking for 3 h. The Tachisorb was pelleted by centrifugation for 30 min at 1,500 *g* at 4°C, washed once with 2.0 ml PBS, and counted in an LKB model 1282 gamma counter. Assays on patient serum were performed in duplicate and at two different dilutions. Using this assay, the normal range of serum EPO levels is 16–38 mU/ml calibrated against the WHO Second International Reference Standard.

Northern Blot Analysis. Total RNA was prepared from cultured cells as described by Chirgwin et al. [7]. The RNA was denatured in formaldehyde, electrophoresed on a 1% agarose gel containing 2.2 *M* formaldehyde and a trace amount of ethidium bromide, and transferred to a GeneScreen Plus filter (New England Nuclear) using $10\times$ standard saline citrate (1.5 *M* NaCl, 0.15 *M* sodium citrate) [8]. EPO cDNA in an SP65 plasmid was digested with the restriction enzyme EcoR1, the EPO insert isolated by agarose gel electrophoresis, followed by electroelution [8] and ^{32}P labelled to a specific activity of between 3×10^8 and 1.2×10^9 cpm/μg of cDNA [9]. The radiolabeled cDNA was then mixed with carrier salmon sperm DNA, denatured by boiling for 10 min, and hybridized to the filter at 5×10^5 cpm/ml of hybridization solution (50% formamide, 1 *M* NaCl, 1% SDS, 10% dextran). Hybridization was performed at 42°C for 20 h. The final washing was done in $0.5\times$ standard saline citrate (0.075 *M* NaCl, 0.0075 *M* sodium citrate) at 65°C. Autoradiography was performed with intensifying screens at –80°C using Kodak X-Omat AR film.

Mouse β-actin cDNA was also radiolabeled and hybridized to the same filters in order to provide an internal control for the efficiency of RNA transfer to the filters.

EPO mRNA Stability. Hep 3B cells were placed in either a 1 or 21% O_2 containing atmosphere for 18–24 h at 37°C. At '0 time' the O_2 content of the atmosphere was manipulated as described below and either actinomycin D or cycloheximide was added to final concentrations of 5 or 20 μg/ml, respectively. After varying periods of incubation, total cellular RNA was isolated from the cells and Northern blot analysis were performed. Densitometric scanning was performed with a Molecular Dynamics Model 300A computing densitometer. Relative EPO mRNA levels represent arbitrary units normalized relative to β-actin mRNA levels.

Patient Population. Patients entering the Brigham and Women's Hospital, Dana-Farber Cancer Institute, and the Beth Israel Hospital for either autologous or allogeneic bone marrow transplantation (BMT) were enrolled in the study. Serum samples were collected on the first hospital day (prior to the initiation of cytotoxic therapy), within 24 h of completing cytotoxic therapy (hereafter designated day 0), and on days 7, 14, and 28 following BMT. Preparative regimens varied according to the protocols used by each participating institution and the patient's diagnosis. All patients had an initial serum creatinine less than or equal to 2.0 mg/dl. In general, patients received red blood cell transfusions to maintain a hematocrit in the vicinity of 25%.

Reference Population. Eleven volunteers with normal hematocrits and normal renal function served as controls. Sixteen patients with well-documented aplastic anemia or myelo-dysplastic anemia who had normal renal function and had never received chemotherapy served as a comparison group. Together these 27 subjects comprised the reference population.

Statistical Methods. Of the 31 patients completing the study, 1 patient was eliminated from the analysis. This patient suffered an acute massive gastrointestinal hemorrhage during the fourth week of hospitalization which produced a marked increase in EPO level and transfusion requirement.

The data base therefore consisted of (a) hematocrit and serum EPO measurements made on each of 30 BMT patients at the five time intervals noted above, and (b) hematocrit and EPO measurements made at a single point in time on the 27 subjects in the reference population. The hematocrits tended to be normally distributed, and therefore were correctly represented by the arithmetic mean ± 1 SD, and analyzed by parametric methods. The EPO distributions were log normally distributed and better represented by the geometric mean, particularly in regression analysis. However, for consistency of reporting and discussion, and because outcome is not affected by use of the less efficient central measure, the mean ± 1 SD was used for all distributions. Comparison of the hematocrit and EPO data between the respective time periods and the reference population was done using appropriate two-sample and multiple-sample comparison tests.

Results

Cell Culture Studies

Experiments were undertaken to investigate posttranscriptional influences on steady-state EPO mRNA levels. Initially, Hep 3B cells were grown in 1% O_2 to increase EPO mRNA levels, and subsequently were switched to 21% O_2. EPO mRNA levels were then determined after varying periods of time by Northern blot analyses. As demonstrated in figure 1, in 21% O_2 EPO mRNA has a rapid rate of decay with steady-state levels falling by 50% within 1.5–2 h. This finding is similar to reported changes in kidney EPO mRNA levels in mice switched from a hypoxic to a nonhypoxic environment [10] and represents a maximal estimate of the in vivo half-life of the EPO mRNA (since new

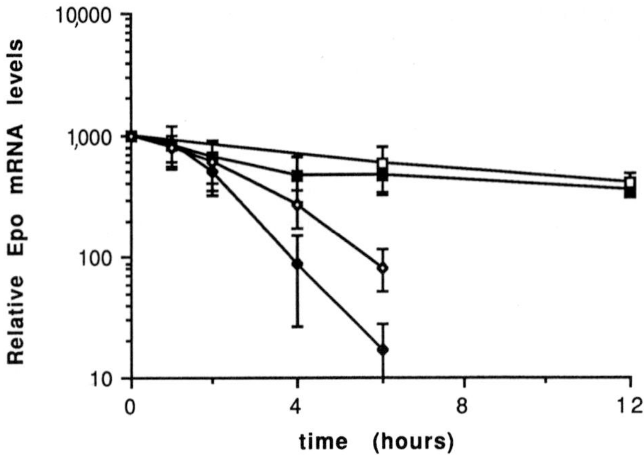

Fig. 1. EPO mRNA stability. Experiments were performed as described in the Methods section. Relative EPO mRNA levels represent arbitrary units normalized relative to β-actin mRNA levels. Each data point is the average (±1 SD) of at least two experiments with most points representing the average of three or more experiments. Closed diamonds, 21% oxygen; open diamonds, 21% oxygen plus 20 μg/ml cycloheximide; closed squares, 21% oxygen plus 5 μg/ml actinomycin D; open squares, 1% oxygen plus 5 μg/ml actinomycin D.

transcription was not blocked). In order to distinguish between transcriptional and posttranscriptional contributions to this observed fall in steady-state EPO mRNA levels, actinomycin D chase experiments were performed. Initial experiments demonstrated that actinomycin D at a concentration of 5 μg/ml blocked greater than 98% of the incorporation of ^{3}[H]-uridine into total cellular Hep 3B RNA under both hypoxic and nonhypoxic conditions. Hep 3B cells were made hypoxic in order to allow an increase in EPO mRNA levels. After the addition of actinomycin D the cells were either kept hypoxic or rapidly equilibrated with a 21% O_2 atmosphere for various periods of time. The stability of the EPO mRNA in the presence of actinomycin D at both O_2 tensions was much greater than that observed in the absence of actinomycin D (fig. 1) and much greater than that reported in vivo. Thus, the addition of actinomycin D itself resulted in an increased stability of EPO mRNA.

If actinomycin D was preventing the transcription of rapidly turning over mRNA whose protein product or products participate in the degradation of EPO mRNA, one would expect cycloheximide to have a similar effect on the stability of EPO mRNA. Hence, parallel experiments were performed using 20 μg/ml cycloheximide instead of actinomycin D. These experiments demon-

Table 1. Mean hematocrits and EPO levels on patients prior to and following BMT (n = 30)

	Hematocrit, %	EPO, mU/ml
Admission	32±5	79±113
Day 0	28±4	213±141
Day 7	28±5	284±190
Day 14	28±3	165±135
Day 28	29±3	75±48

strated a reproducible increase in the stability of the EPO mRNA in the presence of cycloheximide as well (fig. 1). Evidence that the cycloheximide enhances EPO mRNA stability rather than stimulating de novo transcription is provided by the fact that cycloheximide blocks hypoxia and $CoCl_2$-induced increases in EPO mRNA [2] and cycloheximide by itself does not cause an increase in steady-state EPO mRNA levels [unpubl. observation]. However, as seen in Figure 1, the effect of cycloheximide on increasing EPO mRNA stability is not quite as marked as the effect of actinomycin D. This may be due to the inability of cycloheximide to block translation for a sustained period of time as completely as actinomycin D blocks transcription [11].

Patient Studies

Of the 30 patients included in the analysis, 17 underwent allogeneic BMT and 13 received autologous BMT. The EPO levels and hematocrits are summarized in table 1. Mean EPO levels initially increased after patients received cytotoxic therapy from 79±133 mU/ml on the day of admission to a peak value of 284±190 mU/ml measured on day 7 post-BMT. As might be expected, this initial increase in mean serum EPO levels between the day of admission and day 7 corresponded to a significant decrease in mean hematocrit (32±5 vs. 28±5%, respectively; $p < 0.01$). However, while the mean hematocrits were essentially constant on days 7, 14, and 28 post-BMT (28±5, 28±3, and 29±3%, respectively), the mean serum EPO levels fell almost 4-fold during this same period (284±190, 165±135, and 75±48 mU/ml, respectively; $p < 0.01$). This unexpected result suggested a decreased EPO response to anemia between approximately days 14 and 28 post-BMT.

To further evaluate the impact of cytotoxic therapy on serum EPO levels as a function of hematocrit, the mean EPO levels and corresponding hematocrits for the five time points were plotted together with the EPO levels and

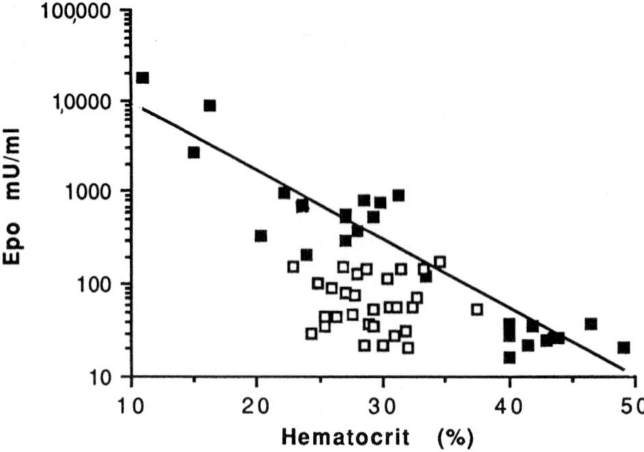

Fig. 2. EPO levels as a function of hematocrit in BMT patients 28 days after BMT versus the reference population. Closed squares represent the reference population. Open squares represent the BMT patients on day 28 post-BMT. Solid line is a linear regression line for the reference population.

hematocrits of the reference population. This enabled us to compare two groups of patients with comparable degrees of bone marrow failure and study the impact of cytotoxic therapy on serum EPO levels. Figure 2 shows that the reference log EPO levels describe a downward linear trajectory as a function of hematocrit. The mean log EPO levels obtained from the transplant patients administered cytotoxic therapy fall below the line generated by the reference population and outside the 95% confidence intervals. The admission and day 14 post-BMT mean EPO levels are 1.2 SD below the regression line (NS) while day 0 and 7 post-BMT levels are 0.84 and 0.44 SD below the line (NS), respectively. However, the day 28 post-BMT mean log EPO level is 2 SD below the line ($p < 0.05$). Thus by day 28 post-BMT, these patients manifest not only a decreased EPO response for a given degree of anemia compared to their own day 7 post-BMT response (table 1), but they also showed a significantly decreased response compared to the reference population (fig. 2).

Discussion

The data presented in this paper suggest that EPO mRNA levels are determined by a complex process involving both the rate of gene transcription and posttranscriptional events. The fact that steady-state EPO mRNA levels increase more than 50-fold in response to hypoxia and $CoCl_2$ while EPO gene transcription increases only about 10-fold in Hep 3B cells suggests that there is a significant posttranscriptional component to EPO gene regulation in this cell line. Numerous examples of posttranscriptional regulation of mRNA have been well documented, particularly at the level of mRNA stability [12, 13]. Although still poorly understood, multiple mechanisms for this regulation of the rate of mRNA degradation have been demonstrated [12]; however, many of these mechanisms seem to share certain common features. In many cases mRNA degradation requires ongoing protein synthesis since stabilization occurs in the presence of various protein synthesis inhibitors [12, 14–17]. Two explanations for the requirement of ongoing protein synthesis have been proposed: (1) certain mRNAs may be degraded by rapidly turning over specific ribonucleases, and (2) the degradation of some mRNAs may be directly coupled to their translation. Cotranslational degradation has been elegantly demonstrated for tubulin and histone mRNAs [15, 16]. On the other hand, although indirect evidence suggests the presence of rapidly turning over specific ribonucleases [12], thus far none of these nucleases have been well characterized.

If the expression of these putative nucleases are themselves regulated at the level of transcription, one would expect that inhibitors of transcription as well as inhibitors of protein synthesis would stabilize the mRNA targets of these ribonucleases. This is not the case for the protein synthesis-requiring degradation of the c-myc [14], c-fos [17, 18], and GM-CSF [19] mRNAs. However, the transcription inhibitor actinomycin D does stabilize poly(I)-poly (C)-induced fibroblast interferon mRNA [20] as well as prevents the decay of human transferrin receptor mRNA [21]. Furthermore, recent studies by Shyu et al. [18] demonstrate two independent determinants of c-fos mRNA instability, one of which appears to be dependent upon ongoing transcription. EPO is another case in which mRNA instability requires both ongoing transcription and protein synthesis. However, unlike many of the other known examples, EPO's biogenesis [22, 23] and its biological actions [24] are extremely tissue specific. The data presented here support a mechanism in which EPO mRNA degradation requires both the transcription and translation of a rapidly turning over mRNA (or mRNAs) whose protein product(s) participates in the degradation of EPO mRNA. In addition, this phenomenon clearly demonstrates a potential pitfall in relying on actinomycin D chase experiments alone to estimate mRNA half-lives.

The evidence presented here suggesting the existence of a rapidly turning over EPO mRNA degrading protein raises the possibility that the concentration and/or the activity of this protein may be decreased during hypoxia or $CoCl_2$ exposure. However, direct demonstration of pO_2-dependent changes in EPO mRNA stability in intact Hep 3B cells is impossible using actinomycin D since the actinomycin D itself alters the mRNA stability by blocking synthesis of the presumptive EPO mRNA destabilizing protein.

In the case of EPO gene regulation, the finding that steady-state EPO mRNA levels may be significantly influenced by a rapidly turning over EPO mRNA degrading protein is particularly intriguing because it may have biological significance. The combination of the hypoxia-induced increased EPO gene transcription coupled with increased EPO mRNA stability permits a marked amplification of EPO mRNA levels. A modest increase in the rate of EPO gene transcription and a modest increase in EPO mRNA stability acting in synergy can explain how the cell is able to regulate EPO mRNA levels such that during hypoxia, circulating levels of EPO protein can increase by three orders of magnitude.

We have prospectively measured endogenous serum immunoreactive EPO levels in 31 patients receiving intensive chemotherapy and combination chemotherapy and radiation therapy in preparation for autologous or allogeneic bone marrow transplantation. Similar to several previous studies [25, 26], we noted a characteristic pattern of increasing serum EPO concentrations following cytotoxic therapy. These previous reports suggested that the EPO increase was caused by a mechanism other than increasing anemia and triggering of the oxygen sensor in the kidney. By comparing the data to our reference population we found that the observed fall in the hematocrit during this period appeared to be enough to explain the rise in EPO levels. However, within the study group it must be noted that there did appear to be a small but statistically significant increase in mean serum EPO levels between days 0 and 7 post-BMT (213 ± 140 vs. 284 ± 184 mU/ml, $p < 0.05$) which occurred without a significant change in hematocrit (28.3 ± 4.0 vs. $27.5\pm4.6\%$, NS). Possible explanations include cytotoxic therapy (a) causing direct injury to the EPO producing cells in a manner which mimics hypoxia, (b) altering blood flow to the kidney and/or liver in such a way as to expose the EPO producing cells in these organs to an increased degree of hypoxia, or (c) disrupting the usual EPO degradation pathway(s) and thereby extending the serum half-life of the protein. Chemotherapy and radiation therapy may clearly interfere with ongoing protein synthesis and gene transcription. Given the findings presented above that ongoing protein synthesis and gene transcription are necessary for the normal degradation of EPO mRNA, it is possible that this increase in serum EPO levels may be a reflection of enhanced EPO mRNA stability following such cytotoxic therapy. In vivo animal studies would be necessary to confirm this hypothesis.

The etiology of the decreased EPO response to anemia that these patients demonstrated remains open to speculation. The onset of the blunted response occurring about 2 weeks after cytotoxic therapy is similar in timing to the myelosuppression following such therapy. Although the exact nature of the EPO producing cells in the kidney and liver is controversial, it is possible that the EPO producing cells are damaged by the chemotherapy and radiotherapy. This has been suggested as the etiology of the anemia associated with cisplatin chemotherapy [27], though direct erythroid marrow toxicity may also play a role [28]. Furthermore, since most of these patients are exposed to multiple potential nephrotoxic drugs during their hospital course, one cannot completely exclude the potential contributions of these agents.

While the etiology is open to speculation, it is clear that during the first 4 weeks after BMT, these patients treated with large doses of cytotoxic therapy manifested not only a decreased EPO response for a given degree of anemia compared to their own day 7 post-BMT response, but they also showed a decreased response compared to the reference population. Thus, clinical trials assessing the efficacy of rhEPO in the treatment of anemias associated with intensive cytotoxic therapy appear warranted.

Acknowledgements

This work was supported in part by NIH Grant Nos. DK01401, CA39542, and PO1CA38493 as well as by HRSA Grant No. PE91000–02, the Lillian L. and Harry A. Cowan Foundation, and the Larry Lawrence Foundation. Data organization and analysis were performed using the data analysis facilities of the Beth Israel Hospital Clinical Research Center. We wish to give special thanks to the bone marrow transplantation nurses at all the participating institutions. Mr. Thomas Schneider provided excellent technical assistance in performing the EPO RIAs.

References

1   Goldberg, M. A.; Glass, G. A.; Cunningham, J. M.; Bunn, H. F.: The regulated expression of erythropoietin by two human hepatoma cell lines. Proc. Natl. Acad. Sci. USA *84:* 7972–7976 (1987).

2   Goldberg, M. A.; Dunning, S. P.; Bunn, H. F.: Regulation of the erythropoietin gene: Evidence that the oxygen sensor is a heme protein. Science *242:* 1412–1415 (1988).

3   Beru, N.; McDonald, J.; Lacombe, C.; Goldwasser, E.: Expression of the erythropoietin gene. Mol. Cell. Biol. *7.* 2571–2575 (1986).

4 Bondurant, M.; Koury, M.: Anemia induces accumulation of erythropoietin mRNA in the kidney and liver. Mol. Cell. Biol. *6:* 2731–2733 (1986).

5 Goldberg, M. A.; Gaut, C. C.; Bunn, H. F.: Erythropoietin mRNA levels are regulated by both transcriptional events and by changes in RNA stability. Blood *74:* 716A (1989).

6 Egrie, J. C.; Cotes, P. M.; Lane, J.; Gaines Das, R. E.; Tam, R. C.: Development of radioimmunoassays for human erythropoietin using recombinant erythropoietin as tracer and immunogen. J. Immunol. Methods *99:* 235–241 (1987).

7 Chirgwin, J. M.; Przybyla, A. E.; MacDonald, R. J.; Rutter, W. J.: Isolation of biologically active ribonucleic acid from sources enriched in ribonuclease. Biochemistry *18:* 5294–5299 (1979).

8 Maniatis, T.; Fritsch, E. F.; Sambrook, J.: Molecular Cloning: A Laboratory Manual. Cold Spring Harbor, Cold Spring Harbor Laboratory, 1982.

9 Feinberg, A. P.; Vogelstein, B.: A technique for radiolabeling DNA restriction endonuclease fragments to high specific activity. Anal. Biochem. *32:* 6–13 (1983).

10 Schuster, S. J.; Badiavas, E. V.; Costa-Giomi, P.; Weinmann, R.; Erslev, A. J.; Caro, J.: Stimulation of erythropoietin gene transcription during hypoxia and cobalt exposure. Blood *73:* 13–16 (1989).

11 Mullner, E. W.; Neupert, B.; Kuhn, L. C.: A specific mRNA binding factor regulates the iron-dependent stability of cytoplasmic transferrin receptor mRNA. Cell *58:* 373–382 (1989).

12 Cleveland, D. W.; Yen, T. J.: Multiple determinants of eukaryotic mRNA stability. New Biol. *1:* 121–126 (1989).

13 Brawerman, G.: mRNA decay: finding the right targets. Cell *57:* 9–10 (1989).

14 Linial, M.; Gunderson, N.; Groudine, M.: Enhanced transcription of c-myc in bursal lymphoma cells requires continued protein synthesis. Science *230:* 1126–1132 (1985).

15 Pachter, J. S.; Yen, T. J.; Cleveland, D. W.: Autoregulation of tubulin expression is achieved through specific degradation of polysomal tubulin mRNAs. Cell *51:* 283–292 (1987).

16 Sive, H. L.; Heintz, N.; Roeder, R. G.: Regulation of human histone gene expression during the HeLa cell cycle requires protein synthesis. Mol. Cell. Biol. *4:* 2723–2734 (1984).

17 Rahmsdorf, H. J.; Schonthal, A.; Angel, P.; Litfin, M.; Ruther, U.; Herrlich, P.: Posttranscriptional regulation of c-fos mRNA expression. Nucleic Acids Res. *15:* 1643–1659 (1987).

18 Shyu, A.-B.; Greenberg, M. E.; Belasco, J. G.: The c-fos transcript is targeted for rapid decay by two distinct mRNA degradation pathways. Genes Dev. *3:* 60–72 (1989).

19 Shaw, G.; Kamen, R.: A conserved AU sequence from the 2' untranslated region of GM-CSF mRNA mediates selective mRNA degradation. Cell *46:* 659–667 (1986).

20 Cavalieri, R. L.; Havell, E. A.; Vilcek, J.; Pestka, S.: Induction and decay of human fibroblast interferon mRNA. Proc. Natl. Acad. Sci. USA *74:* 4415–4419 (1977).

21 Mullner, E. W.; Kuhn, L. C.: A stem-loop structure in the 3' untranslated region mediates iron-dependent regulation of transferrin receptor mRNA stability in the cytoplasm. Cell *53:* 815–825 (1988).

22 Koury, S. T.; Bondurant, M. C.; Koury, M. J.: Localization of erythropoietin synthesizing cells in murine kidneys by in situ hybridization. Blood *71:* 524–527 (1988).

23 Lacombe, C.; Da Silva, J.-L.; Bruneval, P.; Fournier, J.-G.; Wendling, F.; Casadevall, N.; Camilleri, J.-P.; Bariéty, J.; Varet, B.; Tambourin, P.: Peritubular cells are the site of

erythropoietin synthesis in the murine hypoxic kidney. J. Clin. Invest. *81:* 620–623 (1988).

24   Spivak, J.L.: The mechanism of action of erythropoietin. Int. J. Cell Cloning *4:* 139–166 (1986).

25   Birgegard, G.; Wide, L.; Simonsson, B.: Marked erythropoietin increase before fall in Hb after treatment with cytostatic drugs suggests mechanism other than anaemia for stimulation. Br. J. Haematol. *72:* 462–466 (1989).

26   Piroso, E.; Erslev, A.J.; Caro, J.: Inappropriate increase in erythropoietin titers during chemotherapy. Am. J. Hematol. *32:* 248–254 (1989).

27   Smith, D.H.; Guarneri, C.M.; Whaling, S.M.; Vokes, E.E.: Erythropoietin response in cancer patients receiving cisplatin. Proc. Am. Assoc. Cancer Res. *29:* 52A (1988).

28   Rothmann, S.A.; Paul, P.; Weick, J.K.; McIntyre, W.R.; Fantelli, F.: Effect of *cis*-diaminedichloroplatinum on erythropoietin production and hematopoietic progenitor cells. Int. J. Cell Cloning *3:* 415–423 (1985).

Mark A. Goldberg, MD, Brigham and Women's Hospital, Hematology Division, 75 Francis Street, Boston, MA 02115 (USA)

Gurland HJ, Moran J, Samtleben W, Scigalla P, Wieczorek L (eds): Erythropoietin in
Renal and Non-Renal Anemias. Contrib Nephrol. Basel, Karger, 1991, vol 88, pp 46–47

Discussion

to the Paper by M. A. Goldberg et al.

Goldwasser (Chicago): With regard to your proposed destabilizing protein, the degrading protein that breaks down the EPO message, do you have any data bearing on its possible specificity, that is, are other messenger RNAs either not stabilized or stabilized in the same system?

Goldberg: The only one that we have looked at is actin mRNA, and it doesn't appear to be altered. One thing that would be important to do is to look at some shorter-lived messages and ask that specific question. The other way we're approaching this is by looking at conserved non-coding regions of the EPO transcript to see if they bind a protein in a specific manner.

Miller (Baltimore): We've looked at our bone marrow transplant group as well. We've studied the EPO response in 70 patients after allogeneic and autologous transplantation. We have also seen suppression of the response after transplantation but it appears that when these patients, similar to the renal failure patients, get severely hypoxic or have hepatitis, they have marked increases in their EPO levels, so there doesn't appear to be an absolute inability of these patients to make EPO. We've also followed these patients up to 6 months and about 50% of our allogeneic patients remain anemic after 6 months. They are all on ciclosporin. These patients all continue to have a suppressed EPO response to anemia up to 6 months post-transplant.

Goldberg: Sorry, I forgot to mention the Hopkins' group but I know they've also looked at many patients. We also saw this in 1 patient who had a major GI bleed; although his EPO levels were low, he was able to increase EPO production with severe anemia, again analogous to the renal failure population. Even though they can do that, like the renal failure population, I don't think that implies they won't respond to exogenous rhEPO.

Lacombe (Paris): Coming back to the sensor, I would like to know your opinion about the localisation of the oxygen sensor; do you think it's in the same cell which produces EPO?

Goldberg: I think that the Hep 3B cell represents the fetal liver and that in the liver, the sensor and the EPO producer, if the Hep 3B cells are an indication, are in the same cell. I guess, until we isolate the EPO-producing cell in the kidney, maybe Dr. Caro can tell us the next time we meet, I don't know if we can say that the sensor is in the same cell as the EPO producer. I guess it's possible that it's not. There are no data either way and it would only be speculation.

Baldamus (Cologne): Are you able to pin-point the effect of cytotoxic drugs on the EPO increase to one specific drug or is this a phenomenon common to all cytotoxic agents?

Goldberg: The patients that we saw clinically were treated with several different regimens; some of them received radiation therapy but not all of them. Almost all of them received cyclophosphamide but they received various alkylating agents in various combinations. What we plan to do is to look at some of these agents in the Hep 3B cells, which again are a pure population.

Eschbach (Seattle): There may be other reasons why EPO secretion may remain lower than anticipated, besides being suppressed by cytotoxic drugs. Over 10 years ago, Dr. John Adamson and I developed a sheep model for studying the anemia of chronic renal failure. We obtained EPO-rich plasma from normal sheep which we treated with one dose of phenylhydrazine to produce hemolysis, and then daily phlebotomy to maintain a hematocrit between 10 and 12%. The EPO levels measured by radioimmunoassay were over 1,000 mU/ml for 5–8 days and then, despite persistent severe anemia maintained by periodic phlebotomy for 4 weeks, the EPO levels fell towards baseline values. Nevertheless, once phlebotomy was discontinued, and despite near normal plasma EPO levels, the hematocrit returned within 2–3 months to the sheep's normal level of 30%. The serum albumin decreased from 3.3 to 2.0 g/dl during the phlebotomy period and then returned to normal 1 month later. We never fully understood why the EPO levels returned to near normal values despite the severe anemia, nor why the red cell mass eventually increased in association with near normal EPO levels. This phenomenon was reproducible in many sheep.

Goldberg: That's why I like to work with Hep 3B cells, they are simpler than sheep.

Gurland HJ, Moran J, Samtleben W, Scigalla P, Wieczorek L (eds): Erythropoietin in
Renal and Non-Renal Anemias. Contrib Nephrol. Basel, Karger, 1991, vol 88, pp 48–56

Structure and Function of the Erythropoietin Receptor in Stable Erythropoietin-Dependent Transfectants

Alan D. D'Andrea, Jah-Won Koo

Division of Pediatric Oncology, Dana Farber Cancer Institute, Harvard Medical
School, Boston, Mass., USA

Physiologic Role of Erythropoietin in Erythroid Differentiation

While many of the presentations at this symposium have addressed the
process of erythropoietin (EPO) production, primarily by kidney cells, our
work addresses the process of EPO stimulation of target erythroid cells.
Despite the availability of purified recombinant EPO, little is known about the
interaction of EPO and the EPO receptor (EPO-R) or the physiologic mechanisms by which EPO causes cells to undergo proliferation or differentiation.
This is largely due to the lack of adequate quantities of EPO-R for in-depth
biochemical study. Only small numbers of surface EPO-R (less than 1,000) are
present on normal erythroblasts and erythroleukemia cells. EPO provides a
proliferative signal to BFU-E (burst-forming unit-erythroid, an early EPO-
responsive erythroid progenitor) and a differentiative signal to CFU-E (colony-forming unit-erythroid, a later EPO-responsive erythroid progenitor).
These two classes of EPO-responsive cells are clearly different populations
since they can be separated by unit gravity sedimentation and more recently
have been purified to homogeneity.

Structure of the EPO-R

Investigators have used radiolabeled EPO to demonstrate specific binding to cells derived from the erythroid lineage [1]. These cells include normal
erythroid progenitors, virally transformed spleen cells (i.e., Friend cells),
murine and human erythroleukemia cells, and cells from human fetal liver.

Scatchard analysis has been employed to determine the number of binding sites per cell and the affinity constants for the interaction. Approximately 200 EPO-R are present on the cell surface of purified normal erythroid progenitors. On certain cell lines, that number can increase to about 1,000 per cell. This relatively low number of EPO-R is characteristic of other receptors for hematopoietic cytokines such as G-CSF, GM-CSF, IL-3, and IL-6. Scatchard analysis reveals that certain erythroid cells, such as MEL cells, express only low affinity receptors while other cell lines express high and low affinity receptors. The lower affinity receptor has an affinity constant in the 200 pM range and therefore still represents an intimate interaction between receptor and ligand. Although functional differences between the higher and lower affinity EPO-R have not been determined, the two affinities may account for different cellular responses to EPO. For instance, Friend virus-infected cells which have both high and low affinity receptors for EPO respond to EPO with proliferation and differentiation. In contrast, MEL cells bind EPO only with low affinity and do not appear to respond to the hormone.

Affinity cross-linking experiments using radiolabeled EPO reveal two cross-linked EPO-R complexes. The complexes appear as two bands of sizes 145 and 100 kd. The size of the 100-kd band is the sum of the size of EPO (34 kd) plus the size of the EPO-R (66 kd). Other higher and lower molecular weight species have been documented. There is also disagreement on the effect of reducing agents on the cross-linking experiments. Some investigators have demonstrated one large molecule species of about 250 kd which resolves into two bands when reduced, while others have not demonstrated this high molecular weight band. A relationship between the number of bands and the presence of high and low affinity receptors is not evident.

The recent cloning of the murine EPO-R [2] has provided new insights into the understanding of EPO-induced signal transduction. The EPO-R cDNA was cloned by transfecting pools of recombinant plasmids from a MEL cDNA library into COS cells and screening for uptake of radioiodinated EPO by transfected cells. A single cDNA was isolated which was capable of conferring on COS cells the ability to bind EPO. As inferred from the sequence of the cDNA, the cloned EPO-R is a 507 amino acid polypeptide with a single membrane-spanning domain, or a so-called type I membrane spanning protein. As expected, the EPO-R transcript showed erythroid-specific expression [2]. Surprisingly, the COS cell transfectants, unlike MEL cells, demonstrated both high affinity and low affinity receptors. This result suggested that the cDNA encoded one subunit of the EPO-R, and that a second subunit, or accessory protein, was endogenous to COS cells. The COS cell transfectants also demonstrated two cross-linked complexes. These cross-linked complexes were similar in molecular weight to those observed in normal erythroid progenitor cells.

A New Growth Factor Receptor Superfamily

The EPO-R was initially found to have extensive amino acid homology with the IL-2 receptor beta chain [3]. The IL-2 receptor is an alpha/beta heterodimeric receptor with two receptor affinities. Interestingly, the EPO-R cDNA and the IL-2R cDNA each generate high and low affinity receptors and two radiolabeled cross-linked polypeptides when expressed in stable transfectants.The native EPO-R, therefore, probably interacts with a second chain which may be endogenous to COS cells. Also, the greatest sequence identity (35% amino acid identity) between the EPO-R and the IL-2R beta chain exists in the cytoplasmic region, adjacent to the transmembrane domain. Since no tyrosine kinase catalytic domain is evident, this conserved region is of particular importance and probably denotes common signal transduction mechanisms. Interestingly, both EPO-dependent and IL-2-dependent cell lines have been isolated, suggesting that cell viability and proliferation is conferred by these hormones.

The EPO-R family of receptors, or so-called cytokine receptor superfamily, has now expanded to include several other growth factor receptors. This superfamily includes the ligand binding subunits of the receptors for IL-2, IL-3, IL-4, IL-6, IL-7, GM-CSF, and G-CSF, and the receptors for prolactin and growth hormone (fig. 1) [4]. The most striking similarity among all members of this cytokine receptor superfamily includes the conservation of four cysteines and a tryptophan-serine-X-tryptophan-serine motif positioned just outside the transmembrane region. These sequence homologies probably reflect structural homologies among these receptors which may, in turn, extend to structural homologies among the respective growth factors themselves. For instance, the crystal structure of growth hormone reveals an antiparallel four-helix bundle core. Similarly, modeling of the tertiary structure of EPO and IL-6 reveals a growth hormone-like helix bundle fold. There also exists extensive amino acid identity among the EPO-R, IL-2R, IL-3R, and IL-4R in the cytoplasmic domain suggesting common signaling mechanisms (fig. 1). It is likely that all members of this family are multisubunit receptors and that additional subunits account for the variable hormone affinities and responses observed.

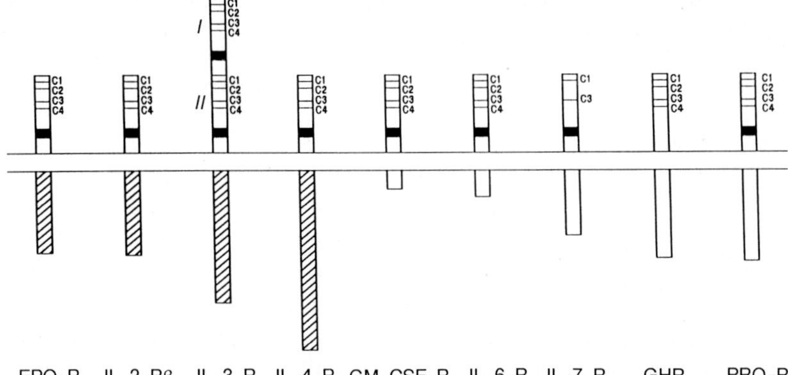

Fig. 1. Schematic representation of a new cytokine receptor superfamily. Homologous domains of the receptors for erythropoietin (EPO), interleukin-2 (IL-2), interleukin-3 (IL-3), interleukin-4 (IL-4), granulocyte-macrophage colony-stimulating factor (GM-CSF), interleukin-6 (IL-6), interleukin-7 (IL-7), growth hormone (GH), and prolactin (PRO) are aligned. The extracellular domains of the receptors share a highly similar 20 amino acid sequence which includes a conserved WS-WS motif (black box), presumed to be involved in protein-protein interaction. Also, four conserved cysteine residues (C1–C4) are aligned. The homologous external domain is duplicated in the IL-3R (regions I and II). The cytoplasmic domain of four of the receptors contain a conserved region, rich in proline, serine, and acidic residues (cross-hatched bars) suggesting a common mechanism of signal transduction.

Although the cytokine receptor superfamily does not share amino acid homology with members of the tyrosine kinase receptor superfamily [5], these two receptor superfamilies do have some common characteristics. Both superfamilies contain member receptors which possess a large glycosylated, extracytoplasmic ligand binding domain, a single hydrophobic transmembrane region, and a variable cytoplasmic tail. Yet, while members of the tyrosine kinase superfamily have a cytoplasmic domain with a tyrosine kinase catalytic domain, the cytokine receptor cytoplasmic domains contain no such enzymatic activity. Due to their configurations, however, members of both superfamilies are considered membrane-associated allosteric enzymes. Ligand binding to the extracytoplasmic region causes an activation which must be translated across the membrane barrier in both cases.

Table 1. Coexpression of gp55 and EPO-R in an IL-3-dependent early B lymphocyte confers growth factor independence

Growth of Ba/F3 lymphocytes after infection with:	RPMI media with		
	IL-3	EPO	none
None	+	−	−
SFFV-gp55	+	−	−
SFFV-EPO-R	+	+	−
SFFV-gp55 + SFFV-EPO-R	+	+	+

Growth of Ba/F3 lymphocytes after infection with a retrovirus expressing the EPO-R or after infection with a retrovirus expressing the gp55. Ba/F3 cells are murine pro-B lymphocytes which have a requirement for IL-3 (multi-CSF) for growth. The cells were infected with retroviral supernatants (SFFV) and assayed for expression of gp55 or EPO-R. Infected cells were then transferred to media with either IL-3, EPO (0.1 unit/ml), or no added growth factor. Cell growth (i.e., the presence of live cells after 2 days in the supplemented growth media) is shown by a + sign. Cells expressing only gp55 still require IL-3 for growth. Cells expressing EPO-R will grow in the presence of IL-3 or EPO, demonstrating that the EPO-R is functional in these cells. Cells expressing both gp55 and EPO-R are growth factor independent. In these cells, there is a physical association between the EPO-R and the gp55 [8].

Transmembrane Signaling by the EPO-R

Several studies have investigated the cellular action of the EPO ligand-receptor complex. Using the intracellular calcium chelators, quin-2 and fura-2, EPO has been shown to induce a rapid increase in intracellular free calcium. EPO has also been demonstrated to activate Mg^{2+}, Ca^{2+}, and Na^+–K^+ATPases. Monesin, a sodium specific ionophore, potentiates erythroid growth, while valinomycin, a potassium-specific ionophore, suppresses growth. Investigators have reported that EPO activates adenylate cyclase and increases cyclic AMP levels, independent of activation by beta-adrenergic receptors. Conflicting results have been found concerning the role of guanidine-nucleotide binding proteins in EPO stimulation. Phospholipase C and phosphoinositol mechanisms do not appear to mediate the noted calcium flux. Also, a protein of 43 kd which is dephosphorylated on serine residues in erythroid cell lines in response to EPO has been described [6].

As discussed previously, the major difficulty encountered in studies of EPO induced signal transduction has been the small number of surface receptors and the unavailability of a purely EPO-dependent cell line. The EPO-R, although expressed in high numbers in COS cell transfectants, is not functional in these cells. The addition of EPO to these transfectants does not change the growth kinetics of the cells or induce erythroid differentiation [D'Andrea, unpubl. observation]. In contrast, transfection of the EPO-R cDNA into Ba/F3 cells, a murine pro-B lymphocyte cell line dependent on the hormone IL-3 (multi-CSF), does confer EPO dependence [7] to these cells. An EPO-dependent clone of Ba/F3 cells (Ba/F3-EPO-R) has been isolated which expresses cell surface EPO-R and which has absolute dependence upon EPO for growth (table 1). The availability of this homogenous, EPO-dependent cell line should greatly facilitate the study of the functional EPO-R structure and signaling mechanisms.

Interaction of the EPO-R with the Friend Virus gp55

Since the EPO-R is a member of a large hematopoietic growth factor receptor superfamily, any molecular insight into the EPO-R subunit structure, generation of its multiple affinities for EPO, or mechanism of signaling may be generalizable to the other family members. Recent insight is derived from the observation that the EPO-R binds to and is activated by the membrane glycoprotein, gp55, of the Friend spleen focus-forming virus (SFFV) [8]. SFFV is a defective murine C-type retrovirus that causes a multistage erythroleukemia in mice and erythroblastosis in bone marrow cultures [reviewed in 8]. The SFFV env gene encodes a membrane glycoprotein, gp55, that is located on the cell surface and within rough endoplasmic reticula and that is essential for the induction of leukemia in vivo and EPO-independent erythroblast proliferation in vitro. By cotransfecting both EPO-R and the gp55 into an IL-3-dependent lymphocyte cell line, it was shown that the physical interaction of these two proteins gives rise to constitutive cell growth. The interaction between the EPO-R and gp55 is shown schematically in figure 2. The EPO-R is a 507 amino acid, type I membrane spanning protein. The gp55 is 409 amino acids, with a carboxy terminal membrane anchor. The interaction between the EPO-R and gp55 could occur at several different sites along the molecules and in several possible subcellular compartments. Through direct binding of the EPO-R, gp55 can stimulate the receptor and bypass the normal requirement for EPO, causing a prolonged growth factor independent proliferation of infected erythroid cells.

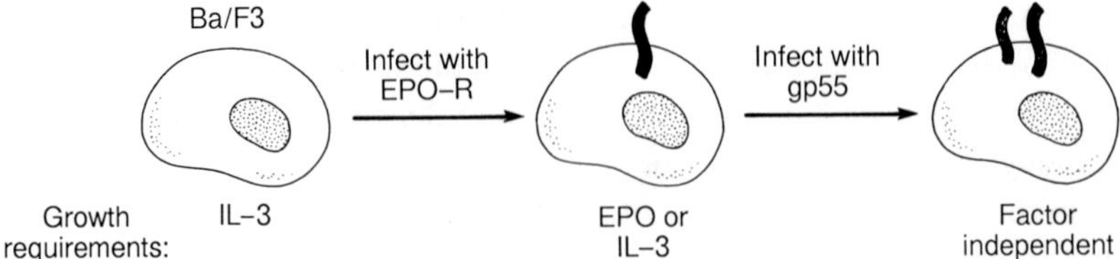

Fig. 2. Schematic model of the physical interaction between the EPO-R and the gp55 of the SFFV. The EPO-R (507 amino acids) and the gp55 (409 amino acids) are type I membrane spanning proteins. Protein-protein interaction may occur either in the membrane spanning regions of the two proteins or in the extracytoplasmic domains of the two proteins. The interaction stimulates EPO-R signaling and thereby mimics EPO binding.

The gp55 may mimic EPO itself, although there is no amino acid homology shared between these two proteins. Alternatively, gp55 may have sequences derived from (and therefore mimic) the normal cellular second subunit of the EPO-R. The interaction between the EPO-R and gp55 is also observed in MEL cells and probably accounts for the absence of high affinity binding sites on MEL cells and for the EPO unresponsiveness of these cells. Recent evidence suggests that the interaction between the EPO-R and the gp55 occurs within the endoplasmic reticulum. The interaction of these two proteins is a novel mechanism of viral transformation leading to growth factor independence. It is possible that analogous retroviruses transform other cell types in a similar manner by using other receptors of the EPO-R superfamily such as the IL-2R or the IL-3R.

Future Directions

The recent cloning of the EPO-R, its membership in a new cytokine receptor family, and its interaction with the gp55, all suggest new directions for erythropoiesis research. The EPO-R, for instance, provides an important stage-specific marker of erythroid differentiation. It is possible that expression of the EPO-R in an early hematopoietic cell (say, BFU-E) actually locks the cell into an erythroid differentiation pattern. Future studies will determine the stage during red cell development that the EPO-R is expressed and how this expression changes during differentiation. Hematopoiesis is likely to be accompanied by the sequential expression and loss of the EPO-R and other growth factor receptors.

It is also possible that the EPO-R plays a role in the pathogenesis of pure red cell aplasia or congenital aplastic anemia (so-called Diamond-Blackfan anemia). With the availability of the human cDNA and gene for the EPO-R [9] and antisera which recognize the normal human EPO-R polypeptide [9], the possible role of EPO-R in the pathogenesis of these anemias will be testable. This will lead to better classification of anemias and could lead to more tailored therapies. Although the EPO-R gene has recently been localized to human chromosome 19p [10], no human diseases suggestive of EPO-R pathology map to this region.

The recent cloning of the EPO-R and the recognition of the new cytokine receptor family will allow a more directed approach to studying EPO-induced signal transduction. Prior to the cloning of the EPO-R, several conflicting studies addressed the question of possible second messengers. The EPO-R has significant amino acid homology (35%) in the cytoplasmic domain with the IL-2R (p75) and the IL-3R, receptors recently shown to transduce signaling through tyrosine phosphorylation. For instance, the IL-2R (p75) subunit activates a tyrosine kinase activity and the p75 subunit is itself tyrosine phosphorylated [11]. It is possible that the cytokine receptors are noncovalently associated with a tyrosine protein kinase in a manner similar to that observed with the T cell surface antigen, CD4 [12]. The cytoplasmic homology of the EPO-R with these other receptors strongly argues for protein phosphorylation as an early component of transmembrane signaling. Also, because the EPO-R, transfected into IL-3-dependent cells, confers EPO dependence on these cells, a common pathway of signaling is likely to be found for these receptors and for other receptors in the cytokine receptor superfamily.

References

1   Sawyer, S. T.; Krantz, S. B.; Luna, J.: Identification of the receptor for erythropoietin by cross-linking to Friend virus-infected erythroid cells. PNAS *84:* 3690–3694 (1987).
2   D'Andrea, A. D.; Lodish, H. F.; Wong, G. G.: Expression cloning of the murine erythropoietin receptor. Cell *57:* 277–285 (1989).
3   D'Andrea, A. D.; Fasman, G.; Lodish, H. F.: Erythropoietin receptor and interleukin-2 receptor β chain: a new receptor family. Cell *58:* 1023–1024 (1989).
4   Bazan, J. F.: A novel family of growth factor receptors. Biochem. Biophys. Res. Commum. *164.* 788–796 (1989).
5   Ullrich, A.; Schlessinger, J.: Signal transduction by receptors with tyrosine kinase activity. Cell *61:* 203–212 (1990).

6   Choi, H.-S.; Wojchowski, D.M.; Sytokowski, A.J.: Erythropoietin rapidly alters phosphorylation of pp43, an erythroid membrane protein. J. Biol. Chem. *262:* 2933–2936 (1987).

7   D'Andrea, A.D.; Szklut, P.; Lodish, H.F.; Alderman, E.: Inhibition of receptor binding and neutralization of bioactivity by anti-erythropoietin monoclonal antibodies. Blood *75:* 874–880 (1989).

8   Li, J.P.; D'Andrea, A.D.; Lodish, H.F.; Baltimore, D.: Activation of cell growth by binding of Friend spleen focus-forming virus gp55 glycoprotein to the erythropoietin receptor. Nature *343:* 762–764 (1990).

9   Simon, S.S.; D'Andrea, A.D.; Haines, A.L.; Wong, C.C.: Human erythropoietin receptor: cloning, expression and biological characterization. Blood (in press).

10 Budarf, M.; Huebner K.; Emanuel, B.; Croce, C.M.; Copeland, N.G.; Jenkins, N.A.; D'Andrea, A.D.: Assignment of the erythropoietin receptor gene to mouse chromosome 9 and human chromosome 19. Genomics (in press).

11 Sorensen, P.; Mui, A.; Krystal, G.: Interleukin-3 stimulates the tyrosine phosphorylation of the 140 kd interleukin-3 receptor. J. Biol. Chem. *264:* 19253–19258 (1989).

12 Veilette, A.; Bookman, M.A.; Horak, E.M.; Bolen, J.B.: The CD4 and CD8 T cell surface antigens are associated with the internal membrane tyrosine-protein kinase p56[lck]. Cell *55:* 301–308 (1988).

Dr. Alan D. D'Andrea, Division of Pediatric Oncology, Dana Farber Cancer Institute, 44 Binney Street, Boston, MA 02115 (USA)

Gurland HJ, Moran J, Samtleben W, Scigalla P, Wieczorek L (eds): Erythropoietin in
Renal and Non-Renal Anemias. Contrib Nephrol. Basel, Karger, 1991, vol 88, pp 57–58

Discussion

to the Paper by A. D. D'Andrea and J.-W. Koo

Goldwasser (Chicago): In the slide showing the hypersensitivity to EPO, did I see the abscissa correctly: the cells appear to respond to as little as 10^{-5} U/ml of EPO?

D'Andrea: No, that is not correct. The hypersensitive mutants respond to EPO in the concentration range of about 10^{-3} U/ml, approximately 10–100 times more sensitive than the wild-type EPO receptor.

Winearls (Oxford): Do your experiments suggest that the EPO maintains viability of cells or just causes them to proliferate or both?

D'Andrea: The Ba/F-3 lymphocyte, transfected with the EPO receptor, clearly require EPO for viability and probably for proliferation. The important thing is that these cells do not differentiate in response to EPO. That is, they do not make any red blood cell antigens. What I am saying is that for these cells, EPO is required for viability, perhaps proliferation, but clearly one cannot make any statement about the differentiation capacities of EPO.

Rich (Ulm): When you transfected the cells with gp55, do you know whether the production of the EPO receptor is in some way inhibited? How do you explain that situation?

D'Andrea: In the cells that are co-expressing EPO receptor and gp55 there is no change in the transcription or translation of the EPO receptor. Also these cells are not making EPO. The gp55 is substituting completely for the effect of EPO.

Halpérin (Geneva): What does the EPO receptor look like in Blackfan-Diamond anemia?

D'Andrea: We have not studied that condition.

Shaldon (Montpellier): In view of the homogeneity of the EPO receptor with several other cell-surface receptors such as IL-2 and IL-3, would you speculate on whether the EPO receptor circulates, or it only cell-associated?

D'Andrea: We have never demonstrated in vivo a circulating form of the EPO receptor. The truncated, secreted mutant of the receptor which I showed was constructed. However, other members of this receptor super family, particularly the interleukin 4 receptor, do appear to exist in a cell-associated form and a secreted form, both found in vivo.

Kurtz (Zurich): I would like to know whether you have any information about the signal transduction mechanism of this EPO receptor. You mentioned that it has no similarity to a tyrosine kinase. Could you speculate about other signal transduction mechanisms? From the literature I know that activation of EPO receptors increases calcium influx in the target cells. Is the EPO receptor perhaps a channel protein?

D'Andrea: We really have very little information along these lines. Studying the EPO receptor structure is a good way to study the very early events of EPO binding and activation, but what second messenger is involved is still not known. For the IL-2 and IL-3 receptors, tyrosine phosphorylation appears to be very important in signalling. Since the EPO receptor is a member of the same family, we are hoping that we can generalize from one receptor to the next in terms of signal pathways.

Goldwasser: Do you have any further thoughts about the great paradox of how you can get two classes of receptors from a single gene transfection?

D'Andrea: It appears that the EPO receptor polypeptide which we have cloned is present in both of those cross-linked complexes. I think there may be an accessory protein which is also present in the larger cross-linked complex which has not yet been identified.

Gurland HJ, Moran J, Samtleben W, Scigalla P, Wieczorek L (eds): Erythropoietin in
Renal and Non-Renal Anemias. Contrib Nephrol. Basel, Karger, 1991, vol 88, pp 59–69

Binding Studies on the Erythropoietin Receptor

Takayuki Hosoi[a], *Stephen T. Sawyer*[a], *W. David Hankins*[b],
Sanford B. Krantz[a]

[a]Division of Hematology, Department of Medicine, Department of Veterans Affairs
Medical Center and Vanderbilt University School of Medicine, Nashville, Tenn., and
[b]National Institutes of Health, Bethesda, Md., USA

In order to study the erythropoietin (EPO) receptor, it is necessary to
have a source of pure EPO and pure erythroid progenitor cells. The advent of
recombinant human EPO provided a plentiful source of the hormone which
could be radioiodinated with retention of biological activity [1]. Highly purified erythroid progenitor cells have been obtained by administering the Friend
virus that produces anemia (FVA) to susceptible mice [2]. This virus elicits a
marked accumulation of erythroid cells (FVA cells) which are arrested at a
stage of development close to the colony-forming unit-erythroid (CFU-E) in
the spleens of infected mice [2]. These cells can be enriched to provide 95%
erythroid progenitor cells with a yield of 5×10^8/spleen. In addition, highly
purified human erythroid progenitor cells [3, 4], and a variety of cell lines,
such as the HCD-57 cells, [5], are now available for studying the EPO receptor.

Cross-linking of ^{125}I-EPO bound to membranes from FVA cells, using
disuccinimidyl suberate (DSS), has shown two radioactive bands with an
apparent molecular mass of 100 and 85 kd when the mass of EPO was sub-
tracted [6, 7]. However, D'Andrea et al. [8] have cloned a cDNA encoding a 55
kd protein which produces an EPO receptor when expressed in COS cells.
When ^{125}I-EPO was cross-linked to transfected COS cells [8], receptor proteins of 105 kd and 65 kd were identified. The relation of the 55–65 kd protein
to the 85–100 kd proteins is still unknown. It is possible that the larger 100 kd
protein arises from the cross-linking of two 55 kd receptor proteins to one
^{125}I-EPO molecule, or of one 55 kd protein and another neighboring protein of
similar size to one ^{125}I-EPO molecule. We have studied this possibility using a
radioiodinated heterobifunctional cross-linker, the Denny-Jaffe (DJ) reagent

[9, 10]. EPO can be chemically attached to one end of the DJ reagent and then, after EPO binding to the receptor, the other end, with a photolabile reactive group, can be activated by ultraviolet light to covalently attach EPO to the receptor. Since this is a monofunctional reagent, EPO is cross-linked to a single protein. In addition, the EPO can be cleaved from the ^{125}I-DJ-EPO receptor complex by the addition of dithionite to break the azo bond in the DJ reagent. With this reagent we have observed cross-linking of EPO to the same 100 and 85 kd EPO receptor proteins identified with DSS, and, after treatment with sodium dithionite to remove the EPO, molecular masses of 105 and 90 kd were directly delineated for these proteins free of the hormone. This shows that the larger proteins identified by EPO cross-linking do not arise from artifactual cross-linking of the 55 kd protein and suggests that the larger bands are either different proteins or consist of 55 kd protein that has been extensively modified.

Methods

Cell Preparation

FVA cells were generated by administering 10^4 FVA spleen focus-forming units intravenously to CD_2F_1 mice [2]. In one experiment the Friend virus that produces polycythemia (FVP) was similarly infused to produce FVP cells [7]. The spleens were removed 2 weeks later and contaminant cells were separated by velocity sedimentation at unit gravity and ammonium chloride lysis of remaining red cells [7]. Murine erythroleukemia (MEL) cells were obtained from W. Le Stourgeon, Vanderbilt University. HCD-57 cells are an EPO-dependent cell line derived from circulating erythroleukemic mice which were infected with Friend murine leukemia virus at birth [5]. Placentas from CD_2F_1 mice were taken at days 14 and 18 of gestation and placentas from Sprague-Dawley rats were taken at 18–20 days of gestation [7]. Placentas were washed and finely minced in phosphate-buffered saline (PBS), pH 7.4, containing a mixture of proteinase inhibitors (2 mM EGTA, 5 mM EDTA, 1 μg leupeptin/ml, 5 mM benzamide, 1 mM iodoacetamide, 10 μg/ml p-tosylamide-2-phenylethylchloromethyl ketone, 10 μg/ml p-tosyl-L-arginine methyl ester, 1 μg/ml n-D-tosyl-L-lysine chloromethyl ketone, 2 μg/ml aprotinin, 1 μg/ml pepstatin, and 0.1 mM phenylmethylsulfonyl fluoride). To prepare membranes the cells or minced placentas were suspended in 10 mM KCl/10 mM Tris-HCl, pH 7.4, with the above mixture of proteinase inhibitors and were broken with a Dounce homogenizer. The homogenates were fractionated by differential centrifugation and the plasma membrane fraction was obtained after equilibrium sedimentation on a discontinuous sucrose gradient [6, 7].

Radiolabelled Recombinant EPO

Pure recombinant human EPO, 129,000 U/mg (Amgen, Thousand Oaks, Calif.), was iodinated using IODO-GEN [1, 3]. One microgram of IODO-GEN in 40 μl of $CHCl_3$ were evaporated onto the wall of a 300-μl conical vial. Two hundred units of the recombinant EPO and 100 µCi of Na^{125}I were incubated in 50 µl of pH 7 buffer for 1 min at 24°C. The mixture was then transferred to a tube containing 0.5 ml PBS, 5 mg KI, and 0.1% gelatin. The ^{125}I-EPO was separated from free ^{125}I by chromatography over a Bio-Gel P6 column equilibrated with PBS containing 0.1% gelatin. The biological activity of ^{125}I-EPO that contained 0.6 molecules of ^{125}I/molecule of EPO had greater than 95% retention of biological activity.

Cross-Linking of ^{125}I-EPO with DSS

^{125}I-EPO was bound to receptors on the plasma membrane fraction and was cross-linked in a similar fashion as described previously [6]. Membranes were incubated with 5.0 units of ^{125}I-EPO/ml in 100 mM phosphate buffer, pH 7.4, containing 1 mM EGTA and 0.1% bovine serum albumin for 15 min at 37°C. The mixture was transferred to an ice bath, and DSS was added to a final concentration of 0.2 mM for 15 min. Tris-HCl, pH 8.0, was added to a final concentration of 150 mM, and the membranes were pelleted by centrifugation at 13,000 g for 30 min. The pellet was resuspended in 10 mM Tris-HCl, pH 7.4, and 100 mM NaCl and washed twice. The pellet was suspended in sample buffer, boiled for 3 min and sonicated briefly. The material was analyzed by NaDodSO$_4$-PAGE as described by Laemmli [11].

Proteolytic mapping of the 100 and 85 kd proteins cross-linked to ^{125}I-EPO was carried out as described by Cleveland et al. [12]. The 100 and 85 kd proteins cross-linked to ^{125}I-EPO were excised from unfixed NaDodSO$_4$-PAGE gels which were frozen and exposed to film [13]. Gel slices and increasing concentrations of *Staphylococcus aureus* V8 protease were loaded into the sample wells of a NaDodSO$_4$-PAGE, and the current was applied until the labeled bands and protease had entered the stacking gel. Following a 60-min incubation in the absence of current to allow the protease to partially digest the proteins in the stacking gel, the current was reapplied to separate the resulting fragments on the separating gel. After fixing and drying, the gel was exposed to x-ray film.

Derivatization of EPO with the DJ Reagent

All of the procedures were done in the dark with a safety light [14]. N-[4-(p-azido-m-(^{125}I)iodophenylazo)benzoyl]-3-aminopropyl-N'-oxysuccinimide ester (DJ reagent) was purchased from New England Nuclear Corp., Boston, Mass. An aliquot of DJ reagent shipped in benzene was put into a conical tube and dried under dry N$_2$ gas. Recombinant EPO (50 units, 0.013 nmol) in 1% dimethyl sulfoxide; 100 mM borate buffer, pH 8.5, was added to the tube coated with the DJ reagent. The solution was kept at room temperature for 120 min to allow the derivatization of a primary amino residue of EPO with the N-hydroxysuccinimide-ester residue of DJ reagent. Tris-HCl (pH 7.4) was then added to quench the reaction, and the solution was kept at room temperature for 15 min. The reaction mixture was applied to a Bio-Gel P6-DG column equilibrated with 0.1% gelatin, 10 mM phosphate, pH 7.4, 150 mM NaCl so that the derivatized EPO (DJ-EPO) was separated from unreacted DJ reagent.

Photoaffinity Labeling of the EPO Receptor

DJ-EPO was incubated with 0.2–0.4 mg HCD-57 cell membrane protein at 37°C for 20 min in the binding/photolysis buffer (1% bovine serum albumin, 1 mM EGTA, 2 µg/ml aprotinin, 10 mM phosphate, pH 7.4, and 150 mM NaCl, degassed and bottled with N$_2$ gas) in 1.5 ml microtubes. Each tube was wrapped with aluminum foil to keep the binding mixture in the dark. The binding mixtures were cooled in ice, transferred into the wells of 24-well culture plate (Costar) and irradiated with ultraviolet light (365 nm) for 15 min on ice using a UVL-56

(Ultra-Violet Products Inc.). The photolyzed samples were washed three times with ice-cold 0.1% bovine serum albumin/100 mM NaCl/50 mM glycine/1 mM EGTA, pH 3.5, and once with ice-cold 1 mM EGTA, 10 mM phosphate, pH 7.2, and 150 mM NaCl by centrifuging at 13,000 g for 15 min at 4 °C. After suspension in the sample buffer containing β-mercaptoethanol, the samples were boiled for 5 min, sonicated briefly and applied to NaDodSO$_4$-PAGE according to the method of Laemmli [11]. The gels were stained with Coomassie brilliant blue, destained, dried, and exposed to Kodak-XAR5 x-ray films for autoradiography.

Cleavage of the DJ Azo Bond

Membranes from HCD-57 cells, which were photoaffinity labeled with ^{125}I-DJ-EPO, were suspended in 2% NaDodSO$_4$, 2 mM EGTA, 100 mM borate buffer, pH 8.0, containing 0.2 M sodium dithionite and were heated at 80 °C for 5 min. Following the addition of the sample buffer, dithionite-treated membranes and control membranes, heated at 80 °C without dithionite for 5 min, were analyzed by NaDodSO$_4$-PAGE and autoradiography.

Results

^{125}I-EPO was bound to membranes prepared from FVA cells, FVP cells, MEL cells, and placentas from mice and rats, and was then cross-linked to the receptor using DSS. With all of these membranes, the ^{125}I-EPO covalently attached to two proteins such that the receptor-EPO complexes migrated at 140 and 125 kd (fig. 1). The results in the presence or absence of reducing agent were identical indicating an absence of disulfide bridges between the two labelled proteins [7]. Similar results were also obtained with purified human CFU-E [7] and subtraction of the molecular mass of EPO led to a calculated mass of 100 and 85 kd for these radioactive bands cross-linked to the hormone.

The cross-linked proteins were analyzed after proteolytic digestion [13]. Figure 2 shows the autoradiograms of the resulting fragments of the 140 kd band (100 kd protein) and 125 kd band (85 kd protein) following degradation with 0.5–100 µg of V8 protease. Identical fragments were generated from both proteins with bands of 26–60 kd predominating. A parallel digestion of ^{125}I-EPO showed only fragments of less than 14 kd [13] and thus almost all of the cleavage products in figure 2 were derived from the receptor proteins.

Since DSS has two N-hydroxysuccinimide esters and might indiscriminately cross-link EPO to more than one neighboring protein, further experiments were performed with the DJ reagent which has only one N-hydroxysuccinimide ester (fig. 3). The format for these experiments is shown in figure 4. EPO was first conjugated to the ^{125}I-DJ reagent (DJ-EPO) in the dark and the DJ-EPO was then separated from unreacted DJ using a gel-sizing column (fig. 4a). The DJ-EPO has a monofunctional reactivity to the receptor and

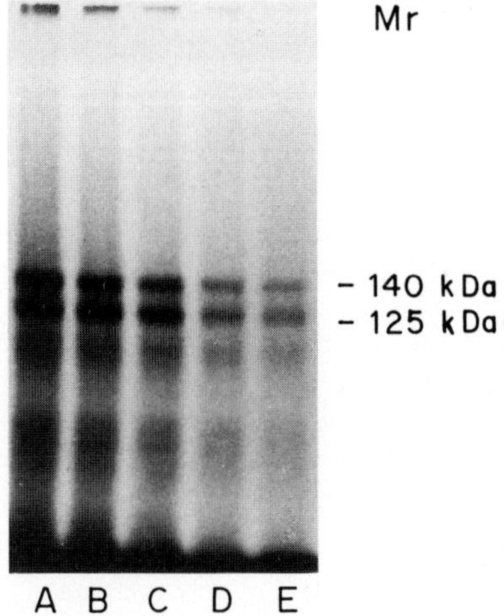

Fig. 1. Cross-linking of ¹²⁵I-EPO to membranes from FVA cells, FVP cells, MEL cells, and placentas from mice and rats. One milligram of membrane protein was incubated with 5 units of ¹²⁵I-EPO for 15 min and cross-linked with 0.2 m*M* DSS. The samples were analyzed by NaDodSO₄-PAGE in the presence of β-mercaptoethanol and autoradiography. Lane A, FVA cells; B, FVP cells; C, MEL cells; D, mouse placenta; E, rat placenta. [Reproduced from 7.]

binds to it through the EPO. Saturable specific binding to HCD-57 cell membranes was confirmed and when the membranes were exposed to ultraviolet light the photoreactive aryl azide formed a single covalent bond with the bound membrane protein (fig. 4b). The photoaffinity labelled receptor was then analyzed by NaDodSO₄-PAGE and autoradiography (fig. 5). Bands of 140 and 125 kd were identified as the same 100 and 85 kd proteins cross-linked to DJ-EPO (lane A) as with ¹²⁵I-EPO and DSS. No labelled bands were observed without photolysis (data not shown) or in the presence of a large excess of unlabelled EPO (lane B), which indicates that specific binding was present. Replicate DJ-EPO membrane preparations were treated with sodium dithionite to cleave the azo bond in the DJ-EPO and remove the EPO (fig. 4B). When these samples were analyzed by NaDodSO₄-PAGE, two new bands of 105 and 90 kd were evident (fig. 5, lane C) and were not seen when DJ-EPO binding was performed in the presence of a large excess of EPO (lane D).

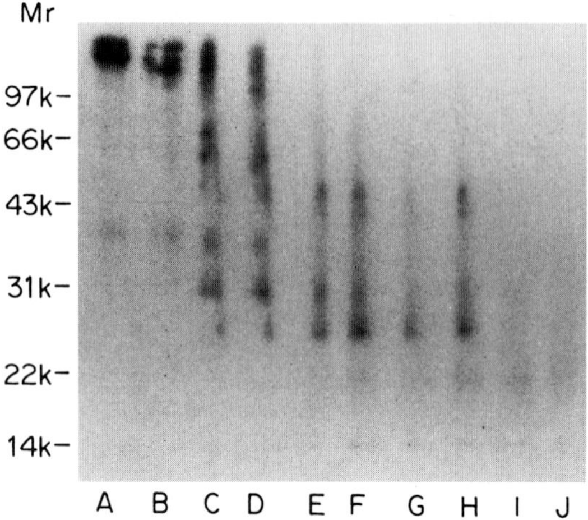

Fig. 2. Peptide mapping of the 100 and 85 kd proteins. The 140 and 125 kd cross-linked bands in FVA cell membranes were excised from a wet unfixed gel which was subjected to autoradiography in the frozen state to identify the bands. The excised slices of gel were digested with V8 protease from *S. aureus* according to the method of Cleveland et al. [12] as described in the Methods section. After digestion in the stacking gel, the resulting fragments were separated on a 10% acrylamide $NaDodSO_4$-PAGE and analyzed by autoradiography. Lanes A, C, E, G, and I, 100 kd protein; lanes B, D, F, and J, 85 kd protein; lanes A and B, 0.5 µg of V8 protease; lanes C and D, 5 µg of V8 protease; lanes E and F, 20 µg of V8 protease; lanes G and H, 50 µg of V8 protease, and lanes I and J, 100 µg of V8 protease. [Reproduced from 13.]

Fig. 3. Chemical formulas for DSS, a homobifunctional cross-linker with two N-hydroxysuccinimide esters, and the DJ reagent, a heterobifunctional cross-linker with one N-hydroxysuccinimide ester for binding ^{125}I-EPO.

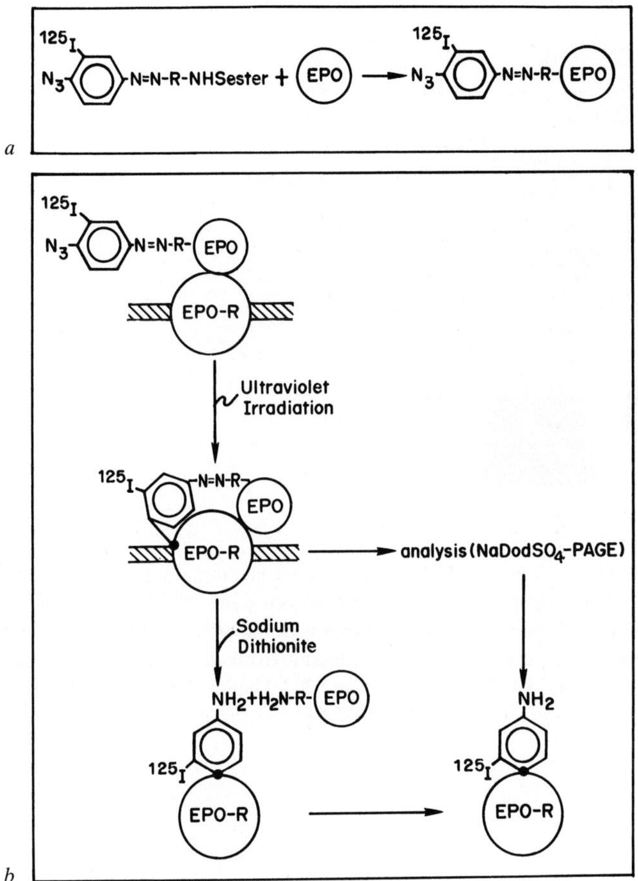

Fig. 4. Experimental plan for use of DJ reagent. *a* A primary amino group of EPO was bound to the DJ reagent through the N-hydroxysuccinimide ester. *b* After specific binding of DJ-EPO to HCD-57 EPO receptors the DJ photoreactive aryl azide group was activated by ultraviolet light for covalent binding (cross-linking) of EPO to the cell membranes. Replicate samples were treated with sodium dithionite to cleave the azo bond and release EPO from the membranes and all samples were analyzed by NaDodSO₄-PAGE and autoradiography.

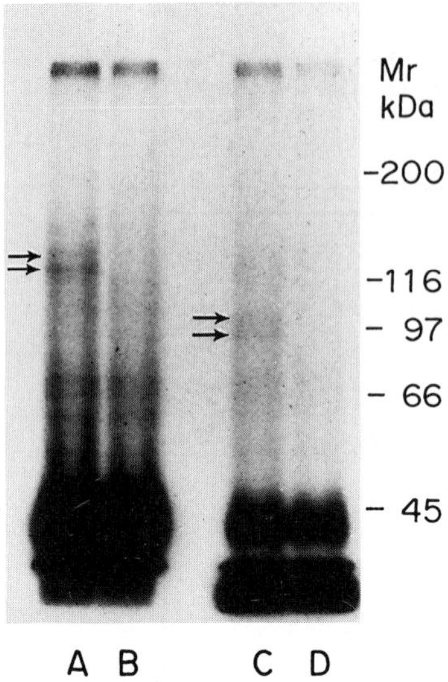

Fig. 5. Cross-linking of EPO to HCD-57 cell plasma membranes using ^{125}I-DJ-EPO. Analysis by NaDodSO$_4$-PAGE showed 140 and 125 kd bands (lane A) and absence of these bands with binding in the presence of a 200-fold excess of unlabeled EPO (lane B). After cross-linking, replicates were treated with sodium dithionite to break the azo bond and release EPO. Analysis by NaDodSO$_4$-PAGE revealed 105 and 90 kd bands (lane C) which were not evident when membranes were bound with ^{125}I-DJ-EPO in the presence of excess EPO (lane D).

Discussion

When ^{125}I-EPO bound to membranes prepared from FVA cells, FVP cells, MEL cells and placentas from mice and rats was cross-linked to the EPO receptor with DSS, two radioactive bands of 140 and 125 kd were identified. Subtraction of the apparent molecular mass of EPO on PAGE indicated that the proteins that were cross-linked to the hormone were 100 and 85 kd. The same bands were seen not only with these tissues but with normal murine and human CFU-E as well as an extensive number of murine and human cell lines, by multiple investigators [15]. This has been a repeated and reproducible observation with all cells or membranes that specifically bind EPO irrespective of subsequent erythroid differentiation [15]. While it is possible that the DSS was artifactually cross-linking a nearest neighbor protein to the hormone, the diversity of these tissues would make that possibility somewhat unlikely.

Further characterization of these putative EPO receptor bands by protease digestion demonstrated identical fragments from the 100 and 85 kd proteins, which strongly suggests that the primary amino acid sequence of these two proteins is similar, if not identical. In addition, increasing the number of protease inhibitors, during the preparation of membranes and the binding and cross-linking steps, increased the ratio of radioactive 100 kd protein to 85 kd protein [13]. The 85 kd protein could be an artifact resulting form proteinase activity, or it could result from a posttranslational modification of the 100 kd protein.

The cloned EPO receptor gene encodes a protein of 55 kd and the relation of that protein to the 100 and 85 kd proteins identified by cross-linking is not known. One possibility is that the bifunctional DSS might cross-link two 55 kd proteins to EPO. The present experiments, however, using the monofunctional DJ reagent, demonstrate that EPO is bound to single proteins which have the same apparent molecular mass of 100 and 85 kd shown with the preceding DSS experiments. In addition, cleavage of the azo bond by sodium dithionite, which releases the EPO from the complex, directly demonstrates that the proteins have a molecular size of 105 and 90 kd corresponding very well to the predicted sizes after subtraction of the molecular mass of EPO.

The EP receptor appears to belong to a family of receptors that includes the interleukin 2 receptor β-chain, the interleukin 3, 4, 6, and 7 receptors, and the granulocyte-macrophage colony-stimulating factor (GM-CSF), growth hormone and prolactin receptors [16–22]. Several of these now appear to have well-defined subunits and it is likely that the EPO receptor consists of more than one protein. The 105 and 90 kd proteins may be additional proteins not related to the cloned gene, or the cloned gene product may be modified to form a new protein either by the covalent coupling of two modified 55 kd subunits, or the addition of another gene product. Even though an EPO receptor gene has been cloned, and extensive cross-linking studies have provided information on the size of the EPO receptor binding proteins, the precise organization of the EPO receptor and the identity of the second messenger remain unknown.

Acknowledgements

The authors would like to acknowledge support from Veterans Health Services and Research Funds and from National Institutes of Health Grants R01 DK 15555, R01 DK 39781 and T32 DK-07186. Dr. Sawyer is a Scholar of the Leukemia Society of America. We also want to thank Ms. Pat Hofmann for her assistance in the preparation of the manuscript and Dr. Eugene Goldwasser for information on the chromatography of EPO on reversed phase HPLC.

References

1 Sawyer, S.; Krantz, S.; Goldwasser, E.: Binding and receptor mediated endocytosis of erythropoietin in Friend virus-infected erythroid cells. J. Biol. Chem. *262:* 5554–5562 (1987).

2 Koury, M.; Sawyer, S.; Bondurant, M.: Splenic erythroblasts in anemia-inducing Friend disease: A source of cells for studies of erythropoietin-mediated differentiation. J. Cell. Physiol. *121:* 526–532 (1984).

3 Sawada, K.; Krantz, S.; Kans, J.; Dessypris, E.; Sawyer, S.; Glick, A.; Civin, C.: Purification of human erythroid colony-forming units and demonstration of specific binding of erythropoietin. J. Clin. Invest. *80:* 357–366 (1987).

4 Sawada, K.; Krantz, S.; Dai, C.-H.; Koury, S.; Horn, S.; Glick, A.; Civin, C.: Purification of human blood burst-forming units-erythroid and demonstration of the evolution of erythropoietin receptors. J. Cell. Physiol. *142:* 219–230 (1990).

5 Ruscetti, S.; Janesch, N.; Chakraborti, A.; Sawyer, S.; Hankins, W.: Friend spleen focus-forming virus induces factor independence in an erythropoietin-dependent erythroleukemia cell line. J. Virol. *63:* 1057–1062 (1990).

6 Sawyer, S.; Krantz, S.; Luna, J.: Identification of the receptor for erythropoietin by cross-linking to Friend virus-infected erythroid cells. Proc. Natl. Acad. Sci. USA *84:* 3690–3694 (1987).

7 Sawyer, S.; Krantz, S.; Sawada, K.: Receptors for erythropoietin in mouse and human erythroid cells and placenta. Blood *74:* 103–109 (1989).

8 D'Andrea, A.; Lodish, H.; Wong, G.: Expression cloning of the murine erythropoietin receptor. Cell *57:* 277–285 (1989).

9 Denny, J.; Blobel, G.: ^{125}I-labeled cross-linking reagent that is hydrophilic, photoactivatable and cleavable through an azo linkage. Proc. Natl. Acad. Sci. USA *81:* 5286–5290 (1984).

10 Jaffe, C.; Lis, H.; Sharon, N.: New cleavable photoreactive heterobifunctional cross-linking reagents for studying membrane organization. Biochemistry *19:* 4423–4429 (1980).

11 Laemmli, U.: Cleavage of structural proteins during the assembly of the head of bacteriophage T4. Nature *227:* 680–685 (1970).

12 Cleveland, D.; Fischer, S.; Kirschner, M.; Laemmli, U.: Peptide mapping by limited proteolysis in sodium dodecyl sulfate and analysis by gel electrophoresis. J. Biol. Chem. *252:* 1102–1106 (1977).

13 Sawyer, S.: The two proteins of the erythropoietin receptor are structurally similar. J. Biol. Chem. *264:* 13343–13347 (1989).

14 Hosoi, T.; Sawyer, S.; Krantz, S.: Photoaffinity labeling of the erythropoietin receptor and its identification in a ligand-free form. Biochemistry (submitted, 1990).

15 Sawyer, S.: Receptors for erythropoietin. Distribution, structure and role in receptor-mediated endocytosis in erythroid cells. Blood Cell Biochem. *1:* 365–402 (1990).

16   Bazan, J.: A novel family of growth factor receptors: A common binding domain in the growth hormone, prolactin, erythropoietin and IL-6 receptors, and the p75 IL-2 receptor β-chain. Biochem. Biophys. Res. Commun. *164:* 788–795 (1989).

17   D'Andrea, A.; Fasman, G.; Lodish, H.: Erythropoietin receptor and interleukin-2 receptor β-chain: a new receptor family. Cell *58:* 1023–1024 (1989).

18   Gearing, D.; King, J.; Gouh, N.; Nicola, N.: Expression cloning of a receptor for human granulocyte-macrophage colony-stimulating factor. EMBO J. *8:* 3667–3676 (1989).

19   Mosley, B.; Bachman, P.; March, C.; Idzerda, R.; Gimpel, S.; Van den Bos, T.; Friend, D.; Alpert, A.; Anderson, D.; Jackson, J.; Wignall, J.; Smith, C.; Gollis, B.; Sims, J.; Urdal, D.; Widmer, B.; Cosman, D.; Park, L.: The murine interleukin-4 receptor: molecular cloning and the characterization of secreted and membrane bound forms. Cell *59:* 335–348 (1989).

20   Harada, N.; Castle, B.; Gorman, D.; Itoh, N.; Schreurs, J.; Barrett, R.; Howard, M.; Miyajima, A.: Expression cloning of a cDNA encoding the murine interleukin-4 receptor based on ligand binding. Proc. Natl. Acad. Sci. USA *87:* 857–861 (1990).

21   Itoh, N.; Yonehara, S.; Schreurs, J.; Gorman, D.; Maruyama, K.; Ishii, A.; Yahara, I.; Arai, K.-I.; Miyajima, A.: Cloning of an interleukin-3 receptor gene: a member of a distinct receptor gene family. Science *247:* 324–327 (1990).

22   Goodwin, R.; Friend, D.; Ziegler, S.; Jerzy, R.; Falk, B.; Gimpel, S.; Cosman, D.; Dower, S.; March, C.; Namen, A.; Park, L.: Cloning of the human and murine interleukin-7 receptors: Demonstration of a soluble form and homology to a new receptor superfamily. Cell *60:* 941–951 (1990).

Sanford B. Krantz, MD, Department of Medicine, C-3101, Vanderbilt Medical Center North, Nashville, TN 37232–2287 (USA)

Gurland HJ, Moran J, Samtleben W, Scigalla P, Wieczorek L (eds): Erythropoietin in
Renal and Non-Renal Anemias. Contrib Nephrol. Basel, Karger, 1991, vol 88, p 70

Discussion

to the Paper by T. Hosoi et al.

Goldwasser (Chicago): We have recently done experiments with both FVA cells and
some of the transformed cell lines that we've been studying, putting the solubilized receptors
on an EPO column and then looking at the size of what is retained in the column by iodinating
it and running it on a gel. To our surprise, we found a protein of the order of 55–60 kD, so we
have more confusion in the whole situation.

Krantz: We think that there are two proteins involved: one is the 65-kD protein and the
other is the 100-kD protein. Different assays and different techniques find one or the other,
and it's possible that the 100-kD protein is a built-up product from the 65-kD protein, but we
really don't know the precise relationship between these two proteins.

Shaldon (Montpellier): With reversed-phase HPLC, are you sure that the native protein
is not changed in any way by the process?

Krantz: It maintains biological activity and specific binding.

Goldwasser: Whether there might be a subtle conformational change by putting the
EPO on a hydrophobic bonding surface and eluting it in acetonitriltrifluoracetic acid is still
open to question. Your elution pattern showed two peaks of the DJ-labelled EPO. What's the
smaller one?

Krantz: It also behaves like DJ-EPO and it actually behaves exactly like the other peak.
Sometimes we pool them and sometimes we take the last one off the column separately
because it's a little more free of EPO. It may be that DJ blinds on different amino groups and
therefore creates a different hydrophobic structure for each of the peaks.

Treatment of Renal Anemia with Recombinant Human Erythropoietin

Gurland HJ, Moran J, Samtleben W, Scigalla P, Wieczorek L (eds): Erythropoietin in
Renal and Non-Renal Anemias. Contrib Nephrol. Basel, Karger, 1991, vol 88, pp 72–80

The Safety of Epoetin-Alpha:
Results of Clinical Trials in the United States

J. W. Eschbach[a], *J. C. Egrie*[b], *M. R. Downing*[b], *J. K. Browne*[b],
J. W. Adamson[c]

[a]University of Washington, Seattle, Wash.; [b]Amgen, Inc., Thousand Oaks, Calif.,
and [c]New York Blood Center, New York, N.Y., USA

Epoetin-alpha (epoetin), the recombinant form of human erythropoietin
produced by the kidney, is a proven therapeutic for correcting the anemia of
chronic renal failure [1–3]. In contrast to many therapeutic agents, epoetin has
been a remarkably safe drug, with a very low risk-benefit ratio. Clinical trials
with epoetin-alpha were initiated in Seattle, in December 1985, to determine
the safety and efficacy of therapy (phase I–II [1]), and expanded in the United
States to a large, phase III, multicenter study [3]. Subsequently, several other
clinical trials related to the safety of epoetin were initiated [4, 5]. This report
will summarize the safety issues related to the use of intravenous epoetin in
493 hemodialysis patients in the United States.

Methods

Amgen, Inc., Thousand Oaks, Calif., the biotechnology firm which first successfully
cloned and expressed the human erythropoietin gene [6, 7], initiated a number of clinical trials
to determine the efficacy and safety of recombinant human erythropoietin in hemodialysis
patients. Five of these trials addressed various potential issues of safety.

The phase I–II trial studied the safety and efficacy of epoetin in 31 patients with
hematocrit values of 25 or less. Fourteen patients failed to respond to doses of 1.5, 5.0 and
15 U/kg of body weight, intravenously (IV), 3 times a week, and all but 4 were discontinued
after 5 weeks of therapy, without any obvious toxicity. The other 4 patients were maintained
on 1.5 (n = 2) and 15 (n = 2) U/kg for 2, 2, 6, and 8 months respectively without any obvious
physical, biochemical or hematological changes. They subsequently were reentered into
studies at higher doses and along with the remaining 17 patients responded to 15, 50, 150, 500
and 1,500 U/kg, IV, 3 times weekly, although 2 had partial responses (at 15 and 50 U/kg) and

had to have dose increases, and 2 others at 50 U/kg dropped out of the study (hyperkalemic death, withdrawal for social reasons) before their hematocrit reached 30. Seventeen of these original patients received epoetin for greater than 3 years [8], and 13 have had 4 years of epoetin therapy.

The phase III clinical trial involving 9 centers, summarized at this meeting a year ago [9], determined the effectiveness and safety in 333 anemic (hematocrit <30) hemodialysis patients, using initial doses of 300 or 150 U/kg, 3 times weekly, IV. Maintenance doses were reduced to 75 U/kg and later adjusted to maintain the hematocrit at 35±3.

A double-blind, placebo clinical trial involving 3 dialysis centers compared the effectiveness and safety of epoetin in 101 anemic (hematocrit <30) hemodialysis patients [4]. Fifty of these patients completed 12 weeks of placebo therapy, failed to respond, and were subsequently treated with epoetin.

Because significant elevations in blood pressure occurred in 35% of the phase III trial, 18 anemic (hematocrit <30), hemodialysis patients had serial hemodynamic studies at either 50 or 150 U/kg, IV, 3 times weekly, to determine whether the dose of epoetin or rate of rise in hematocrit were factors in the blood pressure elevations [10].

Because seizures occurred in several patients in the early clinical trials [1, 2], a study was initiated to determine if epoetin, or a rising hematocrit adversely effected cerebral or cutaneous blood flow. Ten anemic, hemodialysis patients were treated with epoetin, 150 U/kg, 3 times weekly, IV. Five patients had frequent phlebotomy to maintain the baseline hematocrit (25±2) and 5 patients were not phlebotomized and responded by increasing the hematocrit to 33±2 [5].

Safety was evaluated in all patients by serial histories and physical examinations, blood chemistries, hematological values, chest x-rays, electrocardiograms, and determinations of epoetin antibodies. Cerebral blood flow, whole blood viscosity and transcutaneous oxygen tension were measured serially in one subgroup of patients, and serial, noninvasive hemodynamic measurements of cardiac output and peripheral vascular resistance were measured in another subgroup.

An additional group of 117 anemic patients with progressive renal failure not requiring dialysis were treated in the United States with epoetin-alpha, IV, as part of the Ortho Pharmaceutical Corp. study [11]. These patients are not included in this analysis.

Results and Comments

Four hundred ninety-three anemic, hemodialysis patients were treated with epoetin in five clinical trials. Almost all had effective erythroid responses as defined by an increase in hematocrit to 35±3 or a rise of at least 6 hematocrit points.

The adverse effects can be divided into those due to the direct administration of epoetin and those related to the increase in red cell mass. The most common effect of administration is myalgia and/or a flu-like syndrome occurring 60–90 min after IV administration. This can also occur after subcutaneous (SC) administration and after IV administration to normal subjects (personal observation). This has occurred in 4% (16 of 442) of patients analyzed. The reaction is self-limited and does not interfere with the action of epoetin. However, the reaction was so severe that in 2 patients epoetin therapy was discontinued [3].

Miscellaneous direct effects include fever, flank pain and sclerosis of an antecubital vein. There has been no increase in the incidence of headaches and as yet no development of antibodies to epoetin.

Increasing the red cell mass by epoetin therapy has resulted directly or indirectly in most of the perceived adverse effects: iron deficiency, hypertension, seizures, increased dialyzer clotting, and hyperkalemia and hyperphosphatemia.

Iron Stores

Elemental iron is a requirement for adequate hemoglobin formation. Epoetin therapy at the usual doses increases erythropoiesis by 2- to 3-fold [12]. This results in mobilization of reticuloendothelial iron for hemoglobin synthesis and leads to a decrease in serum iron, percent transferrin saturation and serum ferritin. In addition, since red cell transfusions are eliminated, less exogenous iron enters the body, and since hemodialyzers always retain some blood after use, red cell or iron loss continues. As a result of these three mechanisms, iron deficiency is now much more common in the hemodialysis patient than before epoetin therapy. Forty-eight percent (203 of 419) of patients who had adequate iron stores (serum ferritin >100 ng/ml and percent transferrin saturation >20) at the onset of epoetin therapy developed either absolute or relative iron deficiency within the first year of therapy either absolutely or as a functional or relative state. Functional iron deficiency is defined as a normal or slightly elevated serum ferritin coupled with a percent transferrin saturation <20 [2]. Iron deficiency is technically a preventable complication unless the patient is allergic to both intravenous iron dextran and oral iron.

Iron overload can easily develop in the anemic patient with chronic renal failure from frequent red cell transfusions. However, the risks of transfusions are well known and routine transfusions should no longer be necessary in the dialysis patient treated with adequate amounts of epoetin. Eighty-one of 424 (19%) patients had iron overload as defined by a serum ferritin of greater than 1,000 ng/ml. In these patients, after 6 months of therapy, the mean serum ferritin level decreased 38% from 3,387±73 to 2,116±62 ng/ml. Overall, of 354 patients, the mean serum ferritin decreased from 987 to 638 ng/ml within 3 months of epoetin therapy, and in 17 patients treated for at least 3 years, the mean serum ferritin level decreased from 1,139 to 186 ng/ml [8]. This indicates that iron overload, with its associated side effects, will not be a medical problem for dialysis patients in the future.

However, even iron overloaded patients will eventually become iron depleted, and all epoetin-treated patients will eventually require supplemental iron therapy. Because a small percentage of patients have reactions to IV iron dextran [13], and many subjects cannot tolerate oral iron, iron deficiency may be a limiting factor in optimal epoetin therapy. While most patients may be able to maintain minimal iron stores with oral iron, frequent episodes of blood loss in the patient allergic to parenteral iron could result in relative epoetin 'resistance'.

Increasing Blood Pressure

An increase in diastolic blood pressure of $\geq$10 mm Hg or requirement for new or additional antihypertensive medication occurred in 103 of 330 (31%) evaluable patients. Most other groups evaluating recombinant human erythropoietin have also observed that some patients increase their mean arterial pressures in response to a rise in red cell mass. Generally, this elevation in blood pressure can be controlled with ultrafiltration or new or more antihypertensive medications, but occasionally hypertensive encephalopathy, with or without seizures, can evolve. A pressor response does not occur from recombinant human erythropoietin per se [14] and long-term epoetin therapy in normotensive patients with rheumatoid arthritis or acquired immunodeficiency syndrome has not produced a pressor response [15, 16]. While a precise explanation for the pathophysiology of this pressor response is not yet known, patients with chronic renal failure have a high incidence of hypertension and their anemia is more chronic and severe than most chronic anemias. In the epoetin-alpha clinical trials, 68% had hypertension at baseline, and an equal percentage of normotensive and hypertensive patients had a pressor response to an increasing red cell mass. One concern has been whether a more rapid rise in hematocrit or hemoglobin from higher doses of epoetin would accentuate this response. The results of the phase III clinical trial indicated that there was no difference between the incidence of hypertension in those treated with 300 or 150 U/kg [3]. To further evaluate this issue, a subgroup of 18 anemic patients had serial noninvasive hemodynamic studies every month for 6 months. The pressor response in 10 patients receiving 150 U/kg, IV, 3 times weekly, was compared to 8 patients receiving 50 U/kg. Because an earlier study indicated that severe anemia (hematocrit <20) was a risk factor for becoming more hypertensive following epoetin therapy [17], we purposely included more anemic patients in the lower dose group: their baseline hematocrit was 20±2. The baseline hematocrit in the higher dose group was 24±3.

The peripheral vascular resistance increased in both groups associated with normalization of the elevated cardiac output, and mean arterial blood pressure increased equally in both groups. In the 50 U/kg group, new or added antihypertensive medications were required in 4 of the 8 patients after 2 months of therapy, usually associated with a hematocrit that was rising to above 29. Subsequent hemodynamic measurements were difficult to interpret in light of the extra antihypertensive medications.

The pressor response in the higher (150 U/kg) dose group was similar, with one important exception: the response occurred earlier because the red cell mass increased at a brisker rate. This pressor response was so brisk in 2 patients within a month of onset of epoetin therapy, that they were hospitalized for malignant hypertension without seizures [5]. It therefore appears that the pressor response is more a function of an increasing red cell mass than its rate of rise but that if the rate of rise is too brisk, there is less time to intervene successfully with appropriate antihypertensive therapy. Why every dialysis patient does not elicit this response is not clear, but may be because only some have an increased vascular sensitivity to changes in adrenergic tone [18].

Seizures

Eighteen of 424 patients (4%) experienced seizures. Seizures occur at an increased frequency in dialysis patients as reflected by the 8% incidence in 1,111 dialysis patients not receiving epoetin [3]. Since 10 of the 18 seizures occurred within the first 3 months of epoetin therapy when the hematocrit was increasing and when blood pressure may be rising, it is conceivable that some patients are more prone to develop seizures associated with this combination of hemodynamic events. To further assess the role of epoetin and a rising red cell mass in central nervous system function, one clinical trial measured cerebral blood flow, whole blood viscosity and transcutaneous oxygen tension in two groups of anemic patients treated with epoetin. All received 150 U/kg, IV, 3 times weekly for 4 months. Five patients responded by increasing their hematocrit to 33±2, while the other 5 patients had periodic phlebotomy to keep their hematocrit at baseline of 26±2. In those whose hematocrit increased to 33±2, whole blood viscosity increased to normal, cerebral blood flow decreased from above normal to normal and transcutaneous oxygen tension increased. There was no increase in blood pressure. In the group that also received epoetin, but whose hematocrit did not change because of periodic phlebotomies, there was no change in whole blood viscosity, or transcutaneous oxygen tension and cerebral blood flow remained elevated [5]. This study reaffirms that epoetin does not have a direct effect on cerebral blood flow, does not result in microvascular thrombi that would decrease cutaneous, and presumably other small vessel blood flow, and does not directly effect viscosity. Rather, the epoetin-induced improvement in anemia actually has beneficial effects on cerebral circulation and does not lower it to below normal levels.

Effects on Clotting

Forty-seven of 386 patients experienced 72 episodes of access clotting during the initial 6–12 months of epoetin therapy. Although several studies indicate that platelet function improves as reflected by shortening in the prolonged bleeding time when the hematocrit increases to over 30 with either red cell transfusions [19] or epoetin therapy [20], this degree of vascular access clotting is no greater than that observed in 1,111 hemodialysis patients not receiving epoetin [3]. The platelet count may increase slightly, but significantly, but not to above normal levels with partial correction in the anemia, but does not continue to increase with maintenance therapy [3]. In 17 patients treated with epoetin for greater than 3 years, there was no increased incidence of vascular access thromboses: 4 have had no clotting episodes and 6 only one episode [8]. However, increased fibrin formation and clotting in the extracorporeal circuit may occur in approximately one third of epoetin-treated patients when their hematocrit begins to rise. A small increase in heparin is usually sufficient to maintain good dialyzer blood flows and reuse techniques [3, 8]. Epoetin-treated patients, including those with diabetes mellitus, have shown no increased incidence of small or large vessel thromboses, such as strokes, myocardial infarctions or peripheral vascular disease.

Effects on Dialyzer Clearances

The adequacy of hemodialysis is dependent on the dialysis of solutes present in the plasma water. Since this is a function of the hematocrit, it would be anticipated that increasing the red cell mass by epoetin therapy would have a deleterious effect on dialyzer clearances of creatinine, phosphate and potassium. The clearance of urea, being contained mainly in the red cell, is unaffected by the rise in hematocrit. Serial measurements of predialysis serum creatinine, phosphorus and potassium concentrations in 326 epoetin-treated patients disclosed slight, but significant increases (p<0.0005) in creatinine and phosphorus. From a baseline hematocrit of 22.3±0.2 (SE) to 34.0±0.2 after 12–24 weeks of epoetin therapy, the serum creatinine rose from 13.3±0.3 to

13.9±0.4 mg/dl, the serum phosphorus rose from 5.5±0.1 to 6.3± 0.2 mg/dl and serum potassium rose slightly from 5.1±0.04 to 5.2±0.06 mEq/l. While the last solute only rose slightly, it is the most critical, and hyperkalemia has resulted in the deaths of 3 epoetin-treated patients in the clinical trials, due to dietary noncompliance. In 17 patients treated for more than 3 years, there was an increase in predialysis serum creatinine and phosphorus levels within 1 year of therapy which remained stable thereafter [8]. Therefore, dialyzer potassium must be adjusted downward and dietary counseling may be required more frequently in some epoetin-treated patients, especially during the first 6–9 months of epoetin therapy.

Other Effects

In over 4 years of epoetin therapy, there has been no consistent changes in liver function tests, serum uric acid, lipids, calcium, or alkaline phosphatase, white blood count or electrocardiograms. Serial chest x-rays have demonstrated no changes in pulmonary status, but the transverse diameter of the heart has decreased in most patients who had baseline cardiomegaly [17].

Conclusion

The experience in clinical trials with over 493 hemodialysis patients treated with therapeutic doses of epoetin-alpha for the anemia of chronic renal failure, indicates that the recombinant hormone is a remarkably safe drug with a very low risk-benefit ratio. While the most frequent problem is iron deficiency which can result in decreased epoetin effectiveness, the potentially most serious complication is hypertensive encephalopathy related to a sudden rise in blood pressure during the induction phase of therapy when the anemia is being corrected toward the target range. Because of the seriousness of this potential complication, all patients must have their blood pressures and dry weight monitored and assessed carefully and treated accordingly. Neither vascular clotting nor decreased dialyzer clearance have been significant complications of effective epoetin therapy. An additional 50,000 hemodialysis patients have been receiving epoetin since it was approved for use by the United States Food and Drug Administration on June 1, 1989. There have been no new complications reported nor an increased incidence of those reported from the clinical trials. Epoetin-alpha is a safe and effective therapeutic for the uncomplicated anemia of chronic renal failure.

References

1   Winearls, G.; Oliver, D.; Pippard, M., et al.: Effect of human erythropoietin derived from recombinant DNA on the anaemia of patients maintained by chronic haemodialysis. Lancet *ii:* 1175–1178 (1986).
2   Eschbach, J.; Egrie, J.; Downing, M., et al.: Correction of anemia of end-stage renal disease with recombinant human erythropoietin. N. Engl. J. Med. *316:* 73–78 (1987).
3   Eschbach, J. W.; Abdulhadi, M. H.; Browne, J. K., et al.: Results of a phase III multicenter clinical trial with recombinant human erythropoietin in anemic patients with end-stage renal disease. Ann. Intern. Med. *1111:* 992–1000 (1989).
4   Double-Blind Placebo Study: Data on File. Amgen, Inc., Thousand Oaks, Calif.
5   Johnson, W. J.; McCarthy, J. T.; Yanagihara, T.; Osmundson, P. O.; Ilstrup, D. M.; Jenson, B. M.; Bowie, E. J. W.: Effects of recombinant human erythropoietin on cerebral and cutaneous blood flow and coagulability of blood (abstract). Kidney Int. *37:* 303 (1990).
6   Lin, F.-K.; Suggs, S.; Lin, C. H., et al.: Cloning and expression of the human erythropoietin gene. Proc. Natl. Acad. Sci. USA *92:* 7580–7585 (1985).
7   Egrie, J. C.; Strickland, T. W.; Lane, J., et al.: Characterization and biological effects of recombinant human erythropoietin. Immunobiology *92:* 7580–7585 (1986).
8   Eschbach, J. W.; Haley, N. R.; Aquiling, T., et al.: Three years of erythropoietin (rHuEPO) therapy (abstract). Kidney Int. *37:* 237 (1990).
9   Eschbach, J. W.; Downing, M. R.; Egrie, J. C.; Browne, J. K.; Adamson, J. W.: USA multicenter clinical trial with recombinant human erythropoietin (Amgen); in Baldamus, C. A.; Scigalla, P.; Wieczorek, L.; Koch, K. M. (eds): Erythropoietin: From molecular structure to clinical application. Contrib. Nephrol. Basel, Karger, 1989, vol 76, pp. 160–165.
10 Davidson, R. C.; Haley, N. R.; Easterling, T. R., et al.: Serial hemodynamic changes following recombinant erythropoietin (rHuEPO) therapy (abstract). Kidney Int. *37:* 237 (1990).
11 Krantz, S.; Teehan, B.; Abraham, P.; Dauer, A.; Eschbach, J.; Friedman, E.; Greenwald, J.; Lim, V.; McMahon, F. G.; Orringer, E.; Mattern, W. D.; Raja, R.; Rudnick, M.; Cohen, R. M.; Schwartz, A. B.; Shadur, C.; Sheth, A.; Chew, R.; Sullivan, D.; Thompson, D.; Abels, R.: Double-blind, placebo-controlled study of the therapeutic use of recombinant human erythropoietin for anemia associated with chronic renal failure in predialysis patients (submitted).
12 Eschbach, J. W.; Haley, N. R.; Adamson, J. W.: The use of recombinant erythropoietin in the treatment of the anemia of chronic renal failure; in Orlic, D., Molecular and cellular controls of hematopoiesis. Ann. N.Y. Acad. Sci. *554:* 225–230 (1989).
13 Hamstra, R. D.; Block, M. H.; Schocket, A. L.: Intravenous iron dextran in clinical medicine. J. Am. Med. Assoc. *243:* 1726–1731 (1980).
14 Pagel, H.; Jelkmann, W.; Weiss, C.: Erythropoietin and blood pressure. Horm. Metab. *21:* 224 (1989).
15 Means, R. T.; Olsen, N. F.; Krantz, S. B., et al.: Treatment of the anemia of rheumatoid arthritis with recombinant human erythropoietin: Clinical and in vitro studies. Arthritis Rheum. *32:* 638–642 (1989).
16 Fischl, M.; Galpin, J. E.; Levine, J. D.; Groopman, J. E.; Henry, D. H.; Kennedy, P.; Miles, S.; Robbins, W.; Starrett, B.; Zalusky, R.; Abels, R. I.; Tsai, H. C.; Rudnick,

S. A.: Recombinant human erythropoietin for patients with AIDS treated with Zidovudine. N. Engl. J. Med. *322:* 1488–1493 (1990).

17 Buckner, F. S.; Eschbach, J. W.; Haley, N. R., et al.: Hypertension following erythropoietin therapy in anemic hemodialysis patients. Am. J. Hypertens. (in press).

18 Baldamus, C. A.; Pollock, M.; Steffen, H. M., et al.: Adrenergic system in renal anemia, corrected with recombinant human erythropoietin (huEPO) (abstract). Kidney Int. *37:* 208 (1990).

19 Livio, M.; Marchesi, D.; Remuzzi, G., et al.: Uraemic bleeding: role of anaemia and beneficial effect of red cell transfusions. Lancet *ii:* 1013–1015 (1982).

20 Moia, M.; Vizzotto, L.; Cattaneo, M., et al.: Improvement in the haemostatic defect of uraemia after treatment with recombinant human erythropoietin. Lancet *ii:* 1227–1229 (1987).

Joseph W. Eschbach, MD, Department of Medicine, RM-10,
University of Washington, Seattle, WA 98195 (USA)

Gurland HJ, Moran J, Samtleben W, Scigalla P, Wieczorek L (eds): Erythropoietin in
Renal and Non-Renal Anemias. Contrib Nephrol. Basel, Karger, 1991, vol 88, pp 81–86

Quality of Life in
End-Stage Renal Disease Patients during
Recombinant Human Erythropoietin Therapy

Paul A. Keown

On behalf of the Canadian Erythropoietin Study Group[1]

Chronic renal failure is accompanied by profound anemia, necessitating
blood transfusion in more than 60% of patients. Recombinant human erythropoietin (rhEPO) successfully corrects this anemia [1, 2], decreases the likelihood of transfusion-associated infections and iron overload, and in uncontrolled studies appears to improve general well-being, exercise tolerance [3],
and cognitive and sexual function [4].

We have previously evaluated the effect of erythropoietin (EPO) upon
the anemia of renal failure, and determined the dosage and conditions of
administration [5]. We have now also examined its effect upon the quality of
life and exercise capacity of anemic hemodialysis patients in a double-blind,
placebo-controlled trial [6].

Methods

One hundred and eighteen anemic hemodialysis patients in eight Canadian university
centers were randomized to receive: placebo (group 1), EPO at a dose adjusted to maintain
the hemoglobin concentration between 95 and 110 g/l (group 2), and EPO at a dose adjusted to
maintain the hemoglobin between 115 and 130 g/l (group 3). All were between 18 and 75 years
of age, clinically stable for 3 months, with an average hemoglobin <90 g/l, and receiving 3
times weekly hemodialysis. Exclusion criteria were: causes of anemia other than EPO deficiency, factors other than renal failure independently compromising the patients' quality of

[1] The investigators are indebted to the study personnel in the participating centers, and
to Ortho Pharmaceutical (Canada) Ltd. for their invaluable support.

life or exercise capacity (e.g. insulin-dependent mellitus), an inability to perform the study tests, or an unwillingness or inability to give informed consent.

The study drug was injected intravenously as a 10-cm^3 bolus at the end of each dialysis 3 times weekly. The initial dose of EPO in groups 2 and 3 was 100 units/kg/dose (Erythropoietin α; Ortho Pharmaceutical Canada, Ltd) and was adjusted by 25–50 units/kg at weekly intervals as required to maintain a stable hemoglobin within the selected range. Patients with a serum ferritin <250 μg/l received oral or intravenous iron supplementation for 1 month prior to randomization and as necessary throughout the trial.

Two teams of study personnel were established at each center: the unblinded team prescribed the study drug, iron supplementation, and transfusional support, while the blinded team was responsible for routine clinical care, the recording of adverse reactions, and administration of the quality of life and exercise capacity measures.

All patients were followed for 6 months and the outcome measures were assessed prior to randomization and at 2, 4 and 6 months. The two major outcomes assessed were (a) quality of life measured by a special kidney disease questionnaire, the Sickness Impact Profile [7] and the Time Trade-Off technique [8] and (b) exercise capacity, measured by a 6-min walk [9] and a modified Naughton treadmill test [10].

Analysis of the outcome parameters was performed on patients who had completed all four evaluations (baseline, 2, 4 and 6 months) using analysis of variance for repeated measures.

Results

Patient Characteristics and Hematologic Response

Forty patients were randomized to group 1, 40 to group 2, and 38 to group 3. The three treatment groups were comparable at entry (table 1), although patients in group 1 had a shorter mean time on dialysis than the other two groups (p = 0,07).

Nineteen patients were withdrawn during the study; 8 in group 1, 6 in group 2, and 5 in group 3. The principal reasons for withdrawal were transplantation (10), hypertension (3), seizures (3), and pregnancy, transfusion reaction or noncompliance (total 3).

The mean hemoglobin at 6 months was 74 ± 12 g/l (±SD) in group 1, 102 ± 10 g/l in group 2, and 117 ± 14 g/l in group 3. After 8 weeks, 23 patients in group 1, 1 patient in group 2, and 1 patient in group 3 received blood transfusions, the latter two because of gastrointestinal hemorrhage and surgery respectively.

The mean dose of EPO at 6 months was 204 ± 167 units/kg/week for group 2, and 248 ± 146 units/kg/week for group 3. Iron supplementation was given to 34% of patients in group 1, 35% of patients in group 2, and 58% of patients in group 3 (p = 0.10 among groups).

Table 1. Patient baseline characteristics

	Group 1 (n = 40)	Group 2 (n = 40)	Group 3 (n = 38)
Age, years	48±16	44±16	43±15
Male/female	25/15	19/21	26/12
Anephric, %	15	32	26
Time on hemodialysis, years	2.5±3.1	4.6±4.7	4.4±5.1
Transfusions during previous year, n	7.3±8.3	6.6±6.8	5.6±7.4
Hemoglobin, g/l	71±9	69±10	71±12

Quality of Life and Exercise Capacity

The baseline quality of life scores were comparable among the three groups except for time walked on the stress test (p = 0.02). The principal changes in the quality of life and exercise capacity measures in the three groups over time are presented in table 2. In general, the improvements that occurred were apparent by 2 months. There was a marked improvement in the fatigue and physical symptoms dimensions of the kidney disease questionnaire in EPO-treated patients. There were improvements in the relationship and depression dimensions as well, although the magnitude of the changes were smaller. There was no significant improvement in the frustration dimension. Among the patient-specific items there was a highly statistically significant improvement in fatigue and strength in EPO-treated patients.

There was an improvement in both the global and physical scores of the Sickness Impact Profile in EPO-treated patients (table 2). Statistically significant improvements (p <0.05) in the body care and movement, home maintenance, ambulation, communication, and work dimensions of the Sickness Impact Profile were found in EPO-treated patients. There was no improvement in the aggregate psychosocial score or the individual dimensions of sleep and rest, emotional behavior, mobility, social interaction, alertness behavior, recreation and pastimes, or eating. There was no improvement in overall quality of life as measured by the Time Trade-Off technique. The difference in the time walked in the exercise stress test between EPO- and placebo-treated patients was statistically significant, but there was no statistically significant improvement in the distance walked during the 6-min walk test.

There was no statistically significant difference in the change in quality of life or exercise capacity between patients in groups 2 and 3 for any of the outcome measures assessed, expect for the patient-specific item of decreased

Table 2. Effect of EPO on quality of life and exercise capacity

Outcome measure	Statistical significance[1]
Kidney Disease Questionnaire	
Physical	<0.001
Fatigue	<0.001
Relationships	0.001
Depression	0.018
Frustration	NS
Sickness Impact Profile	
Global	0.024
Physical	0.005
Psychosocial	NS
Time Trade-Off	NS
Stress test	0.018
Six-minute walk test	NS

[1]Difference in response between placebo- and EPO-treated groups.

strength (p = 0.02). A statistically significant correlation was found between the change in hemoglobin and the change in the Sickness Impact Profile, the kidney disease questionnaire (except the frustration dimension), and the time walked during the exercise test. However, the Pearson correlation coefficients were relatively low, the highest being observed with the fatigue and physical symptoms dimensions of the kidney disease questionnaire (r = 0.32, p = 0.001 and r = 0.31, p = 0.002, respectively).

Adverse Effects and Clinical Events

There was no statistically significant change in systolic blood pressure throughout the study among the three groups, although diastolic blood pressure was significantly increased in EPO-treated compared with placebo-treated patients (p <0.001). Antihypertensive medications were started or increased in 9% of patients in group 1, compared with 27% of EPO-treated patients (8 patients in group 2 and 10 patients in group 3) (p = 0.06). Four patients were withdrawn from the study for severe hypertension, 2 in group 2 and 2 in group 3. None of the patients were on antihypertensive medications prior to the study.

There was a significant correlation between EPO treatment and both access clotting (p = 0.005) and eye redness (p = 0.04). There were no significant differences in serum potassium, phosphorus, calcium, urea, creatinine or white blood cell count among the groups throughout the study, although the platelet count fell 5,000 ± 39,000 in group 1 and increased by 25,000 ± 64,000 in group 2 and 23,000 ± 47,000 in group 3 (p = 0.005).

Discussion

This randomized, double-blind, placebo-controlled trial demonstrated that patients receiving EPO were less fatigued, felt subjectively better, and had an increased exercise tolerance compared with those in the control group. The magnitude of this improvement was comparable to the difference reported by Hart and Evans [11] between non EPO-treated patients receiving in-center hemodialysis and those with a functioning renal transplant. Although there was no statistically significant difference in quality of life or exercise tolerance between patients randomized to the two EPO treatment groups, there was a modest though statistically significant correlation between the change in hemoglobin and these outcome measures in the treated population during the trial.

The effect of EPO on psychosocial function was less impressive than that on fatigue, physical symptoms and exercise tolerance, with only moderate improvements in depression and relationships with others in the kidney disease questionnaire, and no improvement in the psychosocial dimension of the Sickness Impact Profile.

The two measures of global quality of life employed yielded different results, with an improved quality of life in EPO-treated patients being detected by the global Sickness Impact Profile but not by the Time Trade-Off score. By allowing patients to give their own weighting to the many physical, social and emotional factors that affect their quality of life, the Time Trade-Off is a rigorous and comprehensive assessment, while the Sickness Impact Profile applies fixed weights which may not precisely reflect the concerns of this patient population. The lack of response may therefore indicate that, although EPO causes a significant improvement in quality of life and exercise capacity, many other factors, including the psychological and physical burdens of hemodialysis, also adversely affect the well-being of hemodialysis patients, and may not be substantially improved by EPO.

It is difficult to establish a rigid target hemoglobin level which is satisfactory for all EPO-treated patients. Quality of life and exercise capacity rose linearly throughout the range of hemoglobin achieved, although there was a marked individual variation, and patients in the group with the highest mean hemoglobin had greater problems with hypertension and access clotting than those in the other groups. Selection of the optimal target hemoglobin for each patient must therefore be based on individual clinical criteria in which the quantitative improvement in health status is weighed against the risks and cost of therapy. The hemoglobin range of 100–120 g/l now adopted by many centers would appear to be a reasonable and appropriate compromise.

References

1   Eschbach JW, Egrie JC, Dowing MR, Browne JK, Adamson JW: Correction of the anemia of end-stage renal disease with recombinant human erythropoietin. N Engl J Med 1987;316:73–78.
2   Winearls CG, Pippard MJ, Downing MR, Oliver DO, Reid C, Cotes PM: Effect of human erythropoietin derived from recombinant DNA on the anaemia of patients maintained by chronic haemodialysis. Lancet 1986;ii:1175–1178.
3   Lundin AP: Quality of life: Subjective and objective improvements with recombinant human erythropoietin therapy. Sem in Nephrol 1989;9:22–29.
4   Schaefer RM, Kokot F, Wernze H, Geiger H, Heidland A: Improved sexual function in hemodialysis patients on recombinant erythropoietin: A possible role for prolactin. Clin Nephrol 1989;31:1–5.
5   Canadian Erythropoietin Study Group: A prospective randomized double-blind study of recombinant human erythropoietin (r-Hu-EPO) in chronic hemodialysis (abstract). Kidney Int 1988;33:189.
6   Canadian Erythropoietin Study Group: Association between recombinant human erythropoietin and quality of life and exercise capacity of patients receiving hemodialysis. Br Med J 1990;300:573–578.
7   Bergner M, Bobbitt RA, Carter WB, Gilson BS: The Sickness Impact Profile: Development and final revision of a health status measure. Med Care 1981;19:787–805.
8   Churchill DN, Torrance GW, Taylor DW, et al: Measurement of quality of life in end-stage renal disease: The Time Trade-Off approach. Clin. Invest Med 1987;10:14–20.
9   Guyatt GH, Sullivan MJ, Thompson PJ, et al: The 6-minute walk: A new measure of exercise capacity in patients with chronic heart failure. Can Med Assoc J 1985;132:919–923.
10 Naughton J, Sevelius G, Balke B: Physiological responses of normal and pathological subjects to a modified work capacity test. J Sports Med Phys Fitness 1963;3:201–207.
11 Hart LG, Evans RW: The functional status of ESRD patients as measured by the Sickness Impact Profile. J Chronic Dis 1987;40:117S–130S.

Paul A. Keown, MB, ChB, FRCP(C), FRCP, Professor and Director,
British Columbia Transplant Society, Heather Pavilion, D-10, Rm 19,
855 West 12th Avenue, Vancouver, BC V5Z 1M9 (Canada)

Gurland HJ, Moran J, Samtleben W, Scigalla P, Wieczorek L (eds): Erythropoietin in
Renal and Non-Renal Anemias. Contrib Nephrol. Basel, Karger, 1991, vol 88, pp 87–89

Discussion

to the Papers by J.W. Eschbach et al. and P.A. Keown

Shaldon (Montpellier): I'd like to ask you about the incidence of flu-like and muscle pain symptoms. What was the preparation of the placebo material?

Keown: It was the vehicle for the EPO.

Shaldon: So it would be an albumin-containing solution?

Keown: That's right.

Shaldon: Could you tell me whether it had a monocyte screen for pyrogen contamination or just a LAL test?

Keown: I'm afraid I can't tell you but I can certainly find the answer for you.

Shaldon: I think this is relevant, because it is clearly not an EPO-related phenomenon, and LAL testing of albumin-containing solutions is notoriously unreliable for the detection of endotoxin contamination.

Winearls (Oxford): We described this flu-like syndrome, and sent the EPO from the batch that had caused the syndrome to the National Institute for Biological Standards and Control, which has this monocyte IL-6 release assay. They could not detect any endotoxin in the material.

B. Nielsen (Copenhagen): I have one question for Dr. Eschbach and one comment for Dr. Keown. Do you think the fact that these patients develop more hypertension if they have higher doses is related to the total dose of EPO or to the rate of rise of the hematocrit? And Dr. Keown, I think it is very important that we have had this placebo study before we have had the exact figures. For ethical reasons I think it is a little questionable whether it is permissible to do so in the future.

Keown: Yes, I agree.

Eschbach: I know that many think that the dose and the rate of rise are somehow related to the pressure response. However, as I presented, of over 300 patients in the multicenter trial US using large doses, 300 and 150 U/kg three times weekly, we could show no difference in the incidence of hypertension and the rate of rise of hematocrit. The higher the EPO dose the faster the hematocrit will increase. If there is going to be a pressor response, one may not have time to therapeutically intervene, and that is what is dangerous. But I do not think it is the higher dose per se that causes the pressor response.

Simoes (Lisbon): Dr. Eschbach, the patients who developed hypertension, were they mostly hypertensive before, or not? Were they being treated or not? I think this is a very important point.

Eschbach: In our multicenter trial, 68% had hypertension before they went on EPO therapy. But of those patients who became more hypertensive or developed hypertension, half were normotensive and not on blood pressure medication prior to EPO therapy.

Winearls (Oxford): There is a problem in reconciling the incidence of seizures, which the Canadian study suggests is not above background, and I understand that in US patients not on EPO the level is also about 4%. Am I right in saying that in both these studies patients who had a past history of seizures were specifically excluded?

Eschbach: They were to be excluded, and most were. Amgen found that there was no difference between the incidence of seizures from their survey of over 1000 patients not on EPO and the incidence of seizures when receiving EPO. However, I believe there is an increased incidence of seizures above background, but it occurs only during the induction phase of therapy when the hematocrit is rising and when the blood pressure may suddenly rise.

Winearls: I think that nephrologists in the UK would agree with you because there were 7 seizures in the first 54 patients treated in the UK, all in the phase you are describing, and since the dose has been lowered that incidence has fallen.

Shaldon: It concerns me that you have a new drug that is a physiological replacement drug and that you are using it in pharmacological doses, and there is no question about this. I don't think that you can complacently insist that the pressor effect is not an effect of the drug and is simply an effect of the hematological consequences of the drug. I still reserve judgement. I accept your data, but I am not convinced that you have completely eliminated a possible toxic effect of EPO itself.

Eschbach: There has not been any hypertension in other longer-term EPO studies outside of the dialysis population, such as in patients with rheumatoid arthritis or AIDS.

Winearls: The particularly relevant group were those who were treated with 600 U/kg twice a week for autologous blood transfusion; in the paper by Goodnough in the *New England Journal of Medicine* recently, hypertension was not a problem. This was a dose 12 times that which we are injecting into the hemodialysis population.

Shaldon: I don't think that the normal kidney is a fair comparison, within the context of a diseased kidney and the complexity of hypertension.

Eschbach: There are three reports in the literature, 2 from 50 years ago and another 1 probably 20 years ago, in patients who had severe anemias and normal renal function. Their anemias were corrected by nutritional means and a significant number had an increase in blood pressure. Of course they did not receive exogenous rhEPO.

Ivanovich (Chicago): I'd like to ask a question concerning the incidence of seizures and whether there is a difference between epoetin alpha and beta. In the recent paper in which Dr. Winearls was the senior author [Nephrol Dial Transplant 1990;4:1065–1069] the reported incidence of seizures was quite high in the UK group, whereas it was much lower in a similar European multicenter study. Was that difference related to the type of EPO or to some other factor?

Eschbach: I do not know. Dr. Winearls, do you?

Winearls: Those patients were all treated with epoetin alpha. They were the most anemic patients, they were the transfusion-dependent UK patients who were treated with what was considered a relatively high dose, 150 U/kg 3 times a week. Again, it mostly occurred at the time of rapid increase in hematocrit and was associated with very labile blood pressure. One would have to ask those who analyzed the Boehringer studies whether they have seen the same phenomenon.

Helmers (Stockholm): I would like to ask if you have seen any patient who has had a rise in blood pressure without having a rise in hematocrit when treated with EPO?

Eschbach: Yes, but many dialysis patients have a rise in blood pressure unrelated to treatment with EPO.

Helmers: Yes, but with reference to a primary pressure effect of EPO, we had an elderly woman with myelodysplastic syndrome and normal renal function. She had a blood pressure of about 135–140 systolic and it rose to about 180–200 mm Hg systolic, without any rise in hematocrit at all. And then when the EPO was withdrawn blood pressure went down. That is a response which is difficult to explain.

Eschbach: I don't know what it is, but there are different effects that happen when you give drugs to patients and that's why you need placebo-controlled studies.

Macdougall (Cardiff): As with the incidence of seizures, we have an apparent inconsistency between the two presentations regarding the incidence of vascular access clotting in EPO-treated patients. We have a large multicenter American trial which does not show an incidence above what would be expected in the hemodialysis population, and then we have a well-conducted placebo-controlled study which suggests that there is an increased incidence which appears to be hematocrit related. Can either of the two presenters explain why this is so, and what we are to believe regarding this at the moment?

Keown: My feeling is that there is an increase in seizures, often associated with hypertension, and an increase in vascular access clotting. And the more high-risk individuals you treat the greater will be that increase. It's quite true that in the initial Canadian studies we selected individuals who were not at high risk. The same study is now underway with the remainder of the population and I would predict that there will be an increase in these problems.

Eschbach: I would have expected more clotting, because the bleeding time shortens when dialysis patients are transfused to hematocrits above 30, or when the hematocrit increases from EPO therapy. Part of the problem is that most hemodialysis patients don't have autologous fistulas but vascular access grafts which have an increased incidence of clotting without EPO. So it may be difficult to separate these factors in the individual patient. In the past year, since rhEPO has been available in the US, our vascular access surgeons in Seattle have not seen an increased incidence of clotting.

Gurland HJ, Moran J, Samtleben W, Scigalla P, Wieczorek L (eds): Erythropoietin in
Renal and Non-Renal Anemias. Contrib Nephrol. Basel, Karger, 1991, vol 88, pp 90–106

Morbidity and Mortality in Hemodialysis Patients with and without Erythropoietin Treatment: A Controlled Study

J. Bahlmann[a], *K.-H. Schöter*[i], *P. Scigalla*[i], *H. J. Gurland*[b],
M. Hilfenhaus[a], *K. M. Koch*[a], *F. A. Muthny*[h], *H. H. Neumayer*[c],
W. Pommer[d], *E. Quellhorst*[e], *H. G. Sieberth*[f], *U. Weber*[g]

[a]Abteilung Nephrologie, Zentrum Innere Medizin, Medizinische Hochschule,
Hannover; [b]Abteilung Nephrologie, Medizinische Klinik I, Klinikum Grosshadern,
München; [c]Abteilung Innere Medizin und Nephrologie, Klinikum Steglitz, Berlin;
[d]Innere Medizin III, Nephrologie, Humboldt-Krankenhaus, Berlin;
[e]Nephrologisches Zentrum Niedersachsen, Hannoversch-Münden; [f]Innere Medizin II,
Rheinisch-Westfälische Technische Hochschule, Aachen; [g]Abteilung Dialyse und
Nephrologie, Medizinische Universitätsklinik, Homburg; [h]Psychologisches Institut,
Albert-Ludwigs-Universität, Freiburg i. Br.; [i]Boehringer Mannheim GmbH,
Mannheim, FRG

Recombinant human erythropoietin (rhEPO) is a very effective treatment in nearly all anemic hemodialysis patients and the rise of the hematocrit depends mainly on the dose of rhEPO given [1, 4]. The beneficial effects are obvious. The pivotal points are the elimination of regular blood transfusions and the amelioration of symptoms arising from renal anemia. The long-term treatment with rhEPO is therefore likely to improve morbidity and possibly mortality in hemodialysis patients. Uncontrolled studies of rhEPO treatment [5, 13, 14] reported side effects which may interfere with the aim of reducing morbidity and mortality; these include hypertension, seizure, hyperkalemia and clotting of the vascular access.

The present controlled multicenter study of anemic hemodialysis patients investigates the morbidity and frequency of adverse effects observed in hemodialysis patients undergoing rhEPO treatment in comparison to hemodialysis patients without rhEPO treatment over 6 months.

Table 1. Demographic data (median, range) of enrolled patients and withdrawal during study

	EPO group	Control group
Number of patients in double-blind phase	63	66
Sex, male/female	24/39	31/35
Age, years	56 (21–80)	58 (22–78)
Duration of HD treatment, months	35 (6–68)	44 (6–87)
Number of patients after 6 months	53	46
Number of patients withdrawn	10	20
Death	2	2
Kidney transplantation	4	6
Consent withdrawn	4	12

Patients

129 patients undergoing regular hemodialysis were studied after giving informed consent to participate in the controlled trial of either rhEPO treatment or the conventional treatment of anemia by blood transfusions if necessary. The criteria for admission into the study were: hematocrit (Hct) $\leq 28\%$, regular hemodialysis (HD) for at least 6 months, anemia exclusively caused by end-stage renal disease, no major underlying disease such as infections, epilepsy, cancer and no immunosuppressive therapy. Any hypertension or diabetes mellitus had to be adequately controlled. The blood transfusion requirements should not have exceeded 8 units of packed red cells in the previous year.

All patients underwent hemodialysis 3 times/week in 7 university hospital centers in Germany. The demographic data of the patients admitted to the study and the reasons for withdrawal are given in table 1. The underlying renal disease, the renal status at the start of the study and concomitant cardiovascular diseases, as well as diabetes mellitus, are listed in table 2.

Study Design (table 3)

In the pretreatment period of 2 weeks clinical and laboratory baseline parameters were established. Thereafter, the patients were randomized either into the rhEPO treatment group or the control group. The following 4 weeks were performed in a double-blind fashion using placebo injections in the control group. This was followed by an open controlled study up to 6 months. The double-blind phase was designed to elucidate the side effects of the intravenous injection (e.g. flu-like symptoms) and to gain data on patients' complaints before they could identify their group themselves.

Table 2. Frequency of diseases leading to chronic renal failure, renal status at start of the study and concomitant diseases

	EPO group, %	Control group, %
Renal disease		
Glomerulonephritis	20	27
Pyelonephritis	25	26
Analgesic nephropathy	19	24
Polycystic kidney disease	8	2
Vascular kidney disease	4	4
Diabetic nephropathy	10	4
Unknown	14	13
Renal status at start of the study		
Nephrectomy	9	10
Previous kidney transplantation	14	15
Concomitant diseases		
Hypertension	46	47
Coronary heart disease	22	14
Coronary insufficiency	13	17
Arrhythmias	11	5
Valvular heart disease	2	6
Diabetes mellitus	27	9

Table 3. Protocol of controlled rhEPO study in hemodialysis patients (≥ 6 months on HD and Hct $\leq 28\%$)

Pretreatment period	Recording of baseline parameters (2 weeks)	
	Randomization	
	EPO group (rhEPO)	Control group (placebo)
Correction period	Double-blind phase (4 weeks)	
	Until target Hct 30–35% initial dose: 3×80 U/kg BW/week i.v.	Control period I (8 weeks)
Maintenance period	Hct 30–35% 3×40 U/kg BW/week i.v.	Control period II (12 weeks)

In the rhEPO group the target hematocrit was 30–35% and the initial rhEPO dose 80 U/kg BW/week intravenously at the end of each dialysis session. This regimen was selected from pilot studies with the same rhEPO preparation [1]. From this it was also calculated that the correction period until the target hematocrit was reached would last about 10–12 weeks of which the first 4 weeks were double-blinded because of the small increase of the hematocrit to be expected. During the maintenance period with the hematocrit kept at 30–35%, the rhEPO dose was lowered to 40 U/kg BW/week intravenously.

The control group was investigated during the double-blind phase and further periods of 8 and 12 weeks.

Laboratory Tests

The baseline investigation consisted of a clinical assessment including ECG, chest radiography and laboratory data on complete blood count with white differential and reticulocyte count, coagulation tests, biochemistry profile and parameters related to the anemia (ferritin, transferrin, folic acid, vitamin B_{12}). Complete blood counts and biochemistry were repeated monthly. The ECG was repeated after 3 months and both ECG and chest X-ray after 6 months.

Clinical Course

All clinical events and changes in therapeutic procedures were recorded by the physicians. The patients were asked about possible side effects related to the injection and physical complaints (bone pain, nausea, pruritus, headache, lack of appetite, tiredness, sensation of coldness in the extremities) in weekly intervals. A special questionnaire on physical and psychological symptoms and well-being was answered by the patients in the pretreatment period, at the end of the double-blind phase, and at 3 and 5 months.

Statistical Analysis

The statistical analysis consisted of descriptive methods. Median values and one interquartile to both sides (interquartile range) were calculated. For statistical testing of some variables the Wilcoxon rank sum test for independent groups and Wilcoxon signed rank test for paired samples was used.

Results

Patients at Start

129 patients were randomized to receive either rhEPO (n = 63) or placebo (control, n = 66). The groups were comparable with respect to sex, age and previous dialysis (table 1). The reasons for chronic renal failure were similar but diabetes mellitus and diabetic nephropathy and also polycystic kidneys were more frequent in the EPO group (table 2). Nephrectomy of the patient's own kidneys and kidney transplantation with the patient's return to hemodialysis were performed in a similar number of patients in each group.

In both groups hypertension was the most frequent concomitant disease followed by chronic ischemic heart disease and heart failure. Dependence on blood transfusions in the year before the study was higher in the control group (fig. 2). In the pretreatment period more patients were hypertensive in the EPO group than in the control group (41/63 vs. 32/66). In those patients completing all study periods, hypertension remained more common in the EPO group at the start of therapy (31/53 vs. 23/46; see also figure 3 and 4).

Patients at Follow-Up

30 patients dropped out of the study, 10 in the EPO and 20 in the control group (table 1). Kidney transplantation was performed in 4 patients of the EPO and 6 of the control group. Consent was withdrawn by 4 patients in the EPO and 12 patients in the control group; the latter insisted on receiving rhEPO after serving 12 weeks in the control group and completing the control period I. Only the results of those patients participating in the whole study were evaluated. There were 2 deaths in each group.

Mortality

The 2 deaths in each group reflect the diseased state of the patients and also the complications associated with hemodialysis; they were not related to the rhEPO therapy in that group.

In the EPO group a 68-year-old hypertensive woman died of hemorrhage from a ruptured aneurysm of the ascending aorta after 5 months on rhEPO treatment having a hematocrit of 32% and no change in blood pressure or antihypertensive medication. The second case was a 64-year-old man who succumbed to a septic meningoencephalitis caused by a relapse of mitral valve endocarditis after 2 months of treatment.

In the control group a sudden cardiac death occurred in a 65-year-old woman who had mitral regurgitation and developed heart failure and atrial fibrillation after 5 months in the study. The other death occurred in a 74-year-old man as a result of septic meningoencephalitis caused by an infected dialysis catheter in the third month of the trial.

Changes in Hematological Parameters

The starting hematocrit ranged from 17 to 28 with a median of 23% in the EPO group, and from 18 to 27 with a median of 23% in the control group. The different course of the hematocrit is shown in figure 1. The patients treated with rhEPO responded during the double-blind phase with an increase of the median hematocrit from 23 to 25%, while the control group remained stable at 23%. The target hematocrit was reached within the first 10–12 weeks of the correction period by all patients but 4. In these only a partial response (hema-

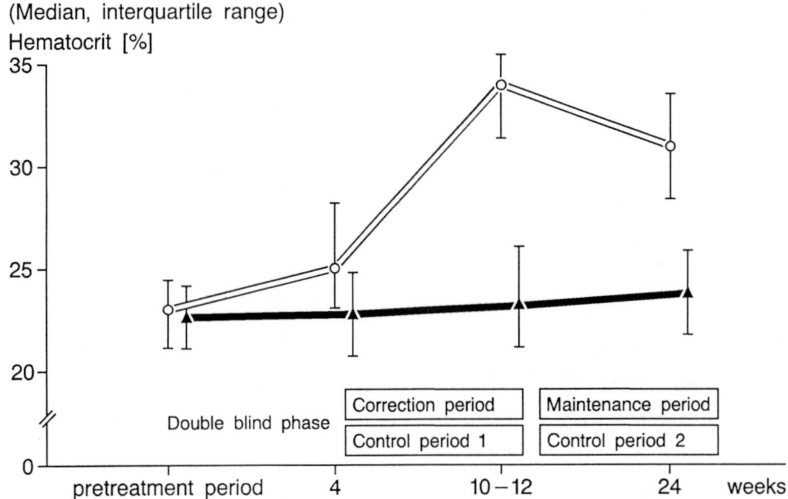

Fig. 1. Hematocrit in patients on hemodialysis with and without rhEPO therapy. ○ = rhEPO (n = 53); ▲ = controls (n = 46).

tocrit 25–29%) was seen. The maximum hematocrit of 34% (median; range 25–42%) was observed at the end of the correction period according to the definition of this study period. During the maintenance period, with the rhEPO dose halved, the hematocrit decreased to 31% (median; range 22–35%).

The median hemoglobin values rose correspondingly from 7.6 to 10.9 g/dl and fell slightly to 10.6 g/dl; the control group values started at 7.5 and ended at 7.8 g/dl. The median changes of hematocrit and hemoglobin during the correction period were significantly different between the groups (p <0.0001). In the control group, blood transfusions were continued at about the same rate as before (fig. 2). In the EPO group after 4 weeks of rhEPO treatment the need for regular blood transfusions was abolished as expected. Thereafter, transfusions were only necessary for acute blood loss or acute exacerbation of systemic lupus erythematosus in 1 patient each.

The white blood count was not altered in both groups. The median platelet count increased with rhEPO treatment from 205 (range 97–466) to 232 (range 103–474) · 10^9/l at the end of the correction period (p = 0.02); in the controls it fell from 233 (range 105–489) to 213 (range 96–456) · 10^9/l (p = 0.001).

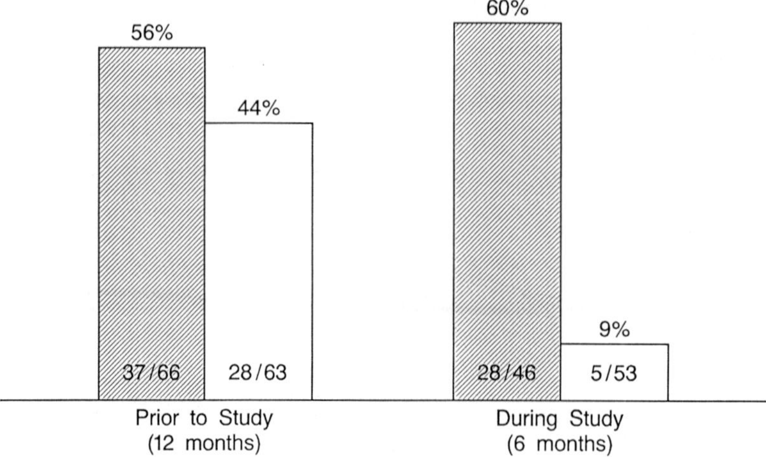

Fig. 2. Number of patients receiving blood transfusions. ▨ = Controls; ☐ = rhEPO.

The serum ferritin at the start was higher in the EPO group; during the correction period it fell from a median of 261 (range 20–6,253) to 120 (range 9–3,380) ng/ml (p = 0.01). In the control group it increased slightly from 163 (7–2,988) to 203 (14–3,715) ng/ml (p = 0.7). Oral iron supplements were given when indicated.

Hypertension and Other Cardiovascular Events
For the evaluation of the frequency of hypertension at the start of the study the blood pressure was measured before three consecutive hemodialyses and averaged. All patients on antihypertensive therapy were labelled hypertensive. The classification into hypotensive, normotensive and hypertensive patients for the pretreatment and different treatment periods is given in figure 3 for rhEPO therapy and in figure 4 for the control patients.

In the EPO group (fig. 3), 2 previously normotensive patients developed hypertension and were started on antihypertensives during the correction period and 3 patients did so during the maintenance period; in the correction period the antihypertensive therapy was increased in another 2 patients. In the maintenance period, 2 other patients needed antihypertensive therapy anew and in 6 it was intensified.

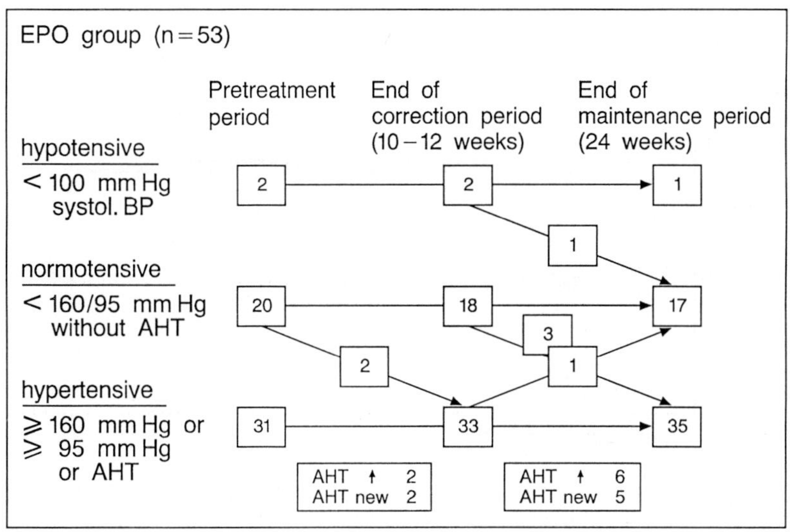

Fig. 3. Changes in blood pressure and antihypertensive therapy (AHT) in patients on hemodialysis with rhEPO therapy.

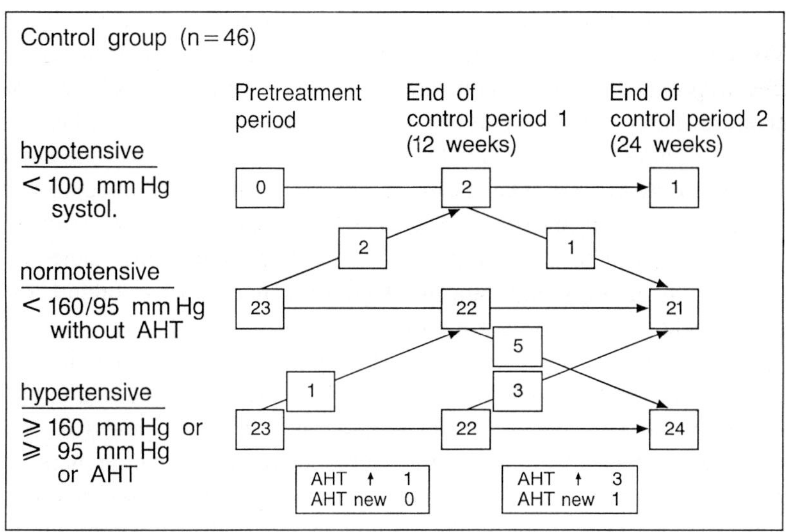

Fig. 4. Changes in blood pressure and antihypertensive therapy (AHT) in patients on hemodialysis without rhEPO therapy.

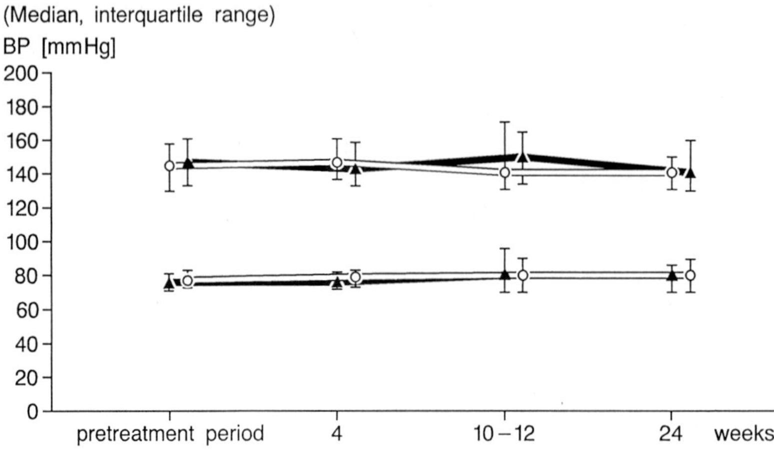

Fig. 5. Systolic and diastolic blood pressure in patients on hemodialysis with and without rhEPO therapy. ○ = rhEPO (n = 53); ▲ = controls (n = 46).

In the controls during period 2 (fig. 4) 5 patients became hypertensive, in 3 of them because of a systolic blood pressure elevation. Antihypertensive therapy was started in 1 patient with an increased systolic and diastolic blood pressure. Three other patients required more antihypertensive medication. In 3 further patients with systolic hypertension the systolic blood pressure fell spontaneously to normal values during the same period. The median systolic and diastolic blood pressure stayed rather constant during the study in both groups (fig. 5). This was the result of a reinforced or newly started antihypertensive therapy, the data of which are summarized in table 4 for the patients who completed the 6 months of the study.

The incidence of hypertensive blood pressure changes classified as intensified and newly started antihypertensive medication amounted to 28% in the EPO and 11% in the control group. The difference points to a clear association between EPO treatment and blood pressure elevation, here represented by the increased antihypertensive therapy. This therapeutic intervention happened mainly during the maintenance period. No patient had to be withdrawn from the study because of uncontrollable hypertension or the other cardiovascular events given in table 5. Seizures were not seen during the study.

Table 4. Changes in antihypertensive therapy (AHT) in patients on hemodialysis with and without rhEPO therapy

	EPO group (n = 53)		Control group (n = 46)	
	start	24 weeks	start	24 weeks
On AHT	27 (51%)	35 (66%)	19 (41%)	20 (43%)
AHT intensified during study	8 (15%)		4 (9%)	
AHT started during study	7 (13%)		1 (2%)	
AHT increased total	15 (28%)		5 (11%)	

Table 5. Cardiovascular events

	EPO group, n	Control group, n
Severe hypertension (BP > 220/100)	3	3
Hypertensive encephalopathy	1	1
Syncope	0	1
Angina pectoris	1	4
Cerebral ischemia	0	1
Stroke	0	1

Clotting of AV Fistula

The groups were comparable in respect to the frequency of clotting of the fistula vessels since beginning hemodialysis treatment and also during the 6 months prior to the study (table 6). During the study, clotting episodes occurred more often in the EPO group; only in 1 patient (No. 53) was it associated with the rise in hematocrit (table 7). Most of the other patients had a higher risk of a thrombotic event resulting from a shunt stenosis known before the study. Clotting of the extracorporeal circuit was prevented by an increase in the mean heparin dose by 20%.

Table 6. Clotting of AV fistula in patients on hemodialysis with and without rhEPO therapy

	EPO group		Control group	
	%	n	%	n
Frequency of patients with clotting				
Since beginning of HD treatment	35		35	
Six months prior to start of study	8		11	
During study (6 months)	9		9	
Numbers during study				
Patients with clotting		5		4
Clotting episodes		8		4
Shunt stenosis known		3		1

Table 7. Clotting episodes of AV fistula in patients on hemodialysis with and without rhEPO therapy

Patient No.	Hct at time of clotting episode %	ΔHct %	Duration of study until clotting days
Control group			
27	25	4	98
117	26	2	115
134[1]	24	–1	19
138	24	2	131
EPO group			
53	32	17	85
39[1]	24	–1	11
48[1]	25	–3	13
	25	–3	36
70	30	3	13
	27	0	22
74[1]	26	–2	78
	29	1	102

[1] Shunt stenosis known.

Table 8. Infections during study

	EPO group, n	Control group, n
Upper respiratory tract infection	12	4
Pneumonia	0	2
Herpes zoster	2	0
Arthritis	2	2
Gastroenteritis	2	1
Urinary tract infection	2	1

Infections

The acute infections recorded are listed in table 8. The actual number of upper respiratory infections was higher in the rhEPO-treated group but pneumonias occurred only in the control group. Additionally, there was one lethal sepsis in each group (see Mortality, p. 94).

Metabolic Data

The efficacy of hemodialysis treatment was not significantly influenced by rhEPO treatment in that group. No significant changes occurred in both groups regarding the duration of dialysis, body weight, serum concentrations of potassium, phosphate, urea and creatinine (table 9). Single episodes of hyperkalemia ($K^+ > 7.5$ mmol/l) without clinical symptoms were more often observed in the EPO group than in the control group (9 vs. 4 patients). A clinically relevant overhydration was also more frequent during EPO treatment (7 vs. 3 patients).

Complaints and Life Satisfaction

The complaints arising from anemia were reduced after the EPO-induced partial correction of anemia. This applied especially to angina, dyspnea and other cardiovascular symptoms. More general complaints such as nausea, lack of appetite and tiredness improved too. The changes in these symptoms were significant after 3 months of rhEPO treatment (table 10).

A score of several physical and psychological symptoms was significantly lower after 3 months of rhEPO treatment compared to the score before treatment and also to the score of the control patients at 3 months. A similar conclusion applies to the significantly increased satisfaction with physical fitness. Sexuality improved slightly in the EPO group. No changes could be

Table 9. Metabolic status of patients on hemodialysis with and without rhEPO therapy (median, range)

	EPO group		Control group	
	pretreatment	24 weeks	pretreatment	24 weeks
Duration of HD, h	4.5	4.5	4.4	4.1
	(2–6)	(2–6)	(2–6)	(2–6)
Body weight, kg	67.3	67.4	61.2	61.4
	(38.5–98)	(39.9–98.4)	(39.2–93.2)	(38.9–93.2)
Potassium, mmol/l	5.7	5.7	5.6	5.7
	(4.03–7.0)	(4.1–11.2)	(4.3–7.6)	(3.6–8.0)
Phosphate, mmol/l	1.96	1.90	2.07	1.81
	(0.9–3.15)	(0.62–2.94)	(1.12–3.33)	(0.9–3.78)
Urea, mg/dl	165.0	160.0	165.0	154.6
	(108–288)	(77–247)	(76–258)	(71–243)
Creatinine, mg/dl	11.3	12.1	11.1	11.3
	(6.3–16.9)	(6.4–17.5)	(4.8–17.9)	(4.9–17.3)

Table 10. Changes in complaints and quality of life in patients on hemodialysis with rhEPO therapy (before vs. 3 months)

	Change	p
Complaints:		
Nausea, lack of appetite, tiredness	↓	<0.05
Score of 22 physical and psychological symptoms	↓	<0.02
Quality of life: satisfaction with:		
Physical fitness	↑	<0.05
Sexual activity	↑	<0.05
Overall quality of life	0	N.S.

demonstrated when considering a score of all life-satisfaction parameters. A separate analysis over 24 weeks gives the variation in the course of the symptom tiredness (fig. 6), which demonstrated a pronounced difference after the rise in hematocrit. Flu-like symptoms were reported during the double-blind phase of this study in about 3% of the rhEPO-treated patients and in about 4% of the control patients.

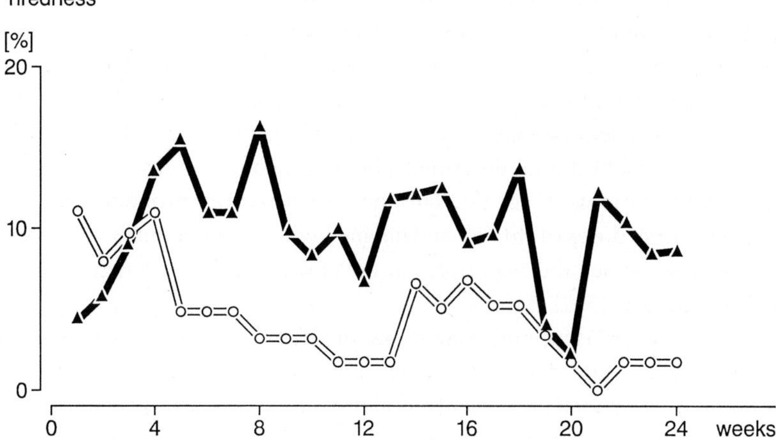

Fig. 6. Complaints of tiredness. ○ = rhEPO (n = 53); ▲ = controls (n = 46).

Discussion

The efficacy and safety of rhEPO treatment in anemic hemodialysis patients is confirmed in this controlled multicenter clinical study. Regular blood transfusions were no longer required by the patients treated with rhEPO. This eliminates the many problems associated with blood transfusions. Several multicenter studies have reported that the intravenous and also subcutaneous administration of rhEPO in anemic dialysis patients is well tolerated [1, 5, 13, 14].

Only the partial correction of anemia with a hematocrit of around 30–35% was aimed at since this achieves sufficient peripheral oxygenation and normalizes the central hemodynamics [3, 8, 9]. This is accompanied by an improvement of the physical symptoms related to renal anemia and a state of general well-being. Exercise ability increased also [7]. It has been shown that no further benefit was attained by increasing the hemoglobin from 95–110 to 115–130 g/l, but the incidence of adverse effects also rose [2].

The successful treatment of anemia with rhEPO is accompanied by some adverse events [4, 10, 12]. Since most of the dialysis patients in these studies had many other medical problems apart from anemia and end-stage kidney disease, it is difficult to judge whether some of the adverse events reported were not just coincidental. For this reason the present controlled study compared the clinical events in a group treated with rhEPO to a control group in which anemia was managed by transfusions as before. An analysis was made of the more common adverse events such as hypertension and fistula clotting which are frequent even in anemic hemodialysis patients.

Most rhEPO studies described a blood pressure increase in about 30% of the dialysis patients [5, 12, 13]. This increase was more pronounced in groups receiving high doses of rhEPO and having higher hemoglobin levels as well [2, 12]. In most cases the hypertension developed during the first 6 months of rhEPO therapy [5, 12–14].

Even when using moderate doses of rhEPO to achieve a hematocrit of 30–35% and comparing this to the control group in the present study, a treatment-associated increase in blood pressure or in the dose of antihypertensive drugs was apparent. The slightly hypertensive patients whose elevated blood pressure was not yet treated before rhEPO needed antihypertensives during therapy with rhEPO. The blood pressure increased mainly during the maintenance period (after 3 months of starting rhEPO) which is at variance with other studies giving an earlier peak [5].

Surprisingly, a similar course was seen in the control group although to a much lesser extent. Taking the spontaneous pressure changes into account, the risk of developing or aggravating hypertension on rhEPO is about 1 in 5 (17%; see table 4). The hemodynamic effects of the correction of anemia in dialysis patients consisted of a decrease in cardiac output and peripheral blood flow and an increase of central and peripheral vascular resistances [8, 9]. This response will be modulated by the vascular adaption to salt and water loading during the dialysis interval [6]. These variables can cause a different response of the blood pressure.

The incidence of fistula clotting seemed higher in rhEPO-treated patients but larger multicenter trials came to the conclusion that it was comparable to hemodialysis patients not receiving rhEPO [5]. Clotting problems occurred mainly in bypass grafts [5, 10] or compromised access sites [13]. In another controlled study clotting of the vascular access was positively associated with rhEPO treatment [2]. In the present study the number of clotting episodes was higher during rhEPO treatment, but these happened in patients with pre-existing anatomical problems. This is in agreement with most other investigations.

Hyperkalemic events and overhydration occurred more often under rhEPO treatment, as described by others. No other metabolic changes were observed, for instance the body weight, serum phosphate and urea remained nearly identical. It is likely that the current knowledge regarding the management of dialysis patients on rhEPO treatment prevented more adverse effects in the study presented.

An improvement in physical performance and physical symptoms was observed in several studies and was also reported in the more formal trials with control groups [2]. Dialysis patients suffer from nonspecific symptoms to a large extent [11], some of which can be ameliorated by the correction of anemia.

It was not unexpected that the controlled trials with rhEPO confirmed its efficacy. This controlled trial puts in the correct setting the adverse events potentially induced by rhEPO treatment in the generally multimorbid hemodialysis patients. The rise in blood pressure and the need for additional antihypertensive treatment remains the most prominent complication. Other adverse events depend very much on the patients' underlying pathology and illnesses. Gradual and limited correction of anemia by rhEPO appears to be the best therapeutic goal in dialysis patients.

References

1   Bommer, J.; Kugel, M.; Schoeppe, W.; Brunkhorst, R.; Samtleben, W.; Bramsiepe, P.; Scigalla, P.: Dose-related effects of recombinant human erythropoietin on erythropoiesis. Contrib. Nephrol., vol. 66, pp. 85–93 (Karger, Basel 1988).

2   Canadian Erythropoietin Study Group: Association between recombinant human erythropoietin and quality of life and exercise capacity of patients receiving haemodialysis. Br. Med. J. *300:* 573–578 (1990).

3   Creutzig, A.; Caspary, L.; Nonnast-Daniel, B.; Bahlmann, J.; Kühn, K.; Brunkhorst, R.; Reimers, E.; Koch, K.M.; Alexander, K.: Skin microcirculation and regional peripheral resistance in patients with chronic renal anaemia treated with recombinant human erythropoietin. Eur. J. Clin. Invest. *20:* 219–223 (1990).

4   Eschbach, J. W.; Egrie, J. C.; Downing, M. R.; Browne, J. K.; Adamson, J. W.: Correction of the anemia of end-stage renal disease with recombinant human erythropoietin: results of a combined phase I and II clinical trial. N. Engl. J. Med. *316:* 73–78 (1987).

5   Eschbach, J. W.; Abdulhadi, M. H.; Browne, J. K.; Delano, B. G.; Downing, M. R.; Egrie, J. C. et al.: Recombinant human erythropoietin in anemic patients with end-stage renal disease: Results of a phase III multicenter clinical trial. Ann. Intern. Med. *111:* 992–1000 (1989).

6   Kim, K. E.; Onesti, G.; DelGuercio, E. T.; Greco, J., Fernandes, M.; Eidelson, B.; Swartz, C.: Sequential hemodynamic changes in end-stage renal disease and the anephric state during volume expansion. Hypertension *2,* 102–110 (1980).

7   Macdougall, I. C.; Lewis, N. P.; Saunders, M. J.; Cochlin, D. L.; Davies , M. E.; Hutton, R. D.; Fox, K. A. A.; Coles, G. A.; Williams, J. D.: Long-term cardiorespiratory effects of amelioration of renal anemia by erythropoietin. Lancet *335:* 489–493 (1990).

8   Neff, M.S.; Kim, K.E.; Persoff, M.; Onesti, G., Swartz, C.: Hemodynamics of uremic
    anemia. Circulation *43:* 876–883 (1971).
9   Nonnast-Daniel, B.; Deschodt, G.; Brunkhorst, R.; Creutzig, A.; Bahlmann, J.; Shal-
    don, S.; Koch, K.M.: Long-term effects of treatment with recombinant human erythro-
    poietin on hemodynamics and tissue oxygenation in patients with renal anemia. Neph-
    rol. Dial. Transplant. *5:* 444–448. (1990).
10 Paganini, E.P.; Latham, D.; Abdulhadi, M.: Practical considerations of recombinant
    human erythropoietin therapy. Am. J. Kidney Dis. *14:* suppl. 1, pp 19–25 (1989).
11 Parfrey, P.S.; Vavasour, H.M.; Henry, S.; Bullock, M.; Gault, M.H.: Clinical features
    and severity of non-specific symptoms in dialysis patients. Nephron *50:* 121–128 (1988).
12 Samtleben, W.; Baldamus, C.A.; Bommer, J.; Grützmacher, P.; Nonnast-Daniel, B.;
    Scigalla, P.; Gurland, H.-J.: Indications and contraindications for recombinant human
    erythropoietin treatment. Contrib. Nephrol., vol. 76, pp 193–200 (Karger, Basel 1989).
13 Sundal, E.; Kaeser, U.: Correction of anaemia of chronic renal failure with recombinant
    human erythropoietin: safety and efficacy of one year's treatment in a European multi-
    center study of 150 haemodialysis-dependent patients. Nephrol. Transplant. *4:* 979–987
    (1989).
14 Winearls, C.G.; Oliver, D.O.; Pippard, M.J., et al.: Effect of erythropoietin derived
    from recombinant DNA on the anemia of patients maintained by chronic hemodialysis.
    Lancet *ii:* 1175–1177 (1986).

Prof. J. Bahlmann, Zentrum Innere Medizin, Abteilung Nephrologie,
Medizinische Hochschule Hannover, Krankenhaus Oststadt, Podbielskistrasse 380,
D–3000 Hannover 51 (FRG)

Gurland HJ, Moran J, Samtleben W, Scigalla P, Wieczorek L (eds): Erythropoietin in
Renal and Non-Renal Anemias. Contrib Nephrol. Basel, Karger, 1991, vol 88, pp 107–116

Side Effects during Recombinant Human Erythropoietin Therapy in 2,000 ESRD Patients

W. Samtleben[a], *B. Ehmer*[b], *Isolde Lutz-Knochenhauer*[b],
Christa Hagmann[b], *P. Scigalla*[b], *H. J. Gurland*[a]

[a]Nephrology Division, Medical Clinic I, Klinikum Grosshadern, Ludwig-Maximilians-
Universität, München, and [b]Boehringer Mannheim GmbH, Mannheim, FRG

Adverse events observed during the evaluation of a new drug in phase I, II and III studies constitute the expected risk profile, which should be known before the drug's general clinical use. Hypertension, seizures and fistula occlusions have been noted in the early reports on the treatment of renal anemia with recombinant human erythropoietin (rhEPO) [1–7]. The aim of this paper is to analyze the serious adverse events observed during treatment of a large population of hemodialysis patients with intravenous rhEPO.

Materials and Methods

The data analyzed are from 2,160 stable chronic hemodialysis patients who entered one of the following multicenter studies using Boehringer Mannheim rhEPO: (1) MF 3787: a dose-finding study in nontransfusion-dependent patients with stable renal anemia (n = 95); (2) MF 3911: a study of the treatment of iron-overloaded or transfusion-dependent patients (n = 589); (3) MF 3981: a randomized controlled study which has been described in detail elsewhere (n = 107) [8]; (4) MF 4028-D: a long-term observation study for drug safety, which included most of the patients (n = 1,347).

Of the initial 2,160 patients who entered the four protocols, data from 2,138 patients were available for evaluation. At this time (June 1990) some patients have been on intravenous treatment for 3 years. The average observation time for all patients is 11 months, giving a total of 1,955 patient years of treatment.

The analysis is based on those serious adverse events reported to the main clinical investigator. An adverse event was defined as serious when it met one or more of the following criteria: (1) the event was fatal or life-threatening; (2) it required hospitalization or prolonged the hospital stay; (3) the patient became permanently disabled, or (4) a previously unrecognized disease was diagnosed during the treatment period. The recording of an adverse event does not of course establish any causal relation to the rhEPO treatment. The reported adverse

Table 1. Causes of death during rhEPO treatment of 2,138 patients

Causes of death	Patients, n	
Cardiac	65	
Myocardial insufficiency		30
Myocardial infarction		18
Arrhythmia		13
Others		4
Cerebrovascular	25	
Cerebral hemorrhage		8
Subarachnoid hemorrhage		5
Cerebral infarction		5
Others		7
Infectious	20	
Septicemia		15
Pneumonia		3
Other		2
Pulmonary embolism	3	
Others	25	
Total	138	

events will be analyzed with respect to deaths, CNS morbidity (with special attention to convulsions), fistula occlusions, infections and to the incidence of certain specific conditions, including hematological abnormalities, malignancies and immune disorders.

Results

Deaths

A total of 138 deaths have been reported in the study population. The causes are listed in table 1. Heart disease is the most common with 65 deaths, followed by 25 deaths due to cerebrovascular causes, 20 due to infections, 5 due to malignancies, 3 due to pulmonary embolism and 25 due to other reasons. This pattern is not different from that of the general dialysis population [9, 10]. Figure 1 depicts the Kaplan-Meier survival analysis of the patient group aged 15–64 years at the start of rhEPO treatment. During the first 21 months of treatment, 67 of the 1,557 patients in this age group died,

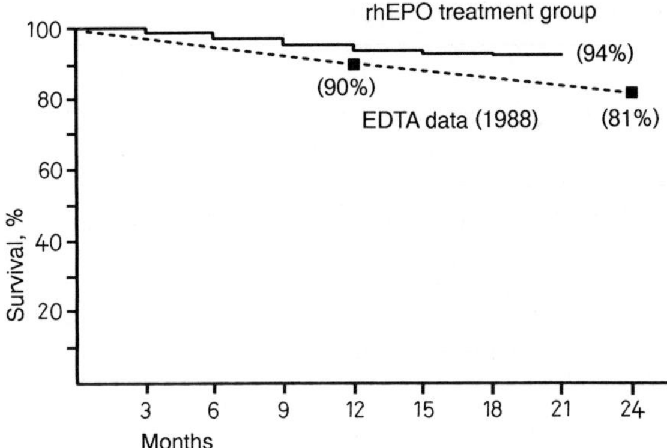

Fig. 1. Patient survival after start of intravenous rhEPO treatment according to Kaplan-Meier. For comparison, EDTA data for the same age group (15–64 years) are shown.

which represents a 94% survival after nearly 2 years of therapy. There is no time period which shows a sharp increase in death rate. To allow a rough comparison, the survival data from the 1988 EDTA report for that age group after commencing hemodialysis [10] are shown as a dashed line. One and 2 years after start of renal replacement therapy, 90 and 81% of the patients, respectively, were still alive in the EDTA population.

The overall survival of the rhEPO-treated group appears to be a little better than that seen in the EDTA population. However, this is not surprising, as severely ill patients, for example those with malignancies, were excluded from all rhEPO studies. These data do not allow the conclusion, therefore, that rhEPO decreases the mortality of dialysis patients. On the other hand, an excess mortality due to rhEPO treatment is also very unlikely. To prove this conclusively, controlled studies including thousands of patients would be necessary.

Adverse CNS Events

Seizures have been reported in 1987 as a side effect of rhEPO therapy [2, 3, 7]. In our patient population only 30 convulsions have occurred in 28 patients, a figure which represents one event every 65 patient years. Table 2 lists the clinical settings in which convulsions have been observed. The incidence of convulsions is very low. However, figures from a comparable

Table 2. Analysis of convulsions during rhEPO therapy

Clinical condition	Events, n
During dialysis without evident cause	5
Due to cardiovascular or other specified reasons	10
Due to pre-existing focal CNS disease (e.g. previous infarction)	8
Associated with hypertension	7
Total	30

Table 3. Serious adverse CNS events without convulsions

Condition	Events, n	Patients, n
Hypertensive encephalopathy	5	5
PRIND/TIA	40	38
Cerebral hemorrhage	19	17
Disturbed conscious state (no reason given)	36	32
Total	100	92

dialysis population not on rhEPO therapy are not available. Grand mal epilepsy was not a cause of convulsions in our study population. This is not surprising, as this condition was an exclusion criterion in all of the studies.

Table 3 lists another 100 CNS events without convulsions reported in a total of 92 patients, which represents an incidence of one nonconvulsive episode every 20 patient years. As with convulsions, figures from a similar patient population are not available.

Fistula Clotting

The possibility of an increased risk of fistula clotting during rhEPO therapy was recognized very early [1, 3, 7]. In this patient population, 221 fistula occlusions have been noted in 160 patients. 43 of the 160 patients experienced more than one occlusion (table 4). The 221 occluded fistulas represent one occlusion in 9 treatment years. This figure seems very low and may reflect more patient selection rather than the real incidence of fistula

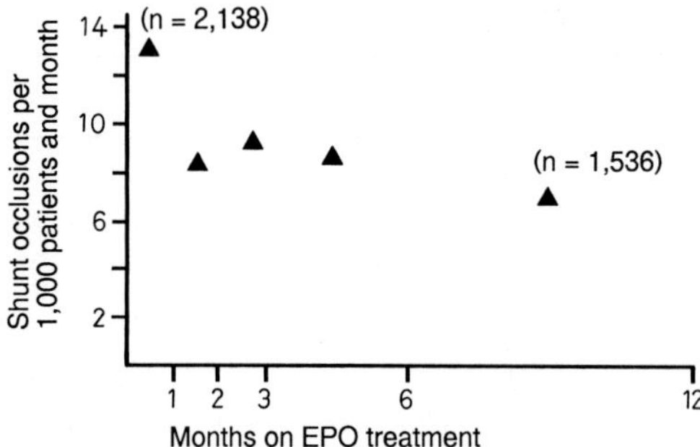

Fig. 2. Shunt occlusions during intravenous rhEPO treatment per 1,000 patient months. Figures in parentheses indicate the number of patients available for evaluation at that particular period.

Table 4. Frequency of fistula occlusions during rhEPO treatment

Patients, n	Episodes of fistula occlusion, n	Episodes, total
1	5	5
2	4	8
11	3	33
29	2	58
117	1	117
160		221

thromboses in an unselected population. Unfortunately, comparable data concerning fistula clotting are not available. The greatest frequency has been observed in the first treatment month (fig. 2), thereafter the incidence is very low at 7–10 fistula occlusions per 1,000 patient-months.

Infections

Infections are another common complication in long-term dialysis patients. 261 infections have been reported in the study population. The organ distribution is shown in table 5. A more detailed analysis of the pulmonary infections is given in table 6 and of the viral infections in table 7.

Table 5. Site of infections during rhEPO treatment

Site	Cases, n
Respiratory tract	63
Skin	59
Septicemia	44
Fistula/shunt	28
Viral	16
Others	51
Total	261

Table 6. Pulmonary infections during rhEPO treatment

Condition	Patients, n
Pneumonia	36
Legionella pneumonia	2
Atypical pneumonia	1
Reactivated tuberculosis	1
Total	40

Table 7. Viral infections during rhEPO treatment

Type of infection	Patients, n
Herpes zoster	10
Hepatitis B	2
Non-A-non-B hepatitis	2
CMV	1
Not specified	1
Total	16

Table 8. Adverse hematological events during rhEPO treatment

Condition	Patients, n
Thrombocytosis	2
Leukocytosis	1
Myelodysplasia	1
Bone marrow aplasia	1
Total	5

Adverse Hematological Events

No specific hematological condition occurred in the study population with a high incidence. Five adverse events have been reported (table 8). An increase in platelets has previously been observed during the correction phase of the renal anemia in dialysis patients treated with high doses of rhEPO [4]. A case from our study population with rhEPO-associated thrombocytosis has been described in detail elsewhere [11]. There is a probable association between iron deficiency and thrombocytosis [12], a mechanism which may also be operative in rhEPO-treated hemodialysis patients [13].

The 1 case with bone marrow aplasia (proven by multiple bone marrow aspirates) came from our center and showed a complete recovery after withdrawal of all medication and after he had overcome a prolonged viral infection. Subsequently he was recommenced on rhEPO, and had a normal hematological response.

Malignancies

Fourteen malignancies were diagnosed during rhEPO treatment (table 9), half located in the gastrointestinal tract. Five patients have died from disseminated disease. The 1988 EDTA report [10] lists a similar organ distribution of malignancies diagnosed after commencing maintenance dialysis. Neither the pattern nor the incidence suggest an increased risk of malignancy following rhEPO.

Immune Disorders

A total of ten immune disorders not recognized prior to rhEPO treatment have been reported in our patients (table 10). No excess of immune events has

Table 9. Diagnosis of malignancies during rhEPO treatment

Site of malignancy	Patients, n	
Gastrointestinal tract	7	
Colon/rectum		2
Stomach		1
Pancreas		1
Liver		2
Gallbladder		1
Renal tumors	3	
Organ not stated	2	
Plasmacytoma	1	
Gynecological tumors	1	
Total	14	

Table 10. Diagnosis of immune disorders during rhEPO treatment

Immune disorder	Patients, n
Rheumatoid arthritis/polyarthritis	4
Lupus erythematosus	2
Wegener's granulomatosis	2
Temporal arteritis	1
Myasthenia	1
Total	10

been observed. However, the study population is obviously too small to accurately assess the incidence of these disorders.

Conclusion

Survival in patients treated with rhEPO is superior to the EDTA population [10], a feature which may be related to patient selection. Convulsions in patients not known to be epileptic are rare, with one event every 65 patient treatment years. CNS events other than convulsions are also rare with one event every 20 patient years. Fistula clotting is a problem in patients with fistulas at risk, as soon as their hematocrit rises; however, one thrombosis every 9 patient years in the four studies available for evaluation is surprisingly low. The 14 malignancies diagnosed during the time of rhEPO treatment represent an incidence and pattern which does not differ from that in the EDTA population [10]. Alarming hematological events and the diagnosis of immune disorders are both rare. In summary, rhEPO treatment is obviously not associated with an increased incidence of adverse events.

Acknowledgements

All the data have been elaborated in the four multicenter studies mentioned in the Introduction. Without the cooperation of several hundred nephrologists in the Federal Republic of Germany it would not have been possible to accumulate that bulk of data. Therefore, the authors would like to thank all those colleagues who have contributed their time and effort to allow an overview of those serious adverse events which may occur in the long-term rhEPO treatment of hemodialysis patients.

References

1   Bommer, J.; Alexiou, C.; Müller-Bühl, U.; Eifert, J.; Ritz, E.: Recombinant human erythropoietin therapy in hemodialysis patients – dose determination and clinical experience. Nephrol. Dial. Transplant. *2:* 238–242 (1987).

2   Casati, S.; Passerini, P.; Campise, M. R.; Graziani, G.; Cesana, B.; Peresic, M.; Ponticelli, C.: Benefits and risks of protracted treatment with human recombinant erythropoietin in patients having haemodialysis. Br. Med. J. *295:* 1017–1020 (1987).

3   Eschbach, J. W.; Egrie, J. C.; Downing, M. R.; Browne, J. K.; Adamson, J. W.: Correction of the anemia of end-stage renal disease with recombinant human erythropoietin. Results of a combined phase I and II clinical trial. N. Engl. J. Med. *316:* 73–78 (1987).

4   Grützmacher, P.; Bergmann, M.; Weinreich, T.; Nattermann, U.; Reimers, E.; Pollock, M.: Beneficial and adverse effects of correction of anemia by recombinant human erythropoietin in patients on maintenance haemodialysis. Contrib. Nephrol., vol. 66; pp. 104–113 (Karger, Basel 1988).

5   Samtleben, W.; Baldamus, C. A.; Bommer, J.; Fassbinder, W.; Nonnast-Daniel, B.; Gurland, H. J.: Blood pressure changes during treatment with recombinant human erythropoietin. Contrib. Nephrol. vol. 66; pp. 114–122 (Karger, Basel 1988).

6   Stutz, B.; Rhyner, K.; Vögtli, J.; Binswanger, U.: Erfolgreiche Behandlung der Anämie bei Hämodialyse-Patienten mit rekombiniertem humanem Erythropoietin. Erhaltungsdosis und Serumkonzentration. Schweiz. Med. Wochenschr. *117:* 1397–1402 (1987).

7   Winearls, C. G.; Oliver, D. O.; Pippard, M. J.; Reid, C., Downing, M. R.; Cotes, P. M.: Effect of human erythropoietin derived from recombinant DNA on the anaemia of patients maintained by chronic haemodialysis. Lancet *ii:* 1175–1178 (1986).

8   Bahlmann, J.; Schöter, K. H.; Scigalla, P.; Gurland, H. J.; Hilfenhaus, M.; Muthny, F. A.; Neumayer, H. H.; Pommer, W.; Quellhorst, E.; Siebert, H. G.; Weber, U.: Morbidity and mortality in hemodialysis patients with and without erythropoietin treatment. A controlled study. Contrib. Nephrol., vol. 88, pp. 90–106 (Karger, Basel 1991).

9   Brunner, F. P.; Fassbinder, W.; Broyer, M.; Dykes, S. R.; Ehrich, J. H. H.; Geerlings, W.; Rizzoni, G.; Selwood, N. H.; Tufveson, G.; Wing, A. J.: Combined report on regular dialysis and transplantation in Europe, XVIII, 1987 (Springer, London 1988).

10 Brunner, F. P.; Broyer, M.; Brynger, H.; Challah, S.; Dykes, S. R.; Fassbinder, W.; Oulès, R.; Rizzoni, G.; Selwood, N. H.; Wing, A. J.: Registry report: Survival on renal replacement therapy: Data from the EDTA Registry. Nephrol. Dial. Transplant. *2:* 109–122 (1988).

11 Scigalla, P.; Messinger, D.; Ehmer, B.; Woll, E. M.; Wieczorek, L.: Nebenwirkungen der Therapie der renalen Anämie mit rekombinantem humanem Erythropoietin; in Gurland, H. J.; Koch, K. M.; Schoeppe, W.; Scigalla, P. (eds): Innovative Aspekte der klinischen Medizin, vol. 1: Nephrologie. Neue Perspektiven für Dialysepatienten (Springer, Berlin 1989).

12 Schloesser, L. L.; Kipp, M. A.; Wenzel, F. J.: Thrombocytosis in iron-deficiency anemia. L. Lab. Clin. Med. *66:* 107–114 (1965).

13 Adamson, J. W.: The promise of recombinant human erythropoietin. Semin. Hematol. *2:* suppl. 2, pp. 5–8 (1989).

PD Dr. med. Walter Samtleben, Nephrology Division, Medical Clinic I,
University Hospital München-Grosshadern, PO Box 701 260,
D–8000 München 70 (FRG)

Gurland HJ, Moran J, Samtleben W, Scigalla P, Wieczorek L (eds): Erythropoietin in Renal and Non-Renal Anemias. Contrib Nephrol. Basel, Karger, 1991, vol 88, p 117

Discussion

to the Papers by J. Bahlmann et al. and W. Samtleben et al.

Shaldon (Montpellier): What percentage of the causes of death were confirmed by autopsy in your study?

Samtleben: I don't have this figure.

Shaldon: Is there no way of finding that out? I think it is relevant to attributing the causes of arrhythmia, for example. What surprised me was that there was a relatively high incidence of cardiovascular deaths. One of the hopes in relieving anemia is the improvement of myocardial function. Your results seem a little disappointing.

Ringoir (Ghent): I would like to know if the speakers think that infections are more frequent or less frequent after EPO treatment. I didn't hear it too clearly.

Bahlmann: It was difficult to draw firm clinical conclusions regarding the acute illnesses, including infections, observed in the controlled study. Only viral infections appeared to be more frequent in the EPO-treated group.

Eschbach (Seattle): I'd like to follow-up Dr. Shaldon's comment. In both of your presentations, I missed control data in terms of the cardiovascular deaths. We all know that it is the major cause of deaths in dialysis patients. But, is it your impression that there were more deaths than you expected and, if so, is it because of the 3 patients that died from hyperkalemia?

Samtleben: As I stated at the beginning of my presentation there are no controls available for the data I presented. Concerning the death rate in the study population, it is not higher than would have been expected from the EDTA data.

Gurland HJ, Moran J, Samtleben W, Scigalla P, Wieczorek L (eds): Erythropoietin in Renal and Non-Renal Anemias. Contrib Nephrol. Basel, Karger, 1991, vol 88, pp 118–125

Hypertension as a Possible Complication of Recombinant Human Erythropoietin Therapy

R. Brunkhorst, B. Nonnast-Daniel, K. M. Koch, U. Frei

Abteilung Nephrologie, Department Innere Medizin und Dermatologie, Medizinische Hochschule Hannover, FRG

Various positive effects of partial correction of renal anemia by recombinant human erythropoietin (rhEPO) on cardiovascular performance have been reported: physical work-load capacity increases [3, 16, 23], cardiac inner diameters decrease [14] and hypertrophy of left ventricular mass is reduced [14]. However, many studies and case reports demonstrate that treatment by rhEPO is also accompanied by adverse cardiovascular effects. In addition to minor increments of diastolic or mean arterial pressure which were seen in nearly all patients, in a considerable number of patients the development of hypertension or the aggravation of preexisting hypertension was observed. Data from uncontrolled multicenter trials show a 35–45% incidence of development and a 30–45% incidence of aggravation of hypertension when anemia is corrected by erythropoietin [10, 11, 24, 27]. Furthermore, a recent double-blind randomized placebo-controlled study showed a significantly higher diastolic blood pressure in the rhEPO-treated patients despite an increase of either the dose or the number of antihypertensive drugs used [5].

The hemodynamic changes involved in the development or aggravation of hypertension may also play a role in the pathogenesis of central nervous complications, mainly seizures, observed under rhEPO therapy in up to 12% of patients studied [9]. In most of the observed cases the neurological symptomatology coincided with the development or aggravation of hypertension. Edmunds et al. [9] reported, however, that the 'blood pressure at the time of the event was lower than that usually associated with hypertensive encephalopathy' and that retinal changes typical for accelerated hypertension were very often missing.

In order to understand the hypertensionogenic effect of rhEPO treatment of renal anemia, an analysis of the hemodynamics of anemia and of the changes in hemodynamics accompanying correction of anemia may be helpful.

Anemia and Hemodynamics

In clinical medicine anemia is the most common cause for an increase of cardiac output at rest [29]. Various investigators have found a correlation between the degree of anemia and the increment of cardiac output at rest when hemoglobin levels had dropped below 8 g/dl [2,29]. The increase in cardiac output coincides with a decrease of peripheral resistance, while blood pressure remains nearly unchanged [29]. Experimental studies suggest that the reduction of peripheral resistance is due to a lowered blood viscosity and possibly also to vasodilation induced by ischemia [29]. The degree of cardiac output change depends on individual factors such as age [8] and preexisting cardiac status. After correction of anemia by therapeutic maneuvers such as iron repletion or blood transfusions the hemodynamic parameters return to normal [8].

Chronic stable anemia in patients with end-stage renal disease is associated with increased cardiac output and normal or lowered peripheral vascular resistance [6, 17]. A significant portion of the patient population is hypertensive. As mentioned above, correction of anemia with rhEPO is very often associated with a rise in arterial blood pressure. Underlying changes of hemodynamic parameters were investigated by several groups in hemodialysis patients. Nonnast-Daniel et al. [18] studied the peripheral circulation and found a decrease of calf blood flow and an increase of regional resistance when anemia was corrected by rhEPO. Deschodt et al. [7] demonstrated by dye-dilution techniques an increase of total peripheral resistance and a decrease of cardiac output during correction of anemia. Both investigators found a small but significant increase in mean arterial pressure in their previously normotensive populations. Although qualitatively cardiac output and total peripheral resistance behave as in nonuremic anemic patients, the quantity of change of one or both of these parameters has to be inadequate in many uremic patients in view of the high incidence of hypertension accompanying rhEPO treatment.

*Pathogenesis of Hypertension Accompanying rhEPO Treatment in
End-Stage Renal Disease*

Peripheral Resistance

In general, peripheral resistance may be considered to be determined by
two factors – by the viscosity of blood (the rheological factor) and the cross-
sectional area of the peripheral vascular bed (the geometric factor) [12, 13].

The rheological factor is affected by hematocrit, by red cell abnormalities
and by the composition of the plasma proteins. Whole blood viscosity has
therefore to be considered a potential cause for an inadequate response of
peripheral resistance during correction of anemia by rhEPO. Existing data
indicate that whole blood viscosity at the usual target hematocrit of 30–35% is
lower than that of nonanemic normal persons [26]. Whether whole blood
viscosity after complete correction of anemia is within the normal range so far
has not been studied.

The geometric factor is a result of either structural alteration of the
vascular wall and/or of functional vasopressor effects. Independent of their
actual blood pressure at the start of rhEPO treatment the majority of regular
hemodialysis patients have a history of longlasting hypertension. In hypertensive individuals the cross-sectional area of the peripheral vascular bed is
functionally diminished either by an increased sympathetic tone or by increased release of pressor hormones such as angiotensin II. In longstanding
hypertension a structural adaptation in the vascular wall represents an additional factor [12]. In principle both of these mechanisms may cause a rise in
peripheral resistance which in anemic patients may be diminished or abolished
by reduced blood viscosity and anemia-induced hypoxic vasodilation. When
anemia is corrected the resulting increase in blood viscosity and possibly also a
reduction of hypoxic vasodilation may restore peripheral resistance to its
originally elevated level.

Whether rhEPO itself has vasoconstrictive properties is still controversial. Clinical arguments against such properties are the following: An acute
pressure rise during intravenous bolus administration of rhEPO has not been
observed. In spite of a three times weekly administration and the relative short
half-life of rhEPO, the observed blood pressure elevation is constant and not
fluctuating. So far only one experimental study has dealt with this question:
Pagel et al. [22], using an isolated kidney model, did not see an acute vasoconstrictive effect of rhEPO on the renal vasculature. These clinical and
experimental findings appear to be in contradiction to clinical observations
demonstrating a relation between rhEPO dose and the incidence of hyperten-

Table 1. Development of hypertension during rhEPO treatment: the effect of rhEPO dosage [27]

rhEPO, U/kg/week	Patients, n	New or aggravated hypertension, %
3×40	32	28
3×80	31	32
3×120	32	56

sion. Thus a German multicenter trial showed a correlation between rhEPO dosage and the number of patients developing hypertension (table 1).

Other studies with very low intravenous or subcutaneous rhEPO doses showed either no or a only low incidence of hypertension [21, 28]. The data from these trials however do not permit a conclusion as to whether the cause for the higher incidence of hypertension was the higher rhEPO dose or the greater increment in hematocrit, since patients with higher rhEPO doses also had greater weekly increments of hematocrit in the induction phase of therapy [25].

A relation between the development or aggravation of hypertension and the kinetics of correction of anemia would indicate that the development of hypertension could represent a temporary phenomenon of hemodynamic dysregulation. Indeed this is suggested by a retrospective study we performed in the first group of anemic hemodialysis patients we treated with rhEPO (fig. 1). 6–15 weeks after the induction of therapy 15 of the 24 patients, who all had been normotensive with or without antihypertensive therapy, became hypertensive (de novo or aggravated). When the maintenance phase was reached at approximately 24 weeks after start of treatment only 3 of these patients still were in need of intensified (1 patient) or newly instituted antihypertensive therapy (2 patients). Nevertheless, these observations do not exclude a direct hypertensionogenic effect of rhEPO as doses were much lower in the maintenance than in the induction phase.

Cardiac Output

The physiological response of cardiac output to correction of anemia consists in a decrease towards normal. The same seems to apply for hemodialysis patients as shown by the data from Deschodt et al. [7] and Mayer et al. [15]. In spite of these earlier studies, Akiba et al. [1], Buckner et al. [4] and we have found that in a number of patients normalization of cardiac output did

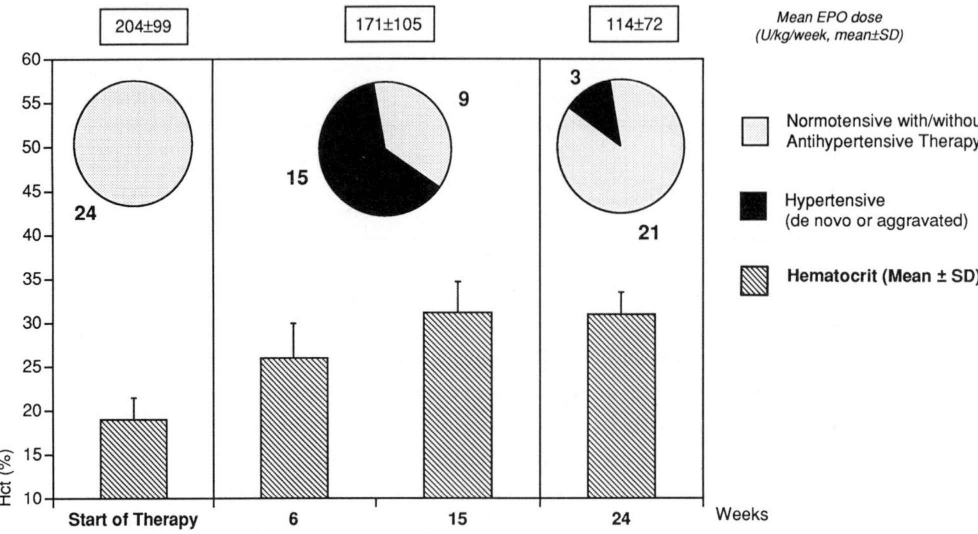

Fig. 1. Development or aggravation of hypertension in 24 regular hemodialysis patients during intravenous (three times weekly) rhEPO therapy.

not take place [19, 20]. When we investigated 7 previously normotensive subjects before and after correction of renal anemia, 2 of them developed hypertension. By use of invasively measured central hemodynamics (Swan-Ganz catheters) we could demonstrate that after the rise of hematocrit peripheral resistance increased in all patients, whereas only in the 2 patients developing hypertension did cardiac output fail to decrease adequately. The same coincidence of a failure of cardiac output to decrease adequately and the development of hypertension was shown by Akiba et al. [1]. Therefore, in some patients an inadequate regulation of cardiac output may be an additional factor in the development of hypertension under rhEPO therapy.

Summary and Conclusion

The analysis of the hemodynamics accompanying correction of renal anemia by rhEPO shows that – although they behave qualitatively as in nonuremic anemic patients – cardiac output and peripheral resistance may change inadequately and thereby cause a rise of blood pressure. The underlying mechanisms are not yet fully understood but to a great part may be related to preexisting pathology due to a history of longlasting hypertension. In some patients the development of hypertension may only represent a temporary phenomenon of hemodynamic dysregulation.

To avoid cardiovascular complications the following should be considered: Patients with a history of hypertension, even if they are normotensive in the anemic state, are at a higher risk of developing hypertension during therapy with rhEPO. Hypertensive complications may be rare events when anemia is corrected slowly. In case of the development or aggravation of hypertension a reduction of the target hematocrit is indicated.

References

1 Akiba, T.; Kurhara, S.; Katoh, H.; Yoneshima, H.; Marumo, F.: Hemodynamic changes of hemodialyzed patients by erythropoietin treatment (abstract). Kidney Int. *35:* 237 (1989).

2 Bishop, J. M.; Donald, K. W.; Wade, O. L.: Circulatory dynamics at rest and on exercise in the hypertonicity states. Clin. Sci. *14:* 329 (1955).

3 Böcker, A.; Reimers, E.; Nonnast-Daniel, B.; Kühn, K.; Koch, K. M.: Effects of erythropoietin on O_2 affinity and performance in patients with renal anemia, in Koch, Kühn, Nonnast-Daniel, Scigalla (eds): Treatment of Renal Anemia with Recombinant Human Erythropoietin. Contrib. Nephrol., vol. 66, pp. 165–173 (Karger, Basel 1988).

4 Buckner, F. S.; Eschbach, J. W.; Haley, N. R.; Davidson, R. R.; Adamson, J. W.: Correction of anemia in hemodialysis patients with recombinant erythropoietin: Hemodynamic changes and risk for hypertension (abstract). Kidney Int. *35:* 237 (1989).

5 Canadian Erythropoietin Study Group: Association between recombinant human erythropoietin and quality of life and exercise capacity of patients receiving haemodialysis. Br. Med. J.*300:* 573–578 (1990).

6 Coleman, G.: Hemodynamics of uremia. Circulation *45:* 510–511 (1972).

7 Deschodt, G.; Granolleras, C.; Alsabadini, B.; Branger, B.; Koch, K. M.; Shaldon, S.: Changes in cardiac output, blood pressure and peripheral resistance following treatment of renal anaemia by recombinant human erythropoietin (abstract). Nephrol. Dial. Transplant *3:* 494 (1988).

8 Duke, M.; Abelmann, W.H.: The hemodynamic response to chronic anemia. Circulation *39:* 503–515 (1969).

9 Edmunds, M. E.; Walls, J.; Tucker, B., et al.: Seizures in hemodialysis patients treated with recombinant human erythropoietin. Nephrol. Dial. Transplant *4:* 1065–1069 (1989).

10 Eschbach, J. W.; Abdulhadi, M. H.; Brown, J. K.: Recombinant human erythropoietin in anemic patients with end-stage renal disease: results of a phase III multicenter clinical trial. Ann. Intern. Med. *111:* 992–1000 (1989).

11 Eschbach, J. W.; Egrie, J. C.; Downing, M. R.; Brown, J. K.; Adamson, J. W.: Correction of the anemia of end-stage renal disease with recombinant human erythropoietin: results of the phase I and II clinical trial. N. Engl. J. Med. *316:* 73–78 (1987).

12 Folkow, B.: The haemodynamic consequences of adaptive structural changes of the resistance vessels in hypertension. Clin. Sci. *41:* 1–12 (1971).

13 Fowler, N. O.; Holmes, J. C.: Blood viscosity and cardiac output in acute experimental anemia. J. Appl. Physiol. *39:* 453–456 (1975).

14 Mcdougall, I. C.; Lewis, N. P.; Saunders, M. J., et al.: Long-term cardiorespiratory effects of amelioration of renal anemia by erythropoietin. Lancet *i:* 489–493 (1990).

15 Mayer, G.; Cada, E. M.; Watzinger, I.; Ludwik, G.; Barnas, U.; Graf, H.: Pathophysiology of hypertension in dialysis patients treated with erythropoietin (abstract). Kidney Int. *35:* 237 (1989).

16 Mayer, G.; Thum, J.; Cada, E. M.; Stummvoll, H. K.; Graf, H.: Working capacity is increased following human erythropoietin. Kidney Int. *34:* 525–528 (1989).

17 Neff, M. S.; Kim, K. E.; Persoff, M.; Onesti, G.; Swartz, C.: Hemodynamics of uremic anemia. Circulation *43:* 876–883 (1971).

18 Nonnast-Daniel, B.; Creutzig, A.; Kühn, K.; Bahlmann, J.; Reimers, E.; Brunkhorst, R.; Caspary, L.; Koch, K. M.: Effect of treatment with recombinant human erythropoietin on peripheral hemodynamics and oxygenation; in Koch, Kühn, Nonnast-Daniel, Scigalla (eds): Treatment of Renal Anemia with Recombinant Human Erythropoietin. Contrib. Nephrol., vol. 66, pp. 185–194 (Karger, Basel 1988).

19 Nonnast-Daniel, B.; Schäffer, J.; Frei, U.: Hemodynamics in hemodialysis patients treated with recombinant human erythropoietin; in Baldamus, Scigalla, Wieczorek, Koch (eds): Erythropoietin: From Molecular Structure to Clinical Application. Contrib. Nephrol., vol. 76, pp. 283–291 (Karger, Basel 1989).

20 Nonnast-Daniel, B.; Frei, U.; Brabant, E. G.; Talartschik, J.; Schaeffer, J.; Daniel, W. G.; Koch, K. M.: Atrial natriuretic peptide and central hemodynamics during correction of anemia by recombinant human erythropoietin in regular dialysis patients (abstract). Nephrol. Dial. Transplant *4:* 478 (1989).

21 Nonnast-Daniel, B.; Frei, U.; Pollok, M.; Granolleras, C.; Shaldon, S.; Koch, K. M.: Correction of renal anemia by daily subcutaneous administration of erythropoietin: An approach to avoid the induction of hypertension. Nephrol. Dial. Transplant *5:* (in press, 1990).

22 Pagel, H.; Jelkmann, W.; Weiss, C.: Erythropoietin and blood pressure. Horm. Metab. Res. *21:* 224 (1989).

23 Rosenlöf, K.; Grönhagen-Riska, C.; Sovijärvi, A., et al.: Beneficial effects of erythropoietin on haematological parameters, aerobic capacity, and body fluid composition in patients on hemodialysis. J. Intern. Med. *226:* 311–317 (1989).

24 Samtleben, W.; Baldamus, C. A.; Bommer, J.; Fassbinder, W.; Nonnast-Daniel, B.; Gurland, H. J.: Blood pressure changed during treatment with recombinant human erythropoietin; in Koch, Kühn, Nonnast-Daniel, Scigalla (eds): Treatment of Renal Anemia with Recombinant Human Erythropoietin. Contrib. Nephrol., vol. 66, pp. 114–122 (Karger, Basel 1988).

25 Samtleben, W.; Baldamus, C. A.; Bommer, J.; Grützmacher, P.; Nonnast-Daniel, B.; Scigalla, P.; Gurland, H. J.: Indications and contraindications for recombinant human erythropoietin treatment; in Baldamus, Scigalla, Wieczorek, Koch (eds): Erythropoietin: From Molecular Structure to Clinical Application. Contrib. Nephrol.; vol. 76, pp. 193–200 (Karger, Basel 1989).

26 Schaefer, R. M.; Leschke, M.; Strauer, B. E.; Heidland, A.: Blood rheology and hypertension in hemodialysis patients treated with erythropoietin. Am. J. Nephrol. *8:* 449–453 (1988).

27   Sundal, E.; Kaeser, U.: Correction of anemia of chronic renal failure with recombinant
     human erythropoietin: safety and efficacy of one year's treatment in a European multi-
     center study of 150 haemodialysis patients. Nephrol. Dial. Transplant *4:* 979–989 (1989).
28   Suzuki, M.; Hirasawa, Y.; Hirashima, k. et al.: Dose-finding double-blind clinical trial
     of recombinant human erythropoietin (Chugai) in Japanese patients with endstage renal
     disease; in Baldamus, Scigalla, Wieczorek, Koch (eds): Erythropoietin from Molecular
     Structure to Clinical Application. Contrib. Nephrol., vol. 76, pp. 179–192 (Karger, Basel
     1989).
29   Varat, M.A.; Adolph, R.J.; Fowler, N.O.: Cardiovascular effects of anemia. Am.
     Heart J. *83:* 415–426 (1972).

Prof. Dr. K.M. Koch, Department Innere Medizin und Dermatologie Abteilung
Nephrologie, Medizinische Hochschule Hannover, Konstanty-Gutschow-Str. 8,
D–3000 Hannover 61 (FRG)

Gurland HJ, Moran J, Samtleben W, Scigalla P, Wieczorek L (eds): Erythropoietin in Renal and Non-Renal Anemias. Contrib Nephrol. Basel, Karger, 1991, vol 88, p 126

Discussion

to the Paper by R. Brunkhorst et al.

Eschbach (Seattle): In the 3 patients that still require antihypertensive therapy, do you know whether they had an appropriate reduction of cardiac output or not?

Koch: Two of the 3 patients who remained hypertensive had only a very small change in cardiac output following correction of anemia.

Shaldon (Montpellier): The maintenance dose was significantly lower than the dose of EPO used during the correction period. Do you think that might also be important in relation to the incidence of hypertension?

Koch: Of course in every study in the maintenance phase, the EPO dose is lower than in the induction phase. So the reduction in blood pressure in the maintenance phase does indeed coincide with the lower EPO doses. This in itself does not prove that EPO is a causative factor in the development of hypertension.

Eschbach: In the United States, a number of nephrologists feel that the hypertension is due to overhydration. One of the previous speakers, I think Dr. Bahlmann, noted that more of the EPO-treated patients were overhydrated than of the control patients. I have not heard anybody from Europe talk about the role of fluid excess in causing hypertension.

Koch: We did not see any correlation between a state of overhydration in the patients and the incidence of hypertension.

Gurland HJ, Moran J, Samtleben W, Scigalla P, Wieczorek L (eds): Erythropoietin in
Renal and Non-Renal Anemias. Contrib Nephrol. Basel, Karger, 1991, vol 88, pp 127–135

Bone Histomorphometry in Recombinant Human Erythropoietin-Treated Patients on Chronic Haemodialysis

Hans-Christof Schober[a]*, Roland Winkler*[a]*, Reinhardt Schmidt*[a]*,
Klaus Abendroth*[b]*, Horst Klinkmann*[a]

[a]Department of Internal Medicine, University Rostock, and [b]Bone Research
Laboratory, Department of Internal Medicine, Friedrich Schiller University, Jena, FRG

Recombinant human erythropoietin (rhEPO) treatment has become a widely accepted therapy in the treatment of anaemia due to chronic renal failure [13]. However, its effects are accompanied by several influences on other systems. There have been reports of altered function of endocrine organs [6, 10]. Increased inorganic phosphorus levels have been described which may stimulate PTH secretion and exacerbate secondary hyperparathyroidism [14]. Therefore, we initiated a study in order to evaluate whether rhEPO treatment would affect renal osteodystrophy (RO). RO occurs in almost all patients on maintenance hemodialysis [1, 7]. Blood (hyperphosphataemia, hypocalcaemia, secondary hyperparathyroidism) [5], as well as histological changes (osteitis fibrosa, osteomalacia) [5, 11] are characteristic features of the disease. More recently, changes due to the therapy of RO, such as aluminium osteodystrophy or adynamic bone disease, have been described [2, 7, 11, 12]. These facts indicate a need to investigate the effect of each drug chronically administered on bone metabolism. The aim of the study was to assess the influence of rhEPO therapy on renal osteodystrophy.

Patients and Methods

Six patients (4 female, 2 male) who had been on chronic haemodialysis for 4–60 months, with an average age of 49.33 ± 19.17 years (range 22–76) were included in the trial after giving informed consent (table 1). Patients were treated with rhEPO (Boehringer Mannheim GmbH) 40 U/kg subcutaneously into the upper arm 3 times weekly before dialysis. During the

Table 1. Patient characteristics in the rhEPO group

Age years	Sex	Duration of dialysis months	Disease	Therapy		
				calcium carbonate	aluminium hydroxide	vitamin D
22	m	12	GN	+	+	+
34	f	60	PN	−	+	−
76	m	8	PN	+	+	−
54	f	4	PN	−	+	+
49	f	4	PN	−	+	+
60	f	14	PN	+	+	−

GN = Chronic glomerulonephritis; PN = chronic pyelonephritis; m = male; f = female.

study the patients were dialyzed 3 times a week for 3–4 h using a hollow-fibre dialyzer (before beginning rhEPO 1.3 m², 1.8 m² while on rhEPO. The standard dialysate solution contained bicarbonate, calcium 1.75 and magnesium 0.75 mmol/l. All patients received aluminium hydroxide, and in 3 cases aluminium hydroxide plus calcium carbonate as phosphate binders. Three patients were supplemented with vitamin D. Calcium, inorganic phosphate, alkaline phosphatase activity, haemoglobin (Hb), haematocrit (Hct), iron and ferritin were measured by standard laboratory methods. PTH(44–68) was determined using a commercial RIA kit (Henning, Berlin).

An iliac crest bone biopsy was performed 8 months after initiating rhEPO by means of a Jamshidi needle (inner diameter 4 mm). After embedding in methyl methacrylate the undecalcified bone specimen was sectioned using a Jung K model. For histomorphometric analysis trichrome-stained sections were utilized. The measurements were performed with the aid of a Merz grid [9]. Separate sections have been stained for aluminium [8].

Six age- and sex-matched patients with previous biopsies served as controls (table 2). Patients with analgesic nephropathy and polycystic kidney disease were excluded because of the different course of RO in such cases. The management of RO therapy was the same in both patient groups. Static histomorphometric parameters of cancellous bone included: bone volume (percentage of tissue volume), osteoid volume (percentage of tissue volume), osteoid surface (percentage of total bone surface), osteoblastic surface (percentage of osteoid surface), eroded (resorption) surface (percentage of total bone surface), osteoclastic surface (percentage of eroded surface), quiescent surface (percentage of total bone surface), trabecular diameter (in μm).

In order to exclude errors caused by differences among the patients we assessed the percentage of deviation from normals [3]. For statistical evaluation all values are expressed as mean ± SD. Double-sided Wilcoxon test and linear regression analysis were performed.

Table 2. Patient characteristics in the control group

Age years	Sex	Duration of dialysis months	Disease	Therapy		
				calcium carbonate	aluminium hydroxide	vitamin D
49	m	47	GN	+	+	+
36	f	36	GN	+	+	+
56	m	6	GN	−	+	+
51	f	51	PN	−	+	−
48	f	48	PN	+	+	+
60	f	59	GN	+	+	+

GN = Chronic glomerulonephritis; PN = chronic pyelonephritis; m = male; f = female.

Table 3. Improvement in anaemic parameters and changes in the iron metabolism in the rhEPO group (n = 6)

	Before rhEPO	After rhEPO	p
Hb, mmol/l	4.38±0.36	6.20±0.32	<0.001
Hct	0.21±0.02	0.29±0.03	<0.001
Iron, μmol/l	28.2±14.3	13.0±5.4	<0.02
Ferritin, μg/l	793 ±183	215 ±101	<0.001

Results

All patients responded to the rhEPO treatment, as shown in table 3 and figure 1. The expected increase in Hb and Hct and the changes in iron metabolism was observed. The effect of rhEPO therapy on calcium, inorganic phosphate and PTH levels and on the activity of alkaline phosphatase is shown in table 4. No significant differences were noted. The slightly increased phosphate level during rhEPO treatment was largely caused by a single elevated value, as shown in figure 2. The static bone histomorphometry revealed similar results for all the parameters measured (fig. 3, 4), except the osteoblastic osteoid surface, which was markedly lower in the control group (table 5). In figure 5 the median values of bone morphometry indicate that there is no difference between the controls and the rhEPO-treated patients. A significant

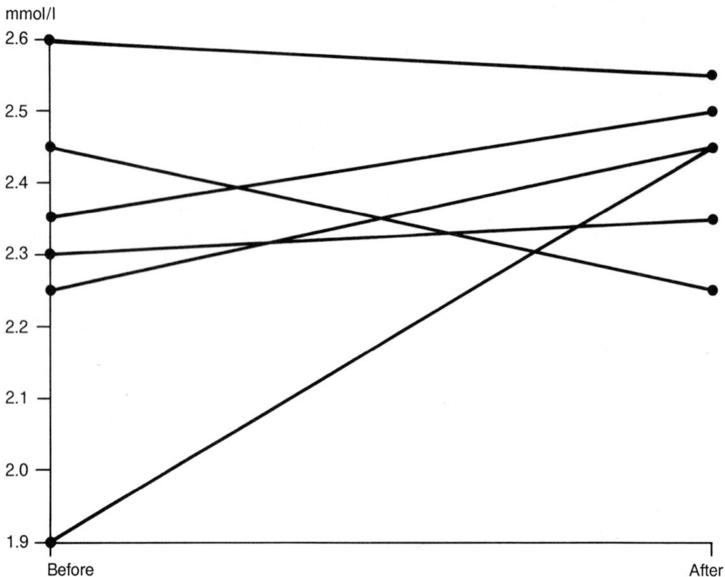

Fig. 1. Calcium changes before and after rhEPO treatment.

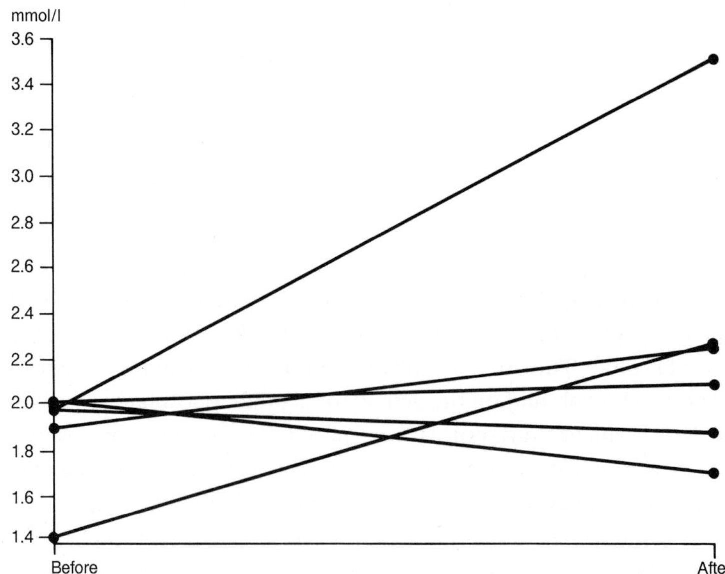

Fig. 2. Inorganic phosphate before and after rhEPO therapy. A general increase was not observed.

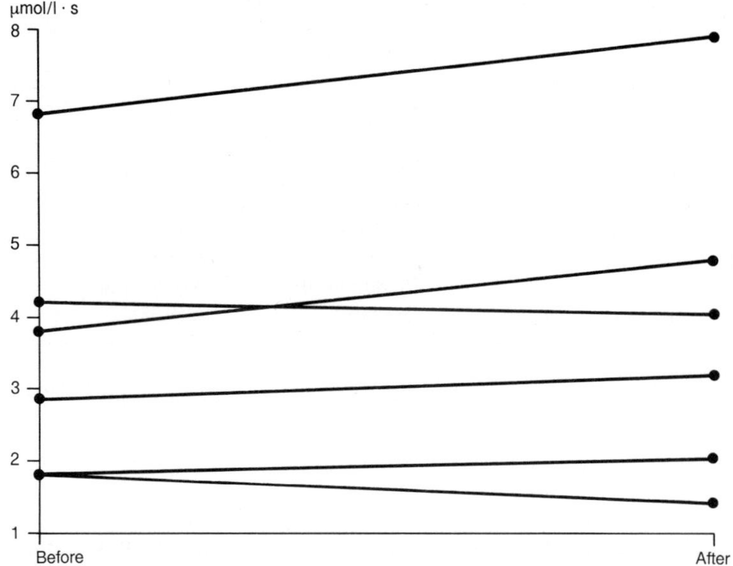

Fig. 3. Alkaline phosphatase activity was not affected by the rhEPO treatment.

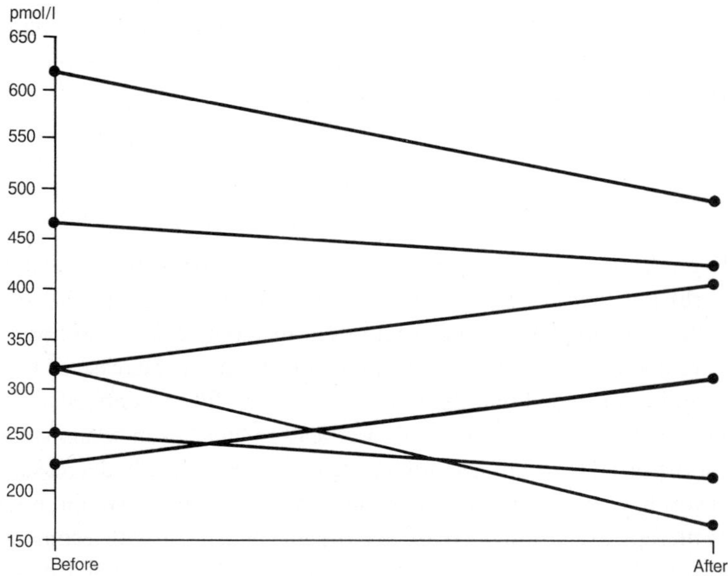

Fig. 4. There seems to be a fall in the PTH levels in most cases who underwent rhEPO treatment.

Table 4. No changes in the parameters of bone metabolism were observed (n = 5)

	Before rhEPO	After rhEPO	p
Ca, mmol/l	2.31±0.24 (2.32)	2.42±0.11 (2.45)	NS
Inorganic phosphate, mmol/l	1.88±0.23 (1.98)	2.28±0.64 (2.17)	NS
Alkaline phosphatase, μmol/l · s	3.54±1.88 (3.32)	3.90±2.32 (3.62)	NS
PTH, pmol/l	367.80±147.03 (321.60)	334.20±126.17 (359.05)	NS

Median values are shown in parentheses.

correlation was found in the control group and in the rhEPO patients for osteoid surface and osteoid volume (EPO, r = 0.89, n = 6, p<0.05; controls, r = 0.82, n = 6, p<0.05). Eroded surface and osteoid surface showed some correlation but this did not reach statistical significance (EPO, r = 0.74, n = 6, NS; controls, r = 0.62, n = 6, NS). Only 1 case in each group showed aluminium on the bone osteoid interface. This finding was not associated with aluminium osteomalacia or adynamic bone disease.

Discussion

To our knowledge there are no publications evaluating bone metabolism during rhEPO therapy. Along with the improvement of anaemia, several other effects of rhEPO have been reported, including changes in hormones which are involved in bone metabolism [6, 10]. From the increase of Hb and Hct it can be concluded that the treatment with rhEPO was effective. Eight months of rhEPO administration did not lead to changes in serum calcium, phosphorus or PTH levels. Slightly increased [6] and slightly decreased [10] PTH levels have been reported after 4 months of treatment. We did not find rhEPO therapy to cause an increase in inorganic phosphate with a consequent increase of calcium phosphorus product, as recently described [14]. Compared to the study of Zehnder et al. [14] the rhEPO dosage given in our population was lower and an intensified dialysis treatment has been applied. Unchanged

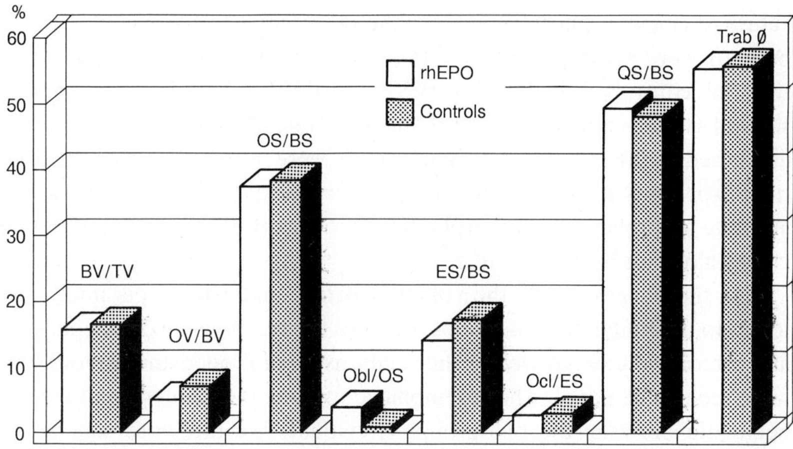

Fig. 5. The median values of bone morphometry are presented. As can be seen, rhEPO did not lead to an alteration of bone morphology. BS = Bone surface; BV = bone volume; ES = eroded surface; Obl = osteoblasts; Ocl = osteoclasts; OS = osteoid surface; OV = osteoid volume; QS = quiescent surface; TV = tissue volume.

Table 5. Static bone histomorphometry; no differences of bone histology were found compared to the controls (n = 6)

	rhEPO	Controls	p
BV/TV, %	15.77±4.77 (15.85)	17.38±8.36 (16.50)	NS
OV/TV, %	4.68±2.02 (5.05)	7.42±4.64 (7.20)	NS
OS/BS, %	36.05±18.01 (37.60)	37.90±13.82 (38.50)	NS
Obl/OS, %	4.13±3.83 (3.90)	1.53±2.11 (0.95)	NS
ES/BS, %	12.80±7.16 (14.25)	16.65±7.09 (17.35)	NS
Ocl/ES, %	4.73±4.57 (2.85)	3.65±3.18 (3.05)	NS
QS/BS, %	51.18±13.54 (49.45)	45.80±11.36 (48.25)	NS
Trabecular diameter, µm	59.17±18.97 (55.50)	59.22±18.89 (56.00)	

Median values are shown in parentheses. For abbreviations see figure 5.

values of calcium, phosphorus, alkaline phosphatase and PTH in the rhEPO patients were accompanied by a bone morphology which was not different from the controls. The duration of 8 months' rhEPO application can be considered as long enough to cause changes in bone morphology, which could be attributed to rhEPO. All static parameters were in the same range within the rhEPO patients and the control group. There were no differences between the absolute and relative histomorphometric results. For that reason the relative values have not been presented.

In the bone not only the volume, surface and cellular parameters were found to be similar in both groups, but also the relationship of osteoid surface and osteoid volume, as well as the relationship of eroded and osteoid surface were seen to be equal. The resemblance in bone morphology and metabolic behaviour between the two groups is evident. We therefore conclude that rhEPO therapy applied in the described manner and dosage did not either improve or worsen the renal osteodystrophy.

References

1   Chan, YL, Furlong TJ, Cornish CJ, Posen S: Dialysis osteodystrophy. A study involving 94 patients. Medicine 1985;64:296–309.
2   Cohen-Solal ME, Westeel PF, Boudaillez B, Moriniere PH, Marie A, Sebert JL, Gueris J, Garabadian M, Fournier A: Non-aluminic adynamic bone disease in non-dialysed patients – A new type of osteopathy due to overtreatment (abstract). Nephrol Dial Transplant 1989;4:467.
3   Delling G: Endokrine Osteopathien, Morphologie, Histomorphometrie und Differentialdiagnose. Veröffentlichungen aus der Pathologie. Stuttgart, Fischer, 1975, p 28.
4   Eschbach JW, Downing MR, Egrie JC, Browne JK, Adamson JW: USA multicenter trial with recombinant human erythropoietin (Amgen). Contrib Nephrol. Basel, Karger, 1989, vol 76, pp 160–165.
5   Kanis JA, Cundy TF, Hamdy NAT: Renal osteodystrophy. Baillière's Clin Endocrinol Metab 1988;2:193–241.
6   Kokot F, Wiecek A, Greszaczak W, Klepacka J, Klin M, Lao M: Influence of erythropoietin treatment on endocrine abnormalities in haemodialyzed patients. Contrib Nephrol. Basel, Karger, 1989, vol 76, pp 257–272.
7   Llach F, Felsenfeld AJ, Coleman MD, Keveny JJ; Pederson JA, Medlock TR: The natural course of dialysis osteopathy. Kidney Int 1986;29(suppl 18):74–79.
8   Maloney NA, Ott SM, Alfrey AC, Coburn JW, Sherrard DJ: Histological quantitation of aluminum in iliac bone from patients with renal failure. J Lab Clin Med 1982;99:206–216.
9   Merz WA, Schenk RK: A quantitative histological study on bone formation in human cancellous bone. Acta Anat 1970;76:1–5.

10   Schaefer RM, Kokot F, Heidland A: Improved sexual function in uremics on erythropoietin. A possible role for prolactin. Kidney Int. 1989;35:263.

11   Sherrard D, Ott S, Maloney N, Andress D, Coburn J: Uremic osteodystrophy: Classification, cause and treatment; in Frame B, Potts JT Jr (eds): Clinical Disorders of Bone and Mineral Metabolism. Amsterdam, Excerpta Medica, 1983, pp 254–259.

12   Smith AJ, Faugere MC, Abreo K, Fanti P, Julian B, Malluche HH: Aluminium-related bone disease in mild and advanced renal failure: evidence for high prevalence and morbidity and studies on etiology and diagnosis. Am J Nephrol 1986;6:275–283.

13   Winearls CG: Treatment of anaemia in haemodialysis patients with recombinant erythropoietin. Nephron 1989;51(suppl 1):26–28.

14   Zehnder C, Glück Z, Descoendres C, Uehlinger DE, Blumberg A: Human recombinant erythropoietin in anaemic patients on maintenance haemodialysis. Secondary effects of the increase in haemoglobin. Nephrol Dial Transplant 1988;3:657–660.

Dr. med. H.-Chr. Schober, Abteilung für Endokrinologie der Klinik
für Innere Medizin der Universität Rostock, Ernst-Heydemann-Strasse,
D-O–2500 Rostock (FRG)

Gurland HJ, Moran J, Samtleben W, Scigalla P, Wieczorek L (eds): Erythropoietin in
Renal and Non-Renal Anemias. Contrib Nephrol. Basel, Karger, 1991, vol 88, pp 136–143

Efficacy Comparison of Intravenous and Subcutaneous Recombinant Human Erythropoietin Administration in Hemodialysis Patients

*J. Bommer, H.-P. Barth, M. Zeier, A. Mandelbaum, G. Bommer,
E. Ritz, H. Reichel, R. Novack*

I. Medizinische Universitätsklinik Heidelberg, FRG

Recombinant human erythropoietin (rhEPO) therapy of renal anemia in dialysis patients is widely used today. In hemodialysis patients, rhEPO can be injected intravenously during hemodialysis sessions 3 times/week. However, in anemic CAPD patients, patients with chronic renal failure or in many other patients suffering from severe anemia, long-term intravenous injections 3 times/week are not suitable. Therefore, alternative routes of administration are of interest.

The pharmacokinetics of rhEPO following intravenous or subcutaneous injection differ markedly [1, 2]. After intravenous injection, the plasma EPO level increases acutely, reaching extreme peak concentrations and decreases with a half-life of 6–9 h. In contrast, after subcutaneous administration, the plasma rhEPO level increases during the first 12–24 h to a more moderate maximum level but decreases very slowly over days. Consequently, more than 100 h after a single subcutaneous injection, the rhEPO level continues to be elevated. After subcutaneous rhEPO administration the bioavailability, calculated as the area under the concentration curve, was less than 50% of that after intravenous rhEPO administration [1, 2]. This raises two questions: First, do more frequent injections improve the efficacy of rhEPO? Second, what is the long-term efficacy of subcutaneous application?

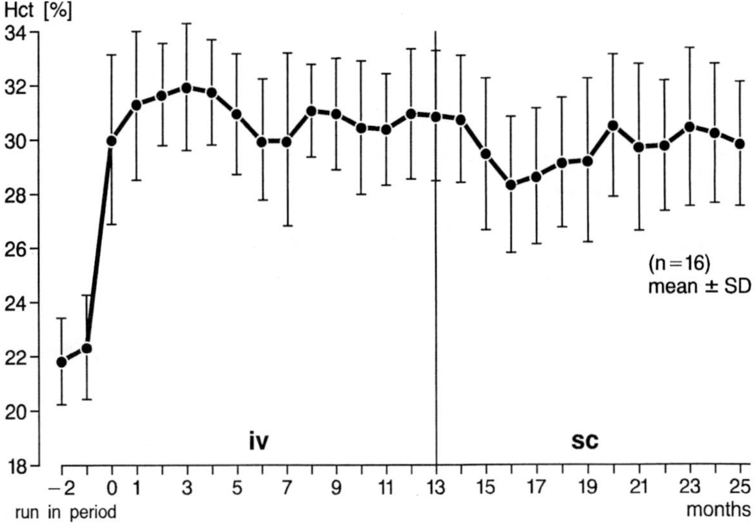

Fig. 1. Hematocrit levels (mean ± SD) in hemodialysis patients treated 1–3 times/week with intravenous or subcutaneous rhEPO (group I).

Material and Methods

Eighty-five patients entered the multicenter trial of rhEPO therapy as chronic hemodialysis patients. At the start of rhEPO therapy all patients had been on hemodialysis for more than 6 months under stable conditions. Patients were dialyzed 3 times/week for 4.5–5 h. In 52 patients uremia was due to glomerular disease and in 35 patients to nonglomerular disease, e.g. reflux nephropathy, nephrolithiasis, analgesic abuse. In 9 patients the primary renal disease was unknown.

For the correction of renal anemia, rhEPO therapy was started with 3 times/week intravenous injection of 40, 80 or 120 U rhEPO (Boehringer Mannheim GmbH, FRG) per kilogram body weight per week. If hematocrit levels were raised to 30–35%, during the following maintenance period in 17 patients (group I) the single rhEPO dose of 40, 80, 120 U/kg/injection was kept constant. However, the frequency of injections per week was reduced to 1–3 times/week with a mean of 1.7–1.9 injections/week. In most of the patients (group II) the rhEPO dose was lowered uniformly to 3×15 U/kg/week. In 16 of the 17 patients (group I), receiving only 1–3 injections/week, maintenance intravenous rhEPO therapy for more than 1 year was followed by subcutaneous rhEPO therapy for another 12 months using a comparable frequency of injection. Twenty-two patients (group II) receiving 3 intravenous rhEPO injections/week during the 1-year maintenance period were also treated with subcutaneous rhEPO for 1 year. At the beginning of subcutaneous rhEPO therapy the dose was reduced to about 50% of the mean intravenous dose given during the last 3 months.

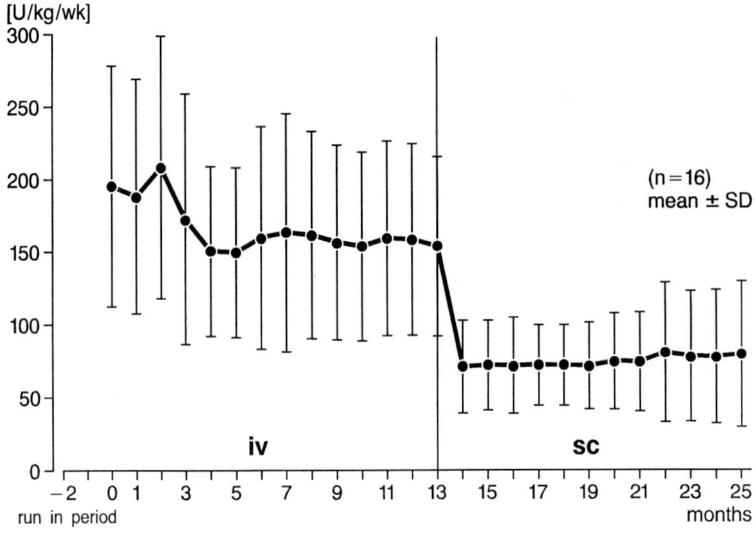

Fig. 2. Weekly rhEPO dose (mean ± SD) in hemodialysis patients treated 1–3 times/ week with intravenous or subcutaneous rhEPO (group I).

Results

After commencing rhEPO therapy, the hematocrit levels increased significantly from 22 to 30–32% during the correction period (fig. 1). During the following 12-month maintenance with intravenous rhEPO therapy in group I, the hematocrit level was rather constant with a mean of 30–32%. After starting subcutaneous rhEPO therapy, the mean hematocrit levels fell by 2%, but rose again during the following 6 months to 30%.

The mean weekly rhEPO dose (fig. 2) was reduced during the first months of the maintenance period. During the last 6 months of intravenous therapy, the mean weekly rhEPO dose was about 155 U/kg/week and the mean frequency of injections per week was 1.7–1.9.

When subcutaneous rhEPO therapy was started, the weekly rhEPO dose was reduced to about 50% of the intravenous dose during the last 3 months. Consequently, subcutaneous therapy was started with a mean of 75 U/kg/ week. The mean subcutaneous rhEPO dose had to be increased by 10% to maintain the hematocrit level during the subcutaneous treatment period.

Serum ferritin levels dropped transiently during the intravenous treatment period, and again after the start of subcutaneous rhEPO therapy (fig. 3).

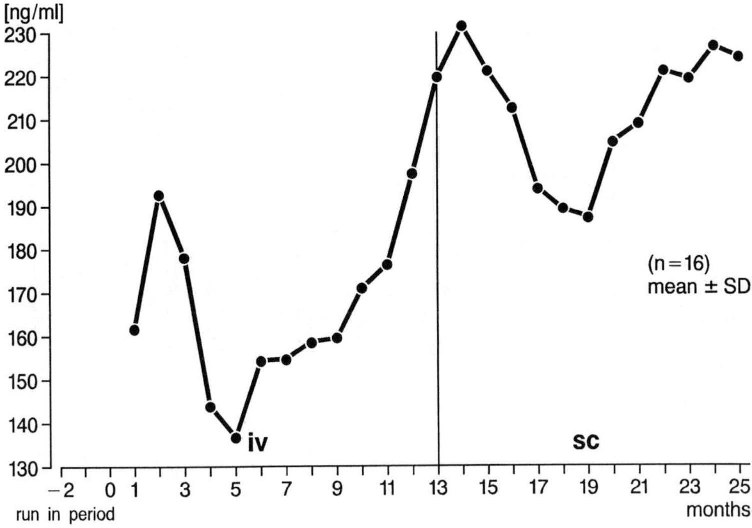

Fig. 3. Serum ferritin levels (mean ± SD) in hemodialysis patients treated 1–3 times/ week with intravenous or subcutaneous rhEPO (group I).

However, such drops in the serum ferritin level are unlikely to explain the variation in hematocrit levels during the study period. Constant absolute reticulocyte counts during the maintenance intravenous and subcutaneous rhEPO therapy periods indicated comparable erythropoiesis during both observations periods.

At the end of the intravenous rhEPO therapy period the median hematocrit levels were not significantly different in groups I and II (fig. 4). In both groups hematocrit levels decreased after the start of subcutaneous therapy, and in contrast to group I, hematocrit levels increased very slowly in group II during the subcutaneous therapy period. The corresponding EPO doses are given in figure 5. Despite the fact that the hematocrit levels tended to be lower in group I than in group II, in group I the median weekly maintenance dose of intravenous rhEPO given by 1–3 injections (mean 1.7–1.9/week) was 155 U/kg/ week, much higher than the dose of 100 U/kg/week in group I (receiving 3 injections/week). In both groups, the rhEPO dose was reduced by 50% when subcutaneous treatment was started. In group I the weekly rhEPO dose had to be increased during the subcutaneous treatment period from 70 to 80 U/kg/ week. In group II, the median intravenous rhEPO dose was about 100 U/kg/ week and the final subcutaneous dose was about 80 U/kg/week. Thus the

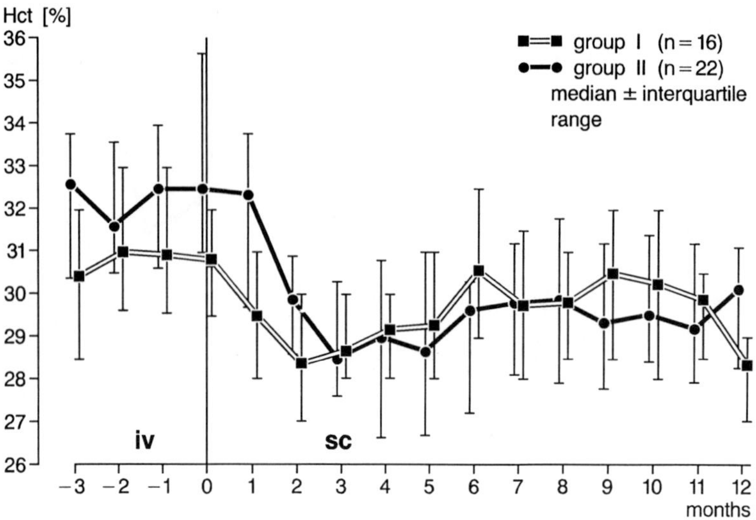

Fig. 4. Hematocrit levels (median ± interquartile range) in hemodialysis patients treated 1–3 times/week (group I) or 3 times/week (group II) with intravenous or subcutaneous rhEPO.

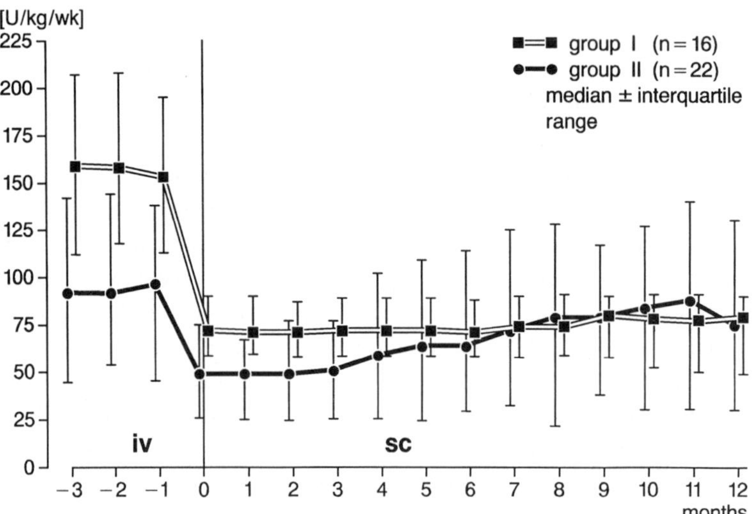

Fig. 5. Weekly rhEPO dose (median ± interquartile range) in hemodialysis patients treated 1–3 times/week (group I) or 3 times/week (group II) with intravenous or subcutaneous rhEPO.

difference between the intravenous and the subcutaneous rhEPO dose was much smaller in group II than in group I.

Discussion

The data confirm our previous results [3] indicating that more frequent intravenous injections improve the efficacy of a given rhEPO dose. At the end of the 1-year intravenous maintenance period, the median rhEPO dose was about 100 U/kg/week in patients receiving 3 injections and 155 U in patients receiving 1–3 injections with a mean of 1.8 injections/week. It must be remembered, however, that patients in group I and group II were not randomized. Furthermore, the 22 patients of group II evaluated in this study remained from more than 50 patients; more than half of the group II patients did not complete the study for various reasons, predominantly transplantation. Therefore, the absolute maintenance doses of EPO used in both groups must be compared with these reservations in mind. However, the data suggest that rhEPO is more effective if given by 3 intravenous injections/week than by 2 intravenous injections at any given weekly dose.

The data confirm our previous observation that subcutaneous rhEPO therapy is more efficient than the intravenous route [3, 4]; in both groups the maintenance subcutaneous rhEPO dose was lower than the intravenous dose. In addition to the hematocrit levels the constant absolute reticulocyte counts under intravenous or subcutaneous rhEPO therapy indicate a comparable erythropoietic effect of 80 U/kg subcutaneous rhEPO and 155 U intravenous rhEPO in group I. Similar results have been obtained in other studies. Stevens et al. [5] found comparable hematocrit levels with 3×25 U/kg s.c. and 3×48 U/kg i.v. doses per week in uremic patients. In predialysis patients with chronic renal failure, Eschbach et al. [6] reported a comparable increase of hematocrit with 3 times 100 U/kg/week s.c. and 3 times 150 U/kg/week i.v. Similarly, Lim et al. [7] reported in preuremic patients a two fold higher efficacy of subcutaneous than intravenous rhEPO.

If patients received only 1–3 instead of a constant 3 injections/week, the difference between subcutaneous and intravenous rhEPO is much more striking. In long-term studies, the efficacy of 155 U of intravenous rhEPO corresponds to 80 U of subcutaneous rhEPO in patients receiving an average of 1.8 injections/week in group I. If patients were treated in group II with 3 injections/week, 100 U/kg/week intravenous rhEPO corresponds to 80 U/kg/week subcutaneous rhEPO. This means that under long-term conditions, the equipotent subcutaneous rhEPO dose was about 60% (using 2 injections/

week) and about 80% (using 3 injections/week) compared to intravenous rhEPO therapy with the same injection frequency. This may be explained by the fact that the higher frequency of injection seems to play a minor role if rhEPO is given subcutaneously; the final maintenance intravenous dose differed markedly in groups I and II, but the final subcutaneous dose of rhEPO was quite similar in both groups (fig. 5).

Iron deficiency seems not to have played a role in this study since the median ferritin levels remained fairly constant except for transient moderate drops. Aluminium intoxication was excluded before rhEPO therapy was started. Accumulation with increasing levels of aluminium during the treatment period cannot be excluded but are unlikely in such long-term hemodialysis patients. Occult intestinal blood loss, subacute viral infection or inflammatory status, conditions well known to interfere with EPO efficacy, were not seen except for transient mild infections. Minor differences of rhEPO resorption after subcutaneous administration at different injection sites can be neglected. The high efficacy of subcutaneous rhEPO is in contrast to the low bioavailability found in pharmacokinetic studies, and therefore difficult to explain. First, it might be speculated that extremely high plasma EPO levels following intravenous injection have no dose-dependent effect, and that much rhEPO is wasted. Second, after kidney transplantation, an acute rise in serum EPO levels from about 20 to 100 U are found for 2–3 weeks. During the following time period only very mild elevation of serum EPO levels were reported, yet the hematocrit levels continue to increase [8]. This suggests that a minor but persistent elevation of serum EPO levels was an effective stimulatory effect on erythropoiesis, and a similar moderate but continuous elevation of serum EPO level results from subcutaneous rhEPO application. Third, the number of receptors per CFU_E cells is quite low at about 400–500 per cell. It cannot be excluded that only a limited number of receptors must be saturated by EPO to induce a maximum proliferation rate. Furthermore, it may be speculated that bioavailability of subcutaneous rhEPO has been underestimated in several experiments because of a high coefficient of variance of serum EPO assays. Consequently, minor changes in serum EPO levels after subcutaneous therapy may be underestimated, especially if the drug is slowly resorbed at the injection site but soon adsorbed at the receptor site preventing a marked rise of serum EPO levels. Recently it has been documented that about 90% of radiolabelled subcutaneous rhEPO was resorbed within 48 h. The highest resorption rate was found after subcutaneous injection in the thigh [9]. Such a high resorption rate suggest that the calculated bioavailability after pharmacokinetic study may underestimate the true efficacy of subcutaneous rhEPO.

In summary, subcutaneous rhEPO seems to be more effective than intravenous. Such subcutaneous administration is more suitable for all patients without intravenous catheters or not having simultaneous intravenous injections of other drugs. Serum EPO levels resulting from subcutaneous injections seem to be more physiological since the high peak concentrations seen after intravenous injections were avoided. The efficacy of intravenous rhEPO can be improved by more frequent injections, e.g. 3 times compared to 2 times/week. Under subcutaneous rhEPO therapy, the maintenance dose was comparable in patients receiving 3 or 2 injections/week. Less frequent subcutaneous injections were preferred by the patients.

References

1 MacDougall, I.C.; Roberts, D.E.; Neubert, P.; Dhamasena, A.D.; Coles, G.A.; Williams, J.D.: Pharmacokinetics of recombinant human erythropoietin in patients on continuous ambulatory peritoneal dialysis. Lancet *i:* 425–427 (1989).
2 Kampf, D.; Kahl, A.; Passlick, J.; Pustelmik, A.; Eckhardt, K.-U.; Ehmer, B.; Jacobs, C.; Baumelou, A.; Grabensee, B.; Gahl, G.M.: Single-dose kinetics of recombinant human erythropoietin after intravenous, subcutaneous and intraperitoneal administration. Preliminary results. Contrib. Nephrol., vol. 76, pp. 106–111 (Karger, Basel, 1989).
3 Bommer, J.; Samtleben, W.; Koch, K.M.; Baldamus, C.A.; Grützmacher, P.; Scigalla, P.: Variations of recombinant human erythropoietin application in hemodialysis patients. Contrib. Nephrol., vol. 76, pp. 149–158 (Karger, Basel, 1989).
4 Bommer, J.; Ritz, E.; Weinreich, T.; Bommer, G.; Ziegler, T.: Subcutaneous erythropoietin. Lancet *ii:* 406 (1988).
5 Stevens, J.M.; Strong, C.A.; Oliver, D.O.; Winearls, C.G.; Cotes, P.M.: Subcutaneous erythropoietin and peritoneal dialysis. Lancet *i:* 1388–1389 (1989).
6 Eschbach, J.W.; Kelly, M.R.; Haley, N.R.; Abels, R.I.; Adamson, J.W.: Treatment of the anemia of progressive renal failure with recombinant human erythropoietin. N. Engl. J. Med. *321:* 158–163 (1989).
7 Lim, V.S.; Kirchner, P.T.; Fangman, J.; Richmond, J.; De Gowin, L.: The safety and efficacy of maintenance therapy of recombinant human erythropoietin in patients with renal insufficiency. Am. J. Kidney Dis. *6:* 496–506 (1989).
8 Sun, C.H.; Ward, H.J.; Wellington, L.P.; Koyle, M.A.; Yanagawa, N.; Lee, D.B.N.: Serum erythropoietin levels after renal transplantation. N. Engl. J. Med. *321:* 151–157 (1989).
9 Macdougall, I.C.; Jones, J.M.; Robinson, M.I.; Miles, J.B.; Coles, G.A.; Williams, J.D.: Subcutaneous erythropoietin therapy: comparison of three different sites of injection. Contrib. Nephrol., vol. 88, pp. 152–156 (Karger, Basel 1991).

Prof. J. Bommer, Medizinische Klinik der Universität, Bergheimer Strasse 58, D–6900 Heidelberg (FRG)

Gurland HJ, Moran J, Samtleben W, Scigalla P, Wieczorek L (eds): Erythropoietin in
Renal and Non-Renal Anemias. Contrib Nephrol. Basel, Karger, 1991, vol 88, pp 144–148

Subcutaneous Erythropoietin: A Comparison of Daily and Thrice Weekly Administration

C. Granolleras[a], *B. Branger*[a], *S. Shaldon*[a], *B. Nonnast-Daniel*[b],
K. M. Koch[b], *M. Pollok*[c], *C. A. Baldamus*[c]

[a]Department of Nephrology, University Hospital, Nîmes, France; [b]Department of
Nephrology, University Hospital, Hannover, and [c]Department of Nephrology,
University Hospital, Cologne, FRG

Since 1986, recombinant human erythropoietin (rhEPO) has been used in
end-stage renal disease. The patient on hemodialysis has had his anemia
treated with predictable success [1]. Initially, the route of administration
suggested was intravenous and the frequency was 3 times weekly. This proposal was universally followed as EPO was easily given to the patient on hemodialysis at the end of each treatment. The possibility that this route and the
frequency were not optimal was suggested [2]. Preliminary data on subcutaneous daily self-administered rhEPO (SADSCEPO) were encouraging in
regard to dose reduction compared to 3 times weekly intravenous rhEPO [3].
This report deals with a comparison of SADSCEPO with 3 times weekly
subcutaneous EPO (TRISCEPO) in the same group of hemodialysis patients.

Material and Methods

Patients. Twelve patients (6 male, 6 female; mean age 33.2 years, range 20–63 years)
were studied. The inclusion criteria were that the patients were nontransfusion dependent
with stable end-stage renal disease maintained on 3 times weekly hemodialysis. They had had
their anemia corrected by SADSCEPO at least 2 months prior to entry and had been
maintained at the target hematocrit (range 31–35 vol%) for the last 2 months on an unchanged
daily dose of rhEPO. Iron deficiency was defined as a transferrin saturation index of <20%
[4], if present it had to be corrected prior to inclusion in the study. The method of correction
was either intravenous or oral.

Study Protocol. The study was performed with lyophilized rhEPO (Boehringer); the
ampoules contained either 1,000 or 2,000 U. The solution was prepared with distilled water

and the volume was kept constant at 1.0 ml. The patients were trained to give subcutaneous rhEPO into their abdomen, thighs or deltoid subcutaneous area. The injection volume did not exceed 0.5 ml and the dose was given via a tuberculin syringe at home in the morning. Blood samples for serum EPO concentration (RIA) and antibodies to EPO were drawn after the longest interval following the last administered dose.

Patients started TRISCEPO after the steady-state dose and hematocrit during SAD-SCEPO was established. On starting, the weekly dose of rhEPO determined during SAD-SCEPO was divided by 3 for the TRISCEPO period. The patients were followed for at least 4 months whilst on TRISCEPO before a comparison with SADSCEPO was made. The basis of the comparison was the hematocrit drawn before treatment on the first day of the week, after the longest interdialytic period. The mean value for the month was obtained from four such readings. If iron deficiency developed during the TRISCEPO period, it was corrected before the comparison was made. All patients were Hb-Ag negative and no evidence of liver disease was observed during the study.

Statistics. The paired t test was used to assess statistical significance.

Results

Overall. The patient training to self-administer rhEPO was not a problem. No local side effects were seen apart from small hematomas in the abdomen without relation to a dialysis day. Heparinization after subcutaneous injection on dialysis days has not produced bleeding in up to 12 months of continuous subcutaneous rhEPO administration. No systemic effects attributable to this method of rhEPO administration have been noted. The patients were all cooperative and compliance was 100%.

SADSCEPO (fig. 1). The median steady-state SADSCEPO dose was 56 IU/kg body weight/week (range 42–112 IU) with a mean hematocrit of 32.3± 1.9 vol%. Transferrin saturation was >25% in all patients studied.

TRISCEPO. After 4 months of 3 times weekly subcutaneous rhEPO on the same weekly total dose as for SADSCEPO, the mean hematocrit had fallen significantly to 29.6±1.8 vol% (p<0.005), whilst the transferrin saturation had not changed. In fact, the monthly mean hematocrit during the fourth month of TRISCEPO decreased in 10/12 patients and remained the same in 1 and increased in 1 patient compared to the SADSCEPO control period (fig. 2).

Serum EPO. The levels measured varied between 40 and 60 mU/ml and did not differ between SADSCEPO and TRISCEPO periods.

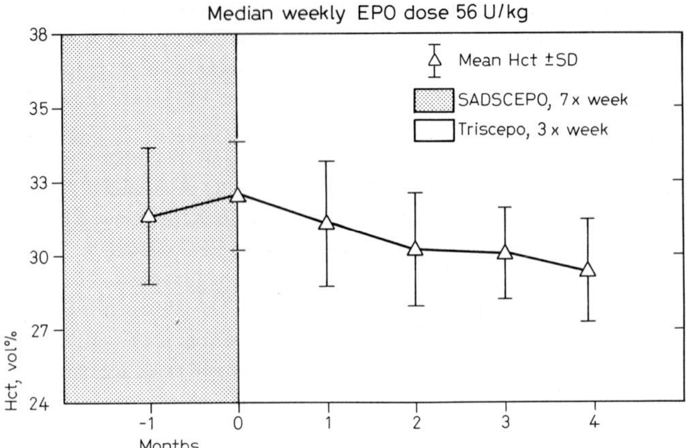

Fig. 1. The mean change in hematocrit ± SD during the 2-months control period of SADSCEPO –1 to 0 months and during the 4-month period of TRISCEPO 1–4 months.

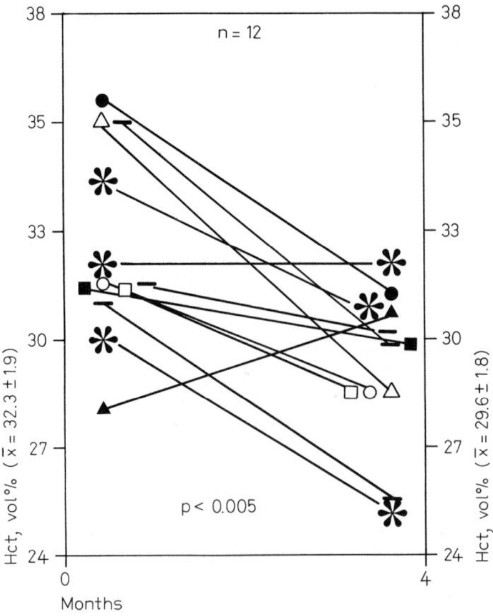

Fig. 2. The individual patient's mean monthly hematocrit response from SADSCEPO at 0 months to TRISCEPO at 4 months.

Circulating Antibodies to EPO. No patient developed circulating EPO antibodies (some of these patients have received subcutaneous rhEPO for 2 years).

Discussion

The observation that 7 times weekly subcutaneous EPO is more effective than 3 times weekly subcutaneous EPO is novel. The mechanism explaining this difference is not clear. It is tempting to speculate on the role of endogenous EPO's contribution to erythropoiesis in these patients. If higher peak levels following TRISCEPO were reached, the suggestion that these higher concentrations might effect either production of endogenous EPO or availability of EPO receptors on the stem cell could be considered. Nevertheless, the serum EPO levels measured during the study showed no difference between the 7 times weekly and the 3 times weekly schedules. The fact that the samples were drawn 72 h after the last TRISCEPO dose compared to 24 h after the last SADSCEPO dose permits the speculation that the peak level of serum EPO during TRISCEPO was in fact higher [5]. However, the overall low serum levels measured in this series will probably preclude accurate pharmacokinetic analysis.

The absence of an adequate explanation for this phenomenon does not prevent the empirical utilization of the technique. It has been suggested [see Koch, this volume] that the target hematocrit is reached more flexibly with SADSCEPO and that there is less overshoot of the target hematocrit and a much reduced incidence of hypertension. If this observation is confirmed, the justification of using the smallest dose of rhEPO to achieve and maintain the partial correction of renal anemia will be established. The potential economic benefits of subcutaneous EPO therapy [6] remain in view of the smallest dose. However, it may prove no cheaper than TRISCEPO as 7 injections weekly may offset the small saving in EPO dose, calculated to be 15–20%.

References

1   Eschbach, J.W.; Egrie, J. C.; Downing, M. R., et al.: Correction of anemia of end-stage renal disease with recombinant human erythropoietin. N. Engl. J. Med. *316:* 73–78 (1987).

2   Bommer, J.; Ritz, E.; Weinreich, T., et al.: Subcutaneous erythropoietin (letter). Lancet *ii:* 406 (1988).

3   Granolleras, C.; Branger, B.; Beau M. C., et al.: Experience with daily self-adminis-
    tered subcutaneous erythropoietin. Contrib. Nephrol., vol. 76, pp. 143–148 (Karger,
    Basel 1989).
4   Macdougall, I. C.; Hutton, R. D.; Cavill, I, et al.: Poor response to treatment of renal
    anaemia with erythropoietin corrected by iron given intravenously. Br. Med. J. *299:*
    157–158 (1989).
5   Macdougall, I. C.; Roberts, D. E.; Neubert, P., et al.: The pharmacokinetics of recom-
    binant erythropoietin in patients on continuous ambulatory peritoneal dialysis. Lancet *i:*
    425–427 (1989).
6   Granolleras, C.; Branger, B.; Deschodt, G., et al.: Two years' experience of daily
    self-administered subcutaneous erythropoietin. Blood Purif. (in press, 1990).

Dr. S. Shaldon, 86, rue de Grézac, F–34080 Montpellier (France)

Gurland HJ, Moran J, Samtleben W, Scigalla P, Wieczorek L (eds): Erythropoietin in
Renal and Non-Renal Anemias. Contrib Nephrol. Basel, Karger, 1991, vol 88, pp 149–151

Discussion

to the Papers by J. Bommer et al. and C. Granolleras et al.

Kurtz (Zürich): Dr. Granolleras, what were the data that made you believe that there is down-regulation of endogenous EPO production by exogenous EPO?

Granolleras: This is a hypothesis. You can imagine that if you inject 120 U intravenously you will get a very high peak in a very short time and this high peak may down-regulate the endogenous production.

Kurtz: But Kai Eckardt in our group has performed a study showing that the injection of high doses of EPO before exposing rats to hypoxia does not change or prevent endogenous EPO production.

Granolleras: It seems logical to imagine that there can be down-regulation. But we need to prove that, and it would seem to be very difficult.

Baldamus (Cologne): I have a question for both speakers. On the slides where you showed the change from intravenous to subcutaneous treatment one saw an initial fall and then a recovery of hematocrit. What is the cause of this phenomenon?

Bommer: That's point I have discussed many times and I have no explanation. It may be that the patient had during intravenous therapy very high peak concentrations, and perhaps the erythroblasts were adapted to such stimulation. The median predialytic serum EPO levels were not different.

Shaldon (Montpellier): May I come back to the question on down-regulation? I think it's not valid to take Eckardt's work on the normal animal species and compare it to the clearly disordered production of endogenous EPO by the anuric kidney. I think you yourself, Dr. Kurtz, suggested this morning that the endogenous production of EPO was not normally regulated in the end-stage renal disease patients. So with all due respect to Eckardt's work I don't think it excludes the possibility that the uremic patient may be down regulating his endogenous EPO.

Eschbach (Seattle): We have clinical evidence that there is not down-regulation: 87 patient received either 50, 150, 300, 500, or 1,500 U/kg i.v. three times a week as initial doses. If there had been down-regulation from the higher doses I would expect that those patients would have required much higher maintenance doses of EPO. In contrast, patients required the same maintenance dose regardless of the initial dose. I'm not convinced that there is 'down-regulation'.

Granolleras: When you have to abruptly stop EPO treatment in a patient, you have a very rapid decrease in hematocrit and you have to wait for a long time until the hematocrit rises again. This may be down-regulation. You all must have experienced this phenomenon.

Unknown participant: I think that you always treated patients with s.c. after having treated them with i.v. EPO. Isn't it time to start treating patients by the s.c. route alone, and not using both methods in the same patient? Because pharmacologically, this becomes extremely confusing.

Bommer: Currently, we start all our patients with s.c. rhEPO because we are convinced that this is much cheaper than i.v. and the cost of rhEPO is very high. Normally, we start with 2 or 3 injections s.c. per week and then reduce the frequency of injection, because we have calculated the costs if you use a high frequency of injection. You may save perhaps 10% with a high frequency of s.c. injections but then you must take into account the amount of EPO you lose during the preparation of each dose. Very frequent injections may be of advantage for the patient. That's still an open question for me. But I think 2 injections per week, or even one, is the cheapest way.

Baldamus: Let me come back to down-regulation. I would like to ask a question of the receptor people like Dr. d'Andrea or Dr. Krantz. Do the EPO receptors on the hemopoietic cells down-regulate in response to the EPO concentration floating around or don't they?

Krantz (Nashville): If you treat the cells in vitro, which is the only way you can do this experiment because you need purified cells to measure EPO receptors, the high-affinity receptors are completely down-regulated within 2 h, and they stay that way through the rest of erythroid development.

Baldamus: Couldn't this be an explanation of your results?

Goldberg (Boston): You've drawn a lot of blood samples to measure these hematocrits, can't you put this whole argument to rest by just taking a little bit of this serum or plasma and measuring their EPO levels? If there is down-regulation you should see a decrease in the serum/plasma EPO level. In answer to Prof. Baldamus, I think you want to know if there is an EPO receptor on the EPO producing cells not on the . . .

Baldamus: . . . no, no, on the EPO responding cells.

Goldberg: If exogenous EPO is down-regulating endogenous EPO production then there must be something telling the EPO-producing cells that there is too much EPO around and they should stop making it. I think Dr. d'Andrea has looked for the presence of EPO receptor message in the kidney or liver and hasn't found it, which would go against down-regulation. But the easiest and most straightforward thing would be to just measure the serum EPO levels.

Granolleras: Are you sure when you measure the same plasma level that you are measuring biologically active EPO? We are not sure!

Winearls (Oxford): There are two points here: there is presumably going to be a reduction in the EPO production after the patient's anemia has been reversed. Prof. Eschbach has shown a very elegant example of this in a patient in whom he measured the erythron transferrin uptake (ETU) before the patient had been treated with rhEPO and then stopped the EPO when the patient had responded and remeasured the ETU. It was much lower than pretreatment, suggesting that the patient's own kidney was no longer producing as much EPO because the hemoglobin had risen. That's a very different situation from what you are suggesting, which is that the hormone acts in its own feedback loop.

Cotes (Harrow): We can answer one of the questions that was posed. In patients with renal disease treated with i.v. rhEPO, which was effective in correcting their anemia, we estimated serum EPO pre-treatment (when the mean hemoglobin was 6.3 g/dl) and after correction of the anemia (mean hemoglobin 12.3 g/dl). We sampled 72 h after the i.v. dose of exogenous EPO, so that rhEPO should not contribute to the estimate of EPO in the serum. There was no change in the serum EPO. Thus, we concluded there was no down-regulation or change in endogenous production of EPO with correction of the anemia.

Bommer: I can absolutely confirm that.

Gurland HJ, Moran J, Samtleben W, Scigalla P, Wieczorek L (eds): Erythropoietin in
Renal and Non-Renal Anemias. Contrib Nephrol. Basel, Karger, 1991, vol 88, pp 152–156

Subcutaneous Erythropoietin Therapy:
Comparison of Three Different Sites of Injection

Iain C. Macdougall[a], *John M. Jones*[c], *Mike I. Robinson*[c],
Janice B. Miles[b], *Gerald A. Coles*[a], *John D. Williams*[a,1]

[a] Institute of Nephrology and [b] Department of Radiology, Royal Infirmary, and
[c] Department of Medical Physics, University Hospital of Wales, Cardiff, UK

The subcutaneous route for administering recombinant human erythropoietin (EPO) is rapidly gaining popularity as the preferred route of administration in both haemodialysis and CAPD patients [1–7]. There is, however, no information as to which is the optimum site for injecting subcutaneous EPO. It has previously been shown that absorption of subcutaneous insulin was fastest from the abdomen, intermediate from the arm, and slowest from the thigh [8, 9]. In view of the cost of EPO, even small differences in bioavailability between different injection sites may result in considerable saving.

The aim of the present study was to compare the absorption kinetics and bioavailability of ^{125}I-labelled EPO injected subcutaneously into the upper arm, the abdomen, and the thigh in normal healthy volunteers.

Subjects and Methods

Eight subjects (4 males, 4 females; mean age 30±5 (SD) years; mean weight 68±14 kg) were studied. Bulkware EPO (Boehringer Mannheim GmbH), which was free from stabilizing and solubilizing agents, was labelled with ^{125}I using the chloramine-T method [10]. The purity and bioactivity of the radiolabelled product was assessed by SDS-polyacrylamide gel electrophoresis, Sephadex G-75 gel permeation chromatography, and polycythaemic mouse bioassay. These procedures confirmed that the radiolabelled material: (a) was homogenous with no evidence of aggregation or fragmentation (fig. 1); (b) had a molecular weight of around 30,000 daltons corresponding to the known molecular weight of EPO [11], and (c) was

[1] Our thanks to Dr. Frieda Houghton of Boehringer Mannheim UK Pharmaceuticals for support and encouragement with this work, and for supplying our bulkware EPO; also to Miss Cheryl Patterson for expert secretarial assistance.

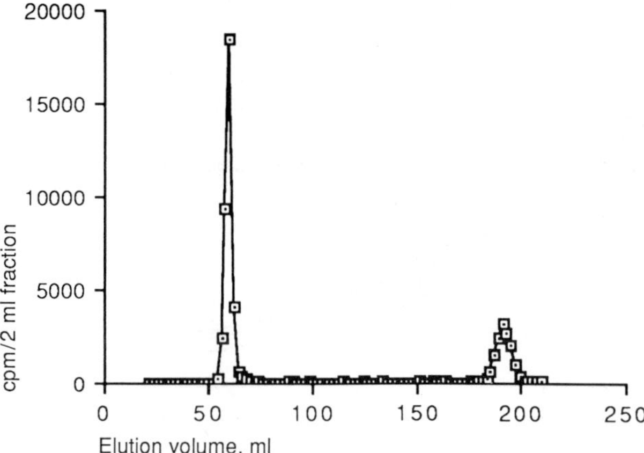

Fig. 1. Elution profile for ^{125}I-labelled EPO in sodium dodecyl sulphate subjected to G-75 Sephadex gel permeation column chromatography. The first peak represents labelled EPO; the second peak constitutes free [125]I.

bioactive. All subjects took oral potassium iodide, 60 mg daily for 7 days, commencing 24 h prior to injection in order to block thyroid uptake of [125]I. 0.5 MBq of ^{125}I-EPO was then injected subcutaneously into the upper arm (mid-deltoid region), the abdomen, and the thigh by the same operator on three occasions, separated by at least 10 days. Absorption of ^{125}I-EPO was monitored in two ways: (a) by its disappearance from the site of injection using an external gamma counter, and (b) by its appearance in the bloodstream. Blood samples were taken at 0, 1, 2, 4, 8, 12, 18, 24, 36, 48, 72, and 96 h after injection, and protein-bound counts determined using a resin which adsorbs free iodide. The thickness of the subcutaneous tissue at each injection site was measured by ultrasound in order to correlate bioavailability with the degree of subcutaneous fat.

Results

The radioactivity monitored externally over the injection site diminished more rapidly following injection into the thigh than for the other two sites (fig. 2). The disappearance profiles for the arm and abdomen were comparable. After 4 days, significantly less ^{125}I-EPO remained in the subcutaneous tissue after thigh injection compared to the other two sites (fig. 2, table 1).

Serum counts (cpm/1 ml of serum) rose faster after injection into the thigh than for the arm or abdomen (fig. 3). Mean peak levels were nearly twice as high for the thigh as for the other two sites (table 1). The time taken to reach peak blood levels was somewhat variable among subjects, and overall there

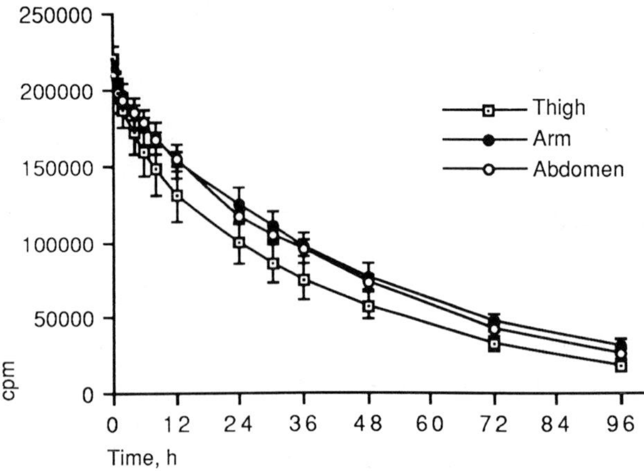

Fig. 2. Disappearance profiles of radioactivity measured externally from three subcutaneous sites following injection of ^{125}I-labelled EPO. Results are expressed as means ± SE.

Table 1. Summary of pharmacokinetic data obtained following subcutaneous injection of ^{125}I-EPO into the thigh, arm, and abdomen (mean ± SD values)

Site	Peak serum level, cpm	Time to peak, h	Elimination constant	AUC to 96 h	AUC to infinity	Percent left at injection site at 96 h
Thigh	809	13.5	0.015	42,376	60,907	8.0
	±354	±6.7	±0.007	±9,751	±13,332	±4.3
Arm	525*	13.5	0.010	33,301**	54,301	14.1*
	±120	±8.8	±0.003	±6,576	±8,853	±5.0
Abdomen	502*	18.8	0.013	31,788***	46,621***	12.2
	±98	±5.9	±0.002	±7,511	±9,451	±4.7

*p<0.05, **p<0.01, ***p<0.005 compared with results for thigh.

was no significant difference between the three injection sites. Likewise, the subsequent elimination from the plasma compartment was fairly comparable for all three sites. The area under the curve (AUC) to 96 h for the serum profile following thigh injection, however, was significantly greater than for the arm (p<0.01) and abdomen (p<0.005). When the AUC was extrapolated to infinity, however, the difference between the thigh and the arm became less

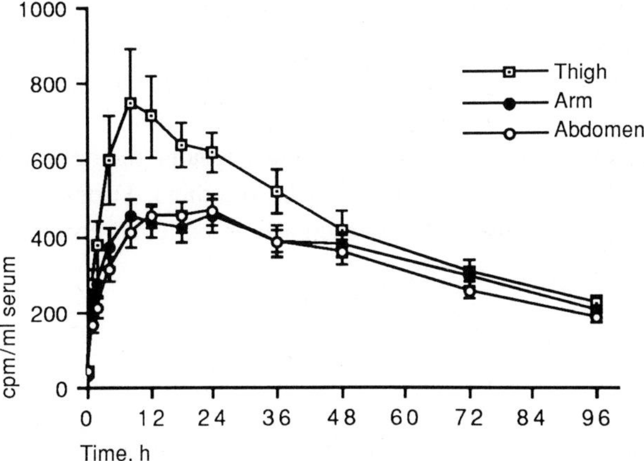

Fig. 3. Serum profiles of radioactivity following injection of ^{125}I-labelled EPO into three different subcutaneous sites. Results are expressed as means ± SE.

marked, both sites being superior to the abdomen (table 1). There was no significant correlation between the thickness of the subcutaneous tissue, as assessed by ultrasound, and the bioavailability (data not shown).

Discussion

Despite increasing usage of the subcutaneous route for administering EPO [1–7], no studies have been published which compare different sites of subcutaneous injection. The results of the present study, which although conducted in normal healthy volunteers rather than patients, suggest that the thigh may be the optimum site of injection. Absorption from this site was more rapid, and higher peak serum levels and bioavailability were obtained. This is in striking contrast to what has been previously reported for subcutaneous insulin where absorption was faster for the abdomen than for the arm, which was, in turn, faster than the thigh [8, 9]. The possible reasons for this discrepancy are not clear at the present time, although EPO is very different in molecular size and composition to insulin, being larger and more heavily glycosylated. Also, the mobility of the subjects in our study was probably greater than for those used in the insulin studies. It is likely that exercising the lower limb, by increasing regional blood flow, would improve absorption from subcutaneous tissue. No restriction was put on our subjects as far as exercise was concerned; they were instructed to carry out their daily activities as usual. It is possible, however, that EPO-treated patients would be less fit, and have correspondingly lower rates of absorption from the thigh, but this requires validation.

In conclusion, on the basis of these preliminary results, the optimum site for subcutaneous administration of EPO may be the thigh. Further studies, however, are required to confirm this, particularly in patients receiving haemodialysis or CAPD.

References

1   Stevens JM, Strong CA, Oliver DO, Winearls CG, Cotes PM: Subcutaneous erythropoietin and peritoneal dialysis. Lancet 1989;i:1388–1389.
2   Macdougall IC, Cavill I, Davies ME, Hutton RD, Coles GA, Williams JD: Subcutaneous recombinant erythropoietin in the treatment of renal anaemia in CAPD patients. Contrib Nephrol. Basel, Karger, 1989, vol 76, pp 219–226.
3   Steinhauer HB, Lubrich-Birkner I, Dreyling KW, Hörl WH, Schollmeyer P: Increased ultrafiltration after erythropoietin-induced correction of renal anemia in patients on continuous ambulatory peritoneal dialysis. Nephron 1989;53:87–88.
4   Bommer J, Ritz E, Weinreich T, Bommer G, Ziegler T: Subcutaneous erythropoietin. Lancet 1988;ii:406.
5   Macdougall IC, Roberts DE, Coles GA, Williams JD: Intraperitoneal erythropoietin. Lancet 1989;i:1389.
6   Granolleras C, Branger B, Beau MC, Deschodt G, Alsabadani B, Shaldon S: Experience with daily self-administered subcutaneous erythropoietin. Contrib Nephrol. Basel, Karger, 1989, vol 76, pp 143–148.
7   Sinai-Trieman L, Salusky IB, Fine RN: Use of subcutaneous recombinant human erythropoietin in children undergoing continuous cycling peritoneal dialysis. J Pediatr 1989;114:550–554.
8   Binder C: Absorption of Injected Insulin: A Clinical-Pharmacological Study. Munksgaard, Copenhagen, 1969.
9   Koivisto VA, Felig P: Alterations in insulin absorption and in blood glucose control associated with varying insulin injection sites in diabetic patients. Ann Intern Med 1980;92:59–61.
10 Hunter WM, Greenwood FC: Preparation of iodine ^{131}I-labelled human growth hormone of high specific activity. Nature 1962;194:495–496.
11 Davis JM, Arakawa T, Strickland TW, Yphantis DA: Characterization of recombinant human erythropoietin produced in Chinese hamster ovary cells. Biochemistry 1987; 26:2633–2638.

I. C. Macdougall, MRCP (UK), Institute of Nephrology, Cardiff Royal Infirmary, Cardiff CF2 1SZ (UK)

Gurland HJ, Moran J, Samtleben W, Scigalla P, Wieczorek L (eds): Erythropoietin in
Renal and Non-Renal Anemias. Contrib Nephrol. Basel, Karger, 1991, vol 88, pp 157–158

Discussion

to the Paper by I. C. Macdougall et al.

Caro (Philadelphia): Did you calculate the actual percentage of recovery in the plasma? In other words what percentage of the dose injected were you able to recover in the plasma? You said that there was left locally about 15–20%; it would be interesting to know the reverse of that, what did actually appear in the plasma?

Macdougall: We didn't actually do that, and I am not at all sure that it is possible to do.

Bommer (Heidelberg): Was there any effect of physical activity in the patient? If he was walking around or he was lying down, is there any effect on the absorption of EPO and/or on the residual activity found at the injection site at the end of the observation period?

Macdougall: I think that's a very valid point. We encouraged all the subjects to carry out their normal daily activities which, as busy hospital staff, involved a fair bit of physical activity, including considerable usage of the lower limbs over the 4-day period of study. I'm sure that is a very relevant factor, especially when one looks at the differences between this and a previous study on absorption of subcutaneous insulin in less-fit diabetic patients. I'm assuming that the dialysis population might also retain a reasonable degree of mobility.

Schaumann (Mannheim): Is it possible to calculate the half-life for the disappearance from the injection site?

Macdougall: Yes, I'm not sure how helpful that would be but if we plot the data on a logarithmic scale it would be easy to calculate the disappearance half-life; I don't have that result to hand, I'm afraid.

Bahlmann (Hannover): The influence of muscular activity has been raised. Did you use the dominant arm in your patients? It has been shown that blood flow in the arm is quite different, depending on whether you are left-handed or right-handed.

Macdougall: In fact, we used the nondominant arm for injection on 5 of the subjects and the dominant arm in 3. It wasn't until after we started the study that we realized we should have standardized the arm selected for injection.

Cotes (Harrow): I found it surprising that as much as 10% of the injected material remained at the injection site at 96 h. Can you give us more evidence that, before administration, this ^{125}I-labelled material still had the same biological activity as the original rhEPO? For example, in terms of the bioassay and its precision, would it have been able to detect perhaps 50% loss of activity.

Macdougall: I think this is a very valid point. What we would have liked to have been able to do was to analyse a number of the serum samples by gel permeation chromatography to check that we still had a single peak of radioactivity with identical elution characteristics to the starting material. Unfortunately, by the time our EPO was diluted in the plasma compartment, the serum counts were too low for us to be able to do that. We therefore have to assume that after injection, the material has remained in exactly the same form as it was prior to injection. There is, however, no reason to suppose otherwise. By determining the protein-bound counts in serum, we at least know that the ^{125}I label was still attached to EPO.

Shaldon (Montpellier): It's really a follow-up to Dr. Cotes' question. What stability does your marker have on your protein? How much of it is coming off as free iodine? Do you have any specific activity measurements?

Macdougall: We do not know.

Gurland HJ, Moran J, Samtleben W, Scigalla P, Wieczorek L (eds): Erythropoietin in
Renal and Non-Renal Anemias. Contrib Nephrol. Basel, Karger, 1991, vol 88, pp 159–168

Self-Administered Daily Subcutaneous Recombinant Human Erythropoietin: An Open Randomised Dose-Finding Study in ESRD Patients Receiving Peritoneal Dialysis

A. Slingeneyer[a], *B. Faller*[b], *B. Laroche*[a], *B. Ehmer*[c], *C. Mion*[a,1]

[a]Service de Néphrologie, Hôpital Lapeyronie, CHU Montpellier, France;
[b]Service de Néphrologie, Hôpital Général, Colmar, France;
[c]Boehringer Mannheim Pharma Laboratories, Mannheim, FRG

The efficacy of recombinant human erythropoietin (rhEPO) in correcting the anemia of hemodialysis patients has been confirmed when this hormone was administered subcutaneously [1–3] rather than using the conventional intravenous route [4]. One possible advantage of daily subcutaneous administration may be a reduction in dosage resulting in substantial economic savings and potentially less toxic dosing [2].

In CAPD, chronic intravenous administration is impractical since a ready vascular access is not available in most patients. The pharmacokinetics of rhEPO suggest that the subcutaneous route is preferable to intraperitoneal administration, as the latter requires a 5- to 10-fold increase in dosage to achieve the same serum profile as that obtained after subcutaneous injection [5].

We present the results of a study designed to assess the efficacy of self-administered daily subcutaneous rhEPO in stable CAPD patients and to find what is the minimum daily dose required to maintain a stable hematocrit in a predefined range.

[1] We thank Dr. K.-U. Eckardt, Physiologisches Institut, Zürich, Switzerland, for his contribution in the measurement of serum rhEPO levels in case B. R. (fig. 5).

Patients and Methods

Patients

Thirty-three patients receiving maintenance peritoneal dialysis in 2 French dialysis centers (15 in Colmar, 18 in Montpellier) were included in the study after informed consent was obtained. There were 13 males and 20 females: 9 patients were on intermittent peritoneal dialysis (IPD), with a mean age of 68.6±7 years, and 24 received CAPD, with a mean age of 57.2±19 years. Primary renal diseases were diabetes mellitus, type I or II, 7; nephroangio-sclerosis, 7; chronic glomerulonephritis, 6; chronic pyelonephritis, 3; polycystic renal disease, 2; unknown, 8.

All patients were in a stable condition and received IPD or CAPD for at least 6 months. Inclusion criteria were persistent anemia with a hematocrit lower than 28%, in the absence of iron, vitamin B_{12} or folic acid deficiencies. Hypertension, a past history of seizures, aluminum intoxication, malignant diseases with or without cytostatic treatment, acute infection or active and extended skin diseases (e.g. psoriasis, scleroderma) were considered as exclusion criteria.

A 2-week pretreatment period preceded the administration of rhEPO during which the following parameters were controlled twice: blood pressure, hemoglobin level, hematocrit, red blood cell and reticulocyte counts, platelet count, blood urea, serum potassium and phosphate levels. From this period onwards, the patients were seen weekly as outpatients for clinical evaluation and control of blood parameters.

During the pretreatment period, patients or their helpers were trained to be self-sufficient in performing the daily subcutaneous administration of rhEPO. Complete dissolution of rhEPO lyophilisate and careful aspiration of the solution into the 1-ml syringe by patients were given special emphasis.

Treatment Protocol

The patient were randomised into 3 groups defined by the individual daily rhEPO dosage prescribed in U/kg body weight: group I: 5 U; group II: 10 U; group III: 20 U. The treatment protocol, designed to achieve and maintain a hematocrit level of 35% (target hematocrit) included two periods: a correction period, during which the rhEPO dose was adapted to the individual patient needs to reach the target hematocrit; and a maintenance period.

Correction Period. After randomisation, the rhEPO dosage was kept constant in each patient during the first 8 weeks. If the hematocrit increase was lower or equal to 4% (i.e. less than 0.5% per week), the daily administered dose was doubled. If after 4 more weeks, the increase in hematocrit was equal or less to 2% by comparison with the week 8 value, another dose doubling was performed. The highest daily dose, however, was limited to a maximum of 40 U/kg body weight.

Maintenance Period. After achieving the target hematocrit, dosage of daily administered rhEPO was reduced uniformly to 50% of the last correction dose. Further dose adjustments were performed once a week depending on the hematocrit behavior. If the hematocrit level did not remain stable at between 30 and 35%, the maintenance dose of rhEPO was either increased or decreased once weekly by 5 U/kg body weight per day. In case of a hematocrit value above 35%, rhEPO administration was discontinued until hematocrit had again reached the desired range.

Statistics

The data are presented as means±SD. Linear regression and correlation coefficients with confidence intervals were computed for mean hematocrit values and rhEPO doses, both during the correction and the maintenance periods.

Table 1. Main characteristics of the three groups of patients obtained after randomisation

	Group I	Group II	Group III
Initial EPO dose, U/kg BW/day	5	10	20
Number of patients	10	12	11
Entry hematocrit, % ($\pm$SD)	22.2$\pm$2.9	22.4$\pm$2.3	22.2$\pm$3.9
Target hematocrit, % ($\pm$SD)	31.8$\pm$1.9	32.3$\pm$1.7	32.1$\pm$2.1
Body weight, kg ($\pm$SD)	63.0$\pm$8.7	64.0$\pm$14.0	63.8$\pm$12.0

Results

Randomisation

As shown in table 1, randomisation resulted in three groups of patients with similar characteristics, including age, body weight, and initial and target hematocrits.

Correction Period

Changes in hematocrit obtained over time according to rhEPO dosage during the correction period are shown in figure 1. A clear dose-dependent increase in hematocrit was observed and the correlation coefficient between dose and hematocrit rise was highly significant in each group. The weekly hematocrit increase was 0.2, 0.6 and 1.1%, respectively, in group I, II and III. The expected times to reach target hematocrit were approximately 31, 17 and 12 weeks, respectively, in groups I, II and III.

Figure 2 shows the increase in rhEPO dosage required to achieve the target hematocrit during the correction period. After 8 weeks, only 3% of the patients had reached the target hematocrit with the initial rhEPO dosage: this percentage increased to 27% at 12 weeks, 50% at 16 weeks and 93% at 28 weeks. The median rhEPO dose (in U/kg body weight/day) remained stable at 10 U during the first 15 weeks, increasing at 20 U between the 15th and 22nd week and reaching 40 U/kg from the 23rd to 28th weeks.

Despite satisfactory ferritin and serum iron levels during the pretreatment period, 88% of the patients needed supplemental iron (administered intramuscularly as ferric hydroxide polymaltose; Fer Lucien, Lucien Laboratories, Paris, France) during the correction period to maintain the serum iron level at above 13 μmol/l and the transferrin saturation coefficients at above 20% (table 2).

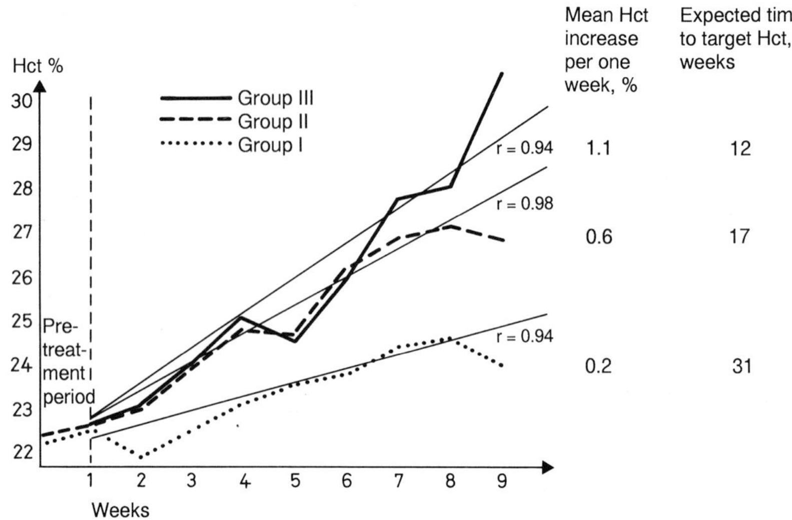

Fig. 1. Rate of anemia correction as a function of initial rhEPO dosage: a comparison of groups I, II and III.

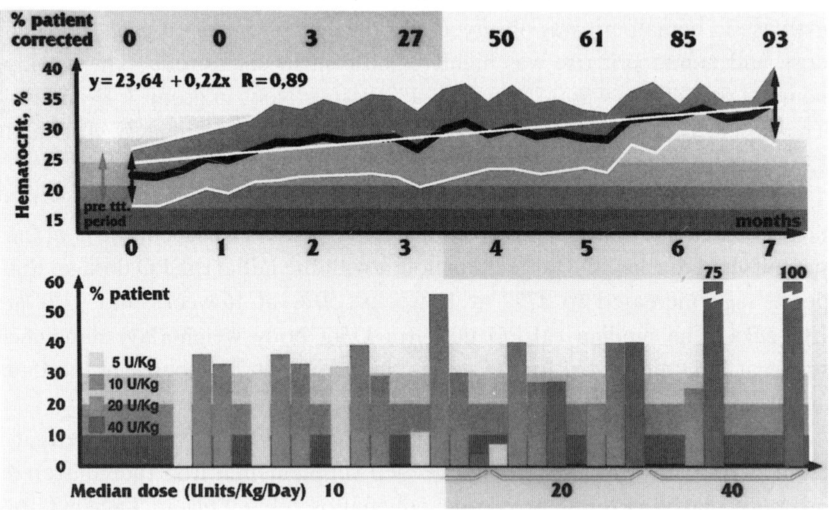

Fig. 2. Correction of anemia with daily subcutaneous rhEPO. The histogram of the lower panel indicates the percentage of patients receiving a given dose of subcutaneously administered rhEPO.

Table 2. Supplemental iron needed during the correction and maintenance periods of daily subcutaneous rhEPO treatment: iron was administered intramuscularly as ferric hydroxide polymaltose

	Correction period	Maintenance period
Number of patients	27	6
Percent of total	84.4	21.4
Mean dose, g ($\pm$ SD)	3.1 $\pm$ 0.7	1.5 $\pm$ 0.7

In 2 female patients, an inadequate response was obtained despite a daily administration of 40 U/kg body weight rhEPO. The first patient was 62 years old and weighed 72 kg; transferred to hemodialysis at her own request at week 32, she was withdrawn from the study. Her hematocrit had increased from 22 to 30% only in spite of adequate increases in rhEPO dosage. The second patient was 60 years old, weighing 72 kg and treated for chronic bronchitis. Her response to rhEPO therapy was delayed and her target hematocrit was reached on week 35 only; during this period her serum ferritin levels ranged from 442 to 1,000 µg/l while the serum iron level was maintained between 9 and 13 µmol/l despite intramuscular administration of 7 g of supplemental iron. At the time of writing, she maintained a hematocrit of 35% while receiving 15 U/kg body weight/day of rhEPO.

Maintenance Period

The observation time beyond the correction period was 7 months in 14 patients, 6 months in 22 patients, 4 months in 26 patients, and 2 months in 27 patients. The results of the maintenance period are shown in figure 3. The hematocrit was maintained within the desired range. As shown in figure 4, a significant decrease in the mean daily dose of rhEPO was obtained, and, eventually, the median dose reached 5 U/kg body weight/day during the 6th and 7th months of maintenance therapy. Intramuscular iron supplement was required in only 6 patients: the mean administered dose was 1.5$\pm$0.7 g of iron (table 2).

In a 56-year-old female patient, the hematocrit level went up to 40% despite the progressive rhEPO reduction in dosage. Administration of the hormone was discontinued at week 19 of the maintenance period: it was resumed 12 weeks later at a daily dose of 2.5 U/kg when the hematocrit had reached the 30% level. At the time of writing, the hematocrit was stabilised at 33%, as shown in figure 5.

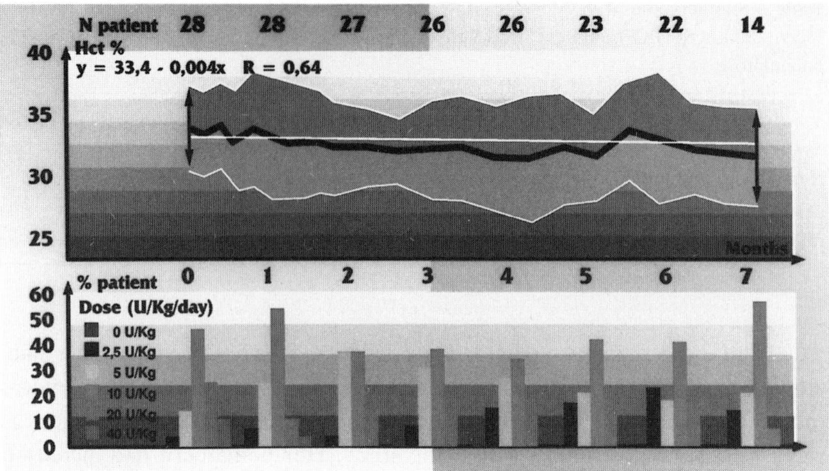

Fig. 3. Evolution of hematocrit levels during the maintenance period. The upper panel indicates the number of patients on rhEPO therapy each month. On the lower panel, the histogram depicts the percentage of patients receiving a given dose of subcutaneously administered rhEPO.

In 13 patients, the maintenance dose had to be increased from 50 to 100% for a few weeks following an acute infection (4 acute bronchitis during an influenza epidemic; 9 CAPD peritonitis). The dose of rhEPO could be reduced to preinfection levels 4–6 weeks later.

Beneficial Effects

The correction of anemia was obtained in 32 of 33 patients. Twenty-five patients described a clear improvement in well-being, while 20 noticed increased appetite. Relief of severe angina pectoris in 4 patients and an improved intermittent claudication of the lower limbs in 3 patients were also noted. In 3 other patients with cerebrosclerosis, cognitive function clearly improved.

Adverse Effects

An elevation in blood pressure level was observed in 9 patients; it was promptly relieved by an adjustment of the dry weight in 2 patients and by an

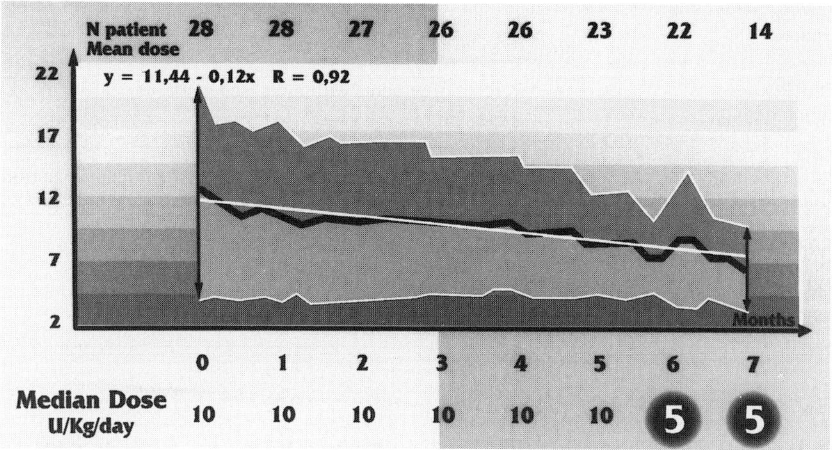

Fig. 4. Progressive reduction in rhEPO dosage during the maintenance period. Note that during the last 2 months of the study, the median rhEPO dose was 5 U/kg body weight/day.

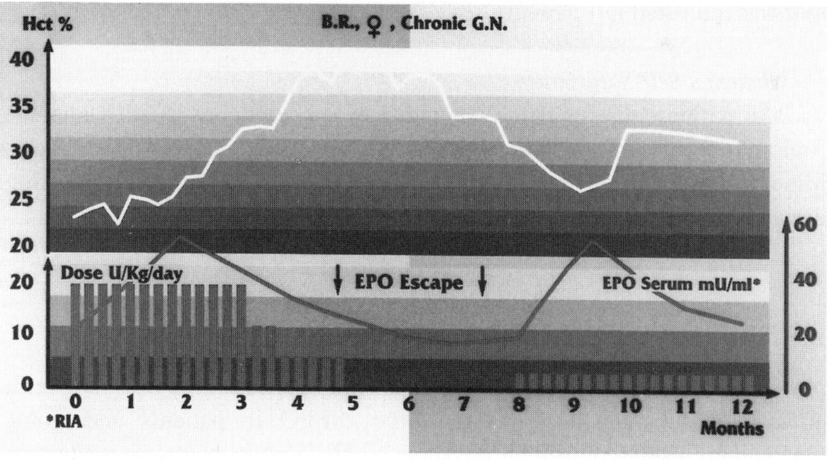

Fig. 5. Hematocrit 'escape' during subcutaneous rhEPO therapy in patient B.R., a 56-year-old female with chronic glomerulonephritis.

Table 3. Percentage of patients in whom an increase of antihypertensive treatment was required

rhEPO dose U/kg BW/day	Percent of patients with increased antihypertensive treatment	
	correction period	maintenance period
5	0	10
10	20	14.3
20	24	0
40	40	0

increase in antihypertensive drug dosage in the others. As shown in table 3, the percentage of patients requiring a change in antihypertensive therapy increased proportionally to the daily administered rhEPO dose.

In 4 patients, 3 with diabetes mellitus, an aggravation of preexisting lower limb distal atherosclerotic arterial disease was observed. In 2 male patients, acute ischemia occurred during the correction period at weeks 6 and 10, respectively, and was complicated with distal gangrene requiring bilateral amputation in 1 case and unilateral sympathectomy in the other; both of them died following surgery. In 2 female patients, foot and leg ulcers of the arteriolar type occurred during the maintenance period; a transtarsal resection of the foot was indicated in 1 patient, while the ulcers were cured in the other.

Patient's Self-Sufficiency

All patients mastered the technique of subcutaneous rhEPO administration without drug spillage. Local tolerance to injections was excellent. Minor subcutaneous hematomas were observed on 3 occasions. No infection occurred at the site of rhEPO injection.

Discussion

To our knowledge, this is the first study reporting on the long-term efficacy of subcutaneously administered rhEPO in patients undergoing CAPD. Our results confirm the advantages of the daily subcutaneous administration of the hormone previously demonstrated in a small group of hemodialyzed patients [2].

During the correction period, a dose-dependent rise in hematocrit was obtained. This dose dependency confirms that, when given by the subcutaneous route, rhEPO retains a similar efficacy to that observed with the intravenous route [4] in spite of large differences in pharmacokinetics [5].

During the maintenance period, the reduction in the daily rhEPO dose was striking: after 6 months of therapy, the median daily dose necessary to maintain the hematocrit in the predefined range was only 5 U/kg. Such a low rhEPO dose amounts to a median weekly dose of 35 U/kg, which is in a sharp contrast with the typical median weekly dose of 200 U/kg required in hemodialyzed patients receiving rhEPO 3-weekly by the intravenous route [4, 5]. There is now no clear explanation for these variations in dosage according to the route of administration.

Twenty-nine of our 33 patients required iron supplementation. None of them, however, presented with clinical signs or abnormal biochemistries suggestive of iron deficiency upon initiation of rhEPO therapy. High iron needs were not expected with CAPD, a dialysis procedure which does not entail repeated blood losses. Two factors may explain the need for iron supplementation in our patients: the lack of blood transfusion before admission on the protocol; the inflammatory state induced by peritonitis and possibly fostered by CAPD itself [7], reducing the availability of tissue iron stores for hemoglobin synthesis. The intramuscular administration of ferric hydroxide polymaltose (0.9 mmol of trivalent iron per ml) was well tolerated and offered a convenient approach to provide the patients with the iron required to restore the full rhEPO efficacy.

In 9 patients, a progressive elevation in blood pressure was associated with the correction of anemia. These changes occurred mainly during the correction period and were observed with a greater frequency in group III patients who received the highest initial rhEPO dose (20 U/kg). In no case were seizures or hypertensive encephalopathy observed, presumably because of the slow pace of hematocrit rise. Hypertension was easily reversed either by lowering the patients' dry weight or by adjusting the dose or modifying the antihypertensive drug prescription. It is noteworthy that in 4 patients, the antihypertensive treatment could be discontinued in spite of the rising hematocrit: a closer clinical surveillance due to the weekly outpatient visit included in the protocol led to a more effective reduction in dry weight followed by an improved blood pressure control without drugs.

Self-administration of rhEPO was well accepted by the patients or their helpers. Two key factors contributed to obtaining an excellent compliance: the lack of pain at the site of subcutaneous injection; the careful training of the patient and/or the helper in the procedures concerning the daily utilisation of rhEPO.

In conclusion, self-administered daily subcutaneous rhEPO was shown to be effective and safe to treat the anemia of patients undergoing CAPD. As the more practical intraperitoneal administration would lead to an unacceptable wastage of a costly drug [5], the subcutaneous route seems the more appropriate in spite of its inconvenience. The extremely low median weekly dose reached during the maintenance period in the present study underscores the usefulness of daily administration. If our results can be reproduced in a larger group of patients, they will stress the dual advantages of this method of rhEPO administration: to bring the prescription closer to the physiology; to cut by half or more the cost of an expensive treatment.

References

1   Bommer J, Weinreich T, Ritz E, Zeier M, Bommer G: Efficacy of subcutaneous or intravenous recombinant human erythropoietin therapy in dialysis patients (abstract). Nephrol Dial Transplant 1989;4:471.
2   Granolleras C, Branger B, Deschodt G, Alsabadani B, Shaldon S: Daily self-administered subcutaneous erythropoietin: The optimal form of erythropoietin for end stage renal disease patients (abstract). Nephrol Dial Transplant 1989;4:473.
3   Stockenhuber F, Loibl U, Jahn C, Manker W, Meissl F, Balcke P: Intravenous versus subcutaneous application of erythropoietin in patients on regular dialysis treatment and CAPD (abstract). Nephrol Dial Transplant 1989;4:478.
4   Eschbach JW, Ergie JC, Downing MR, Browne JK, Adamson JW: Correction of the anemia of end-stage renal disease with recombinant human erythropoietin. Results of a combined phase I and II clinical trial. N Engl J Med 1987;316:73–78.
5   MacDougall IC, Roberts DE, Neubert P, Dharmasena AD, Coles GA, Williams JD: Pharmacokinetics of recombinant human erythropoietin in patients on continuous ambulatory peritoneal dialysis. Lancet 1989;i:425–427.
6   Sundal E, Kaeser U: Correction of anemia of chronic renal failure with recombinant human erythropoietin: Safety and efficacy of one year's treatment in a European multicenter study of 150 haemodialysis-dependent patients. Nephrol Dial Transplant 1989;4:979–987.
7   Beelen RHJ, Vand der Meulen J, Verbrugh H, Hofsmit ECM, Oe PC, Verhoef J: CAPD, a permanent state of peritonitis: A study of peroxidase activity; in Maher JF, Winchester JF (eds): Frontiers in Peritoneal Dialysis, New York, Field Rich, 1989, pp 524–530.

C. Mion, MD, Service de Néphrologie, Hôpital Lapeyronie, CHU,
F–34059 Montpellier Cedex (France)

Gurland HJ, Moran J, Samtleben W, Scigalla P, Wieczorek L (eds): Erythropoietin in
Renal and Non-Renal Anemias. Contrib Nephrol. Basel, Karger, 1991, vol 88, pp 169–179

Long-Term Effects of Recombinant Human Erythropoietin in Patients Treated with Continuous Peritoneal Dialysis: Safety Aspects

Peter Bárány, Anders Tranaeus, Jonas Bergström

Department of Renal Medicine, Karolinska Institute, Huddinge University Hospital,
Stockholm, Sweden

It is established that recombinant human erythropoietin (rhEPO) is efficient in the treatment of anaemia in haemodialysis (HD) patients [1, 2]. In most studies reported rhEPO has been administered intravenously (IV) three times per week. For patients on continuous peritoneal dialysis (CPD), i.e. CAPD or CCPD, who have no vascular access, repeated IV administration is unpractical. Pharmacokinetic studies have demonstrated that subcutaneous (SC) rhEPO seems to be the preferred route of administration compared with IV and intraperitoneal administration [3, 4]. Preliminary data also suggest that smaller weekly doses of SC rhEPO are required when administered daily than when given three times per week [5].

A positive effect of rhEPO in CAPD patients has been observed [6–10] but until now few data on long-term effects of SC rhEPO in CAPD patients have been published [9, 10]. In this communication we report preliminary results of SC treatment with rhEPO in patients treated with CPD (CAPD or CCPD), focusing on possible long-term adverse effects.

Material and Methods

Due to participation in two multicenter studies we followed two different protocols. In one study SC rhEPO was administered three times per week (study 'SC rhEPO 3/w'); an inclusion criterion was that the patients had a stable initial haemoglobin (Hb) concentration below 90 g/l. The target Hb concentration was 100 g/l. In the other study SC rhEPO was administered daily (study 'SC rhEPO daily'); patients with a stable initial haematocrit less than 28% were included and the target haematocrit was 30–35%.

The patient material comprised 14 patients with chronic renal failure who were treated with CAPD or CCPD and had a creatinine clearance of less than 1 ml/min (table 1). Five

Table 1. Clinical characteristics in 14 CPD patients treated with SC rhEPO

Patient	Sex/age	Renal diagnosis	Treatment	Time on CPD months	EPO dose schedule	Hb before EPO g/l	Correction time weeks	Remarks
1	F/66	amyloidosis	CCPD	27	3/week	68	30	
2	F/66	analgesic nephropathy	CCPD	64	3/week	87	24	peritonitis × 1 iron deficiency
3	F/58	carcinoma of renal pelvis, bilateral nephrectomy	CAPD	52	3/week	76	21	
4	F/44	hereditary nephritis	CCPD	46	3/week	60	37	iron deficiency
5	M/44	CGN	CCPD	94	3/week	76	39	peritonitis × 3
6	F/71	DN	CAPD	6	daily	74	16	peritonitis × 1 deceased
7	F/66	DN	CAPD	9	daily	70	15	peritonitis × 1
8	F/50	CPN	CAPD	10	daily	70	16	
9	F/66	DN	CAPD	21	daily	71	–	transplanted
10	F/55	CGN, vasculitis	CAPD	33	daily	87	20	
11	M/60	CGN	CAPD	16	daily	89	10	peritonitis × 1
12	F/79	CRF	CAPD	12	daily	83	10	
13	M/73	CRF	CAPD	6	daily	86	20	
14	F/81	CPN	CAPD	45	daily	80	–	peritonitis × 1 deceased

CGN = Chronic glomerulonephritis; CPN = chronic pyelonephritis; DN = diabetic nephropathy; CRF = chronic renal failure.

patients were treated with SC rhEPO 3/w for a median of 48 weeks (46–50 weeks). Nine patients were treated with SC rhEPO daily for a median of 30 weeks (7–37 weeks). Of these patients, 1 was transplanted 7 weeks after start of treatment (case 9) and 2 elderly patients (cases 6 and 14) with nutritional problems died after 18 und 9 weeks of treatment; the deaths were apparently unrelated to the rhEPO treatment. Case 14 withdrew voluntarily from the study 2 weeks before death. Eight episodes of peritonitis were observed in 6 patients; 1 patient had three episodes and the other 5 had one episode each.

In study SC rhEPO 3/w the initial weekly dose of rhEPO was 60 units/kg body weight (BW); this dose was kept constant during 10 weeks and then individually adjusted to reach the target Hb concentration. In study 'SC rhEPO daily' the patients were randomized to a daily dose of 5, 10 or 20 units/kg BW/day, i.e., a weekly dose of 35, 70 or 140 units/kg BW, respectively, which was kept constant during 8 weeks after which the dose was individually adjusted to reach the target haematocrit.

All patients on SC rhEPO 3/w and 4 patients on SC rhEPO daily injected themselves with rhEPO in the thigh SC tissue. In 5 patients the injections were given by a district nurse. Two of these patients living at home were physically handicapped (case 8 rheumatoid arthritis, case 10 vasculitis with amputated fingers) and 3 of them were elderly and debilitated (case 9, 12 and 14), 2 living in institutions and 1 at home.

The patients volunteered to participate in the studies after having received written and oral information about possible benefits and risks. The protocols were approved by the local ethics committee at Huddinge University Hospital.

Results

Hb concentration and weekly rhEPO dose in the two groups of CPD patients treated with SC rhEPO for more than 6 months are shown in figures 1 and 2; for comparison, data from 25 HD patients treated with IV rhEPO three times per week are included in the figures.

The initial Hb concentration was not significantly different in the three groups. The fastest rise in mean Hb concentration and the highest mean values were observed in the CPD patients receiving SC rhEPO daily, while the slowest rise was observed in the CPD patients on SC rhEPO 3/w. Three of these patients did not reach their target haematocrit within 6 months (table 1); 1 of them developed iron deficiency requiring IV iron therapy and 1 had three episodes of peritonitis. The HD patients showed a slower rise in Hb concentration over 6 months compared with the CPD patients on rhEPO daily.

The weekly maintenance doses of rhEPO after more than 6 months when the target Hb or haematocrit had been reached are shown in figure 3. The lowest mean weekly dose was observed in the patients on daily SC rhEPO. The weekly doses in the HD patients varied within a much larger range and the mean value was higher than in the CPD patients.

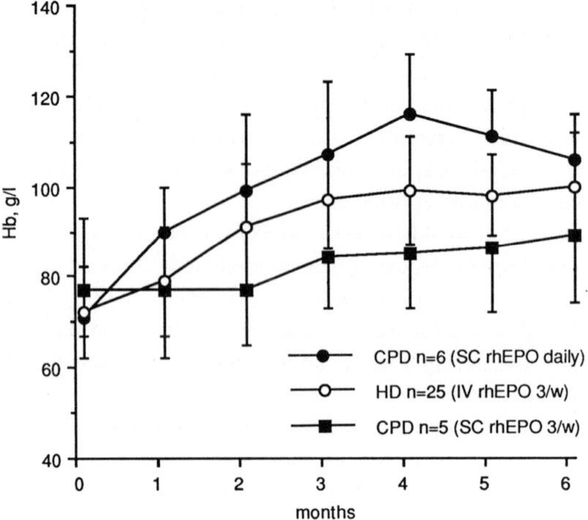

Fig. 1. Hb concentration in CPD patients treated with SC rhEPO for more than 6 months three times per week (SC rhEPO 3/w, n = 5) or daily (SC rhEPO daily, n = 6) and in 25 HD patients on IV rhEPO three times per week (IV rhEPO 3/w). Mean ± SD.

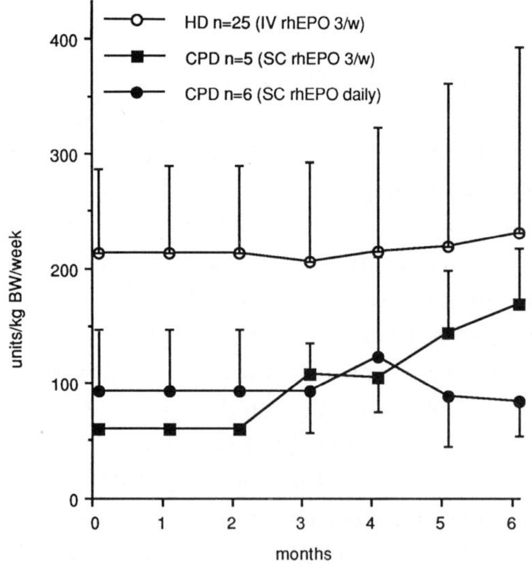

Fig. 2. Weekly dose of rhEPO in CPD patients treated for more than 6 months with SC rhEPO three times per week or daily and in 25 HD patients on IV rhEPO three times per week. For legend, see figure 1. Mean ± SD.

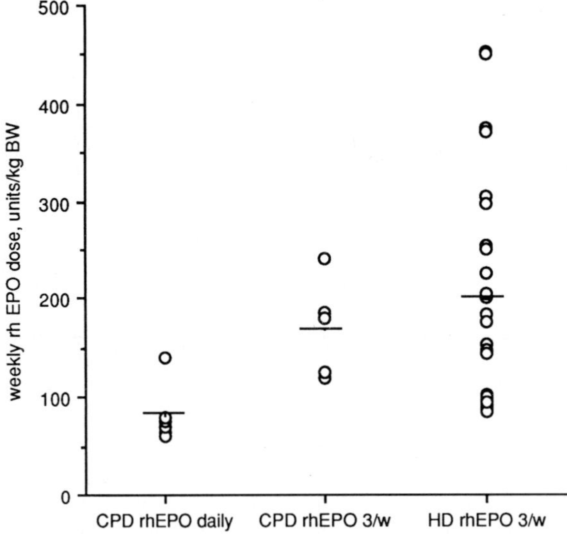

Fig. 3. Weekly maintenance doses in CPD patients receiving SC rhEPO daily or three times per week and in HD patients on IV rhEPO three times per week. Mean ± SD.

No increment was observed in blood platelet counts, nor in serum urea, creatinine, potassium and phosphate levels (fig. 4). None of the patients had any general symptoms in form of seizures, dizziness, headache, shivering, muscle aching, bone pain or fever reactions.

Hypertension: The mean systolic and diastolic blood pressure was not changed in the 11 CPD patients treated with rhEPO for more than 6 months (fig. 5). Only 1 patient (No. 6) was treated for hypertension prior to rhEPO therapy. In this patient the blood pressure rose during rhEPO treatment but could be easily controlled with intensified antihypertensive therapy. None of the other patients developed hypertension. Of 25 HD patients treated with IV rhEPO, 9 had antihypertensive therapy of which 7 patients required increased medication and 2 patients developed hypertension, suggesting that blood pressure control is more problematic in HD than in CPD patients during rhEPO treatment.

Local side effects: One patient had SC haematoma repeatedly at the injection site. Platelet count, prothrombin time and activated partial thromboplastin time were normal in this patient. The patient who had diabetes

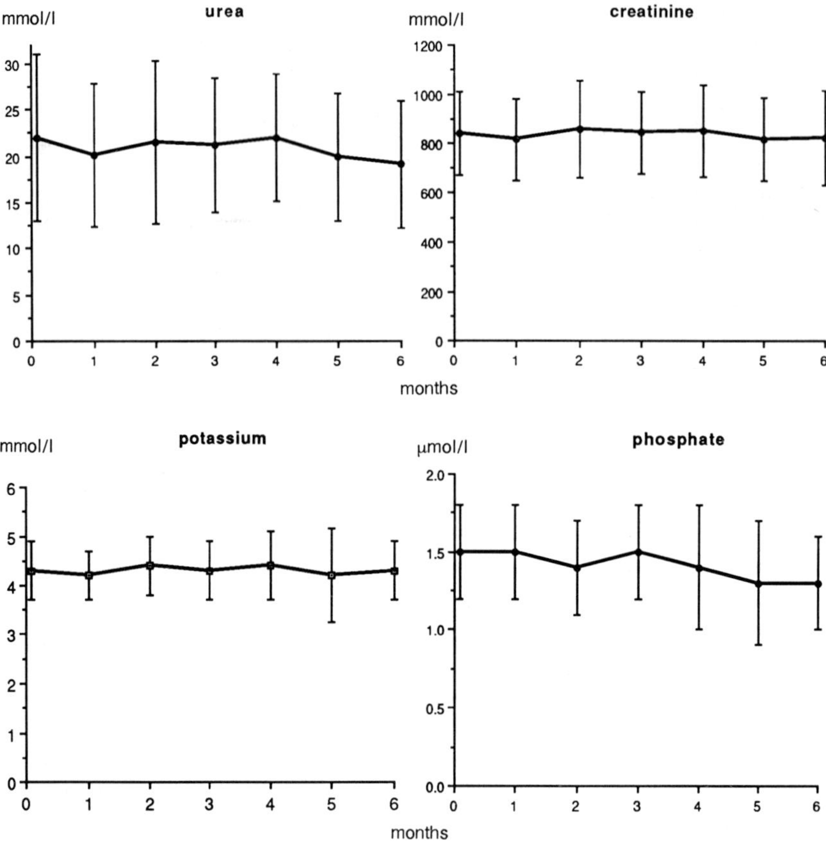

Fig. 4. Serum urea, creatinine, potassium and phosphate in 11 CPD patients treated with rhEPO for more than 6 months. Mean ± SD.

mellitus received insulin SC in the abdominal wall, which was also associated with SC bleeding. Two other patients had minor erythema and itching at the site of injection. The SC rhEPO treatment could be continued in all 3 patients despite these minor problems.

Iron depletion: Mean serum ferritin fell significantly (fig. 6) and 2 patients developed iron deficiency for which they were treated with IV iron. Another 7 patients required oral iron supplementation.

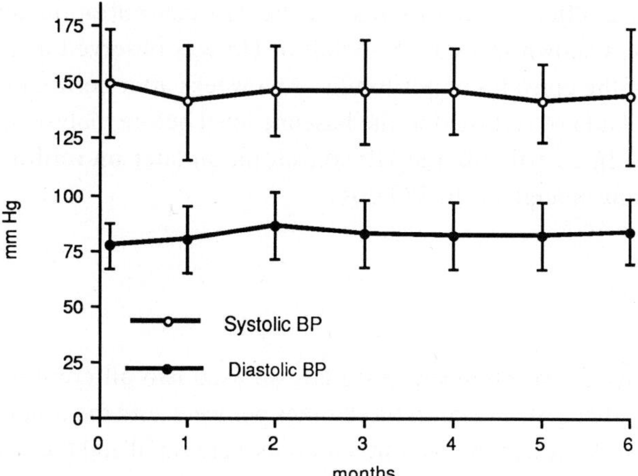

Fig. 5. Systolic and diastolic blood pressure in 11 CPD patients treated with rhEPO for more than 6 months. Mean ± SD.

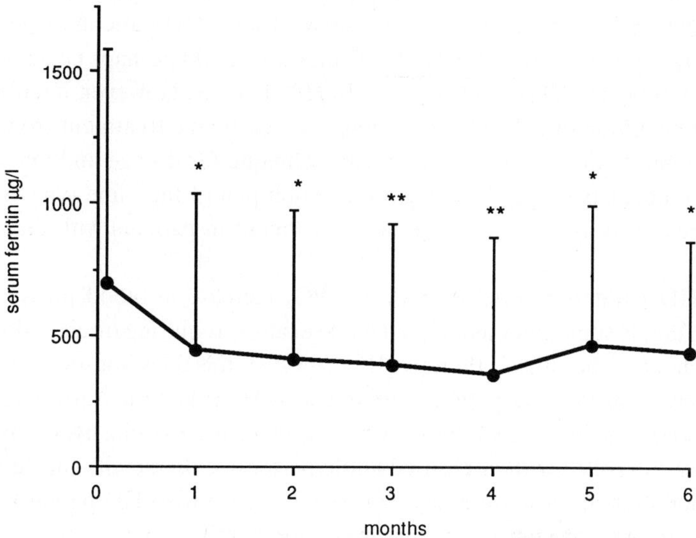

Fig. 6. Serum ferritin in 11 patients treated with SC rhEPO for more than 6 months. Mean ± SD. *$p<0.05$, **$p<0.01$.

Peritonitis: The effect of peritonitis on the Hb concentration during rhEPO treatment is shown in figure 5. A fall in Hb was observed at 1 or 2 weeks after five of the episodes of peritonitis. At 4 weeks after peritonitis the Hb concentration had not returned to the baseline level before dialysis (three episodes studied). In all patients the Hb concentration later on returned to baseline without any change in rhEPO dose.

Discussion

As participants in two multicenter studies we used two different dosing schedules, one involving SC injection three times per week and the other with daily SC injections. Although the patient materials were small and the longest treatment time was only 1 year, the results may still permit some preliminary conclusions, especially when compared with results of IV rhEPO treatment in a larger material of HD patients.

The mean weekly maintenance dose of rhEPO was lower in the patients receiving SC rhEPO daily than in the two other groups of patients, suggesting that this mode of administration is more efficient than either IV or SC administration three times per week. These preliminary data are in keeping with results reported by Granolleras et al. [5] who compared daily SC injection of rhEPO with SC injection three times per week in 4 HD patients, who had previously been on IV therapy. Daily SC therapy should perhaps be advantageous not only in CPD patients but also in HD patients. However, if daily SC self-administration of rhEPO is to become an acceptable treatment from the patient point of view, a more convenient technique for dosage and injection should be developed, e.g. by using an injection pen of the same type as the insulin pen used for multiple dose daily treatment in patients with diabetes mellitus.

In HD patients treated with IV rhEPO, increase in blood pressure is common and is sometimes associated with seizures, requiring interruption or readjustment of the rhEPO therapy [11]. However, this does not seem to be a serious problem in CPD patients treated with SC rhEPO as shown in the present study and in other studies reported in which pre-existing hypertension was easily controlled with intensified antihypertensive therapy [8–10]. In general, blood pressure is more easily controlled in CPD than HD patients who may require antihypertensive therapy more frequently.

Results from a multicenter study demonstrate that hypertension was more common in HD patients receiving higher doses of IV rhEPO with a faster increase in Hb concentration than in patients receiving lower doses with a slower rise in Hb over a more prolonged period of time [12]. In the present study the patients receiving daily SC injections of rhEPO had a faster rise in Hb concentration than in the HD patients on IV treatment, but in spite of those who were normotensive did not develop hypertension *de novo*.

It has been observed in some HD patients that predialysis serum creatinine, potassium and phosphorus increase during treatment with rhEPO [11]. This has been attributed to reduced efficacy of dialysis due to the increase in haematocrit with lowered plasma clearance or to improved food intake. No change in serum urea, creatinine, potassium and phosphate was observed in our CPD patients, suggesting that the efficacy of peritoneal transport was not reduced by the increase in haematocrit. Rise in serum potassium and phosphate observed in CAPD patients after 6 months of SC rhEPO treatment was attributed to improved clinical condition and subsequent dietary changes [10].

Generalized effects (flu-like syndrome) with rising body temperature, shivering, muscle aching and bone pain, have been observed after IV rhEPO in HD patients, although mostly of minor degree [11]. No such side effects were observed by us in the CPD patients treated with SC rhEPO but 2 cases were earlier reported, 1 with generalized myalgia during the first 2 weeks of SC rhEPO therapy which resolved spontaneously [8] and 1 with a flu-like syndrome which disappeared as the treatment progressed [10].

Iron depletion is one of the most important factors that interfere with the therapeutic response to rhEPO in HD patients [11]. That this is also a problem in CPD patients in spite of these patients not losing blood through the dialytic procedure as in HD patients, was demonstrated in 2 of our patients in whom the response to rhEPO was delayed until they received IV iron.

Local side effects of SC EPO at the injection site of minor severity were observed by us in 3 of the 14 patients and have not been a reason for discontinuing therapy. In 2 other studies transient pain at the injection site was reported [8, 10]; this was not considered to be a problem in our patients.

It has been observed that acute or chronic inflammation interferes with the response to rhEPO treatment in HD patients [11] and CAPD patients [8]. Since peritonitis is one of the most common complications in CPD patients it was therefore of interest to see whether episodes of peritonitis negatively influence the response to rhEPO. That this is the case is demonstrated in figure 7, showing decreased Hb concentrations over a period of a few weeks after an episode of peritonitis. However, in all cases the Hb concentration gradually returned to the level before the infection without any increase in rhEPO dose.

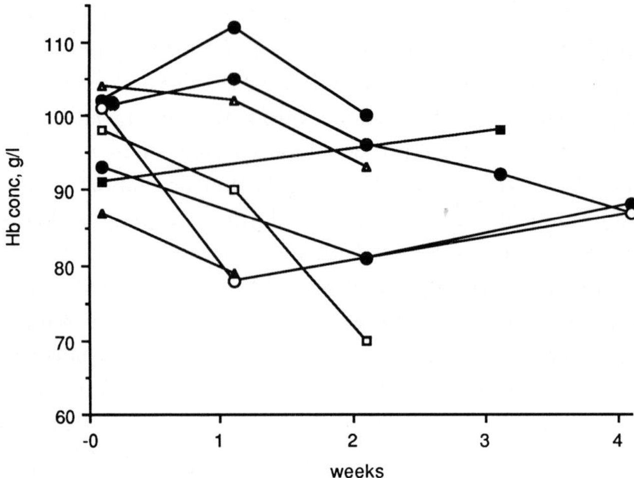

Fig. 7. The effect of peritonitis on the Hb concentration in 6 CPD patients treated with rhEPO. One patient had three episodes of peritonitis, the other 5 patients had one episode each.

In conclusion, SC administration to CPD patients is a safe form of treatment which seems to be associated with less hypertension and other side effects than IV rhEPO treatment in HD patients. With daily SC injections of rhEPO, low maintenance doses are required and this mode of administration may be advantageous in the future provided that the technique for dosage and administration becomes simpler than at present. Iron depletion interferes with the therapeutic response to rhEPO and Hb falls temporarily after episodes of peritonitis.

References

1   Winearls C, Oliver D, Pippard M, Reid C, Downing M, Cotes P: Effect of human erythropoietin derived from recombinant DNA on the anaemia of patients maintained by chronic haemodialysis. Lancet 1988;ii:1175–1178.
2   Eschbach J, Egrie J, Downing M, Browne J, Adamson J: Correction of anaemia of end-stage renal disease with recombinant human erythropoietin. N Engl J Med 1987;316:73–78.

3 Macdougall I, Roberts D, Neubert P, Dharmasena D, Coles G, Williams J: Pharmacokinetics of recombinant human erythropoietin in patients on continuous ambulatory peritoneal dialysis. Lancet 1989;i:425–427.

4 Boelaert JR, Shurgers ML, Matthys EG, Belpaire FM, Daneels RF, DeCre MJ, Bogaert MG: Comparative pharmacokinetics of recombinant erythropoietin administered by the intravenous, subcutaneous, and intraperitoneal routes in continuous ambulatory dialysis patients. Periton Dial Int 1980;9:95–98.

5 Granolleras C, Branger B, Beau MC, Deschodt G, Alsabadani B, Shaldon S: Experience with daily self-administered subcutaneous erythropoietin; in Baldamus CA, Scigalla P, Wieczorek L, Koch KM (eds): Erythropoietin: From molecular structure to clinical application. Contrib Nephrol. Basel, Karger, vol 76, 1989, 143–148.

6 Frenken L, Coppens P, Tigeler R, Koene R: Intraperitoneal erythropoietin (Letter). Lancet 1988;ii:1495.

7 Macdougall I, Cavill I, Davies ME, Hutton RD, Coles GA, Williams JD: Subcutaneous recombinant erythropoietin in the treatment of renal anaemia in CAPD patients; in Baldamus CA, Scigalla P, Wieczorek L, Koch KM (eds): Erythropoietin: From molecular structure to clinical application. Contrib Nephrol. Basel, Karger, 1989, vol. 76, pp 219–226.

8 Piraino B, Johnston JR: The use of subcutaneous erythropoietin in CAPD patients. Clin Nephrol 1990;33:200–202.

9 Sinai-Trieman L, Salusky IB, Fine RN: Use of subcutaneous recombinant human erythropoietin in children undergoing continuous cycling peritoneal dialysis. J Pediatr 1989;114:550–554.

10 Steinhauer HB: Effects of long-term treatment with human recombinant erythropoietin in patients on CAPD. Adv Exp Med Biol 1989;260:157–165.

11 Flaharty KK, Grimm AM, Vlasses PH: Epoetin: Human recombinant erythropoietin. Clin Pharm 1989;8:769–782.

12 Pollok M, Bommer J, Gurland HJ, Koch KM, Schoeppe W, Scigalla P, Baldamus CA: Effects of recombinant human erythropoietin treatment in end-stage renal failure patients; in Baldamus CA, Scigalla P, Wieczorek L, Koch KM (eds): Erythropoietin: From molecular structure to clinical application. Contrib Nephrol, Basel, Karger, 1989, vol. 76, pp 201–211.

Prof. Jonas Bergström, MD, Department of Renal Medicine, Karolinska Institute, Huddinge University Hospital, S–141 86 Huddinge (Sweden)

Gurland HJ, Moran J, Samtleben W, Scigalla P, Wieczorek L (eds): Erythropoietin in
Renal and Non-Renal Anemias. Contrib Nephrol. Basel, Karger, 1991, vol 88, pp 180–181

Discussion

to the Papers by A. Slingeneyer et al. and P. Bárány et al.

Schollmeyer (Freiburg): I have a short comment and a question. We have just finished a study in 14 CAPD patients treated with rhEPO for 1 year. The initial dose we used was 50 U/kg twice weekly. After 1 year the maintenance dose was nearly the same, about 50 U, i.e. 100 U/kg/week. Now the question. We have measured the amount of ultrafiltration in these patients and, in association with the increase in hematocrit, we noticed a significant increase of 20% in ultrafiltration, which persisted after 1 year. We think this increase in ultrafiltration is due to changes in the circulation consequent upon the rise in hematocrit. Have either of you have measured ultrafiltration in these patients and, if so, have you made the same observation?

Bergström: We have not made this observation simply because we have not compiled our data yet. We are doing dwell studies with tagged albumin in some of these patients before and during EPO treatment, but I don't have these data.

Mion: We have no information on this.

Koch (Hannover): Your patients all had the same background, as they were all on peritoneal dialysis, but you had different rates of rise of hematocrit. You had 9 patients with aggravation of hypertension. In which of the groups did they fall? Was there any correlation with the speed of correction of anemia?

Mion: There was a clear correlation with the speed of correction and the hypertensive trend. Most patients with increases in blood pressure fall into groups 2 and 3.

Baldamus (Cologne): I would like to ask Dr. Bergström: you showed a low incidence of hypertension in your CAPD patients, but these data related to patients with a slow increase in hematocrit. You also had a group with a steeper rise in hematocrit. How did they behave?

Bergström: Five of these 6 patients had no change in blood pressure when their hematocrit rose. The sixth patient was already on antihypertensive treatment, and we had to increase the therapy. It was not difficult to control the blood pressure.

Shaldon (Montpellier): I would like to ask Dr. Mion, in view of Dr. Schollmeyer's comment: if I recollect your data your median dose when you had an n of 18 and an n of 14 was 5 U/kg and then you had only 9 patients at the very end, the median dose rose to 10 U/kg. Is that because the long-term survivors suddenly got sicker?

Mion: This might be explained by the difference in attitude of the two physicians in Montpellier and Colmar. I think Dr. Slingeneyer tries harder to reduce the dose than does Dr.

Faller in Colmar. We have to try to see whether there is a difference in policy there. But it is important to stress that it is worthwhile to attempt the maximum dose reduction, as a dose as low as 2.5 U/kg/day in 1 patient seems to be still useful in maintaining a good hematocrit.

Eschbach (Seattle): I want to congratulate both of you on your papers. Of interest to me is that both of you show a mean weekly requirement of around 70 U/kg. Dr. Granolleras showed that the hemodialysis patients also responded to that dose when given daily. Yet there has been an anecdotal story that CAPD patients require much less EPO than do hemodialysis patients. Does either of you or Dr. Granolleras have any comment about the fact that you have equal dose responses?

Bergström: I would like not to comment on that because our data are too limited.

Mion: I have no specific comment regarding this interesting observation that both CAPD and HD patients can benefit similarly from daily subcutaneous rhEPO administration.

Bahlmann (Hannover): Dr. Mion, you introduced a note of caution by mentioning 2 patients with a worsening of peripheral arteriosclerotic disease. Was this really hematocrit-associated, or were these diabetic patients?

Mion: Four patients had a deterioration in their peripheral arteriosclerotic disease. The 2 patients who had acute ischemia with gangrene were not diabetic. On the other hand, the 2 patients with chronic skin ulcers were type II diabetics receiving insulin. It should be stressed, however, that except for 1 patient with acute ischemia, distal ischemic complications of the lower limb occurred only after reaching the target hematocrit.

Shaldon: I'd like to respond to the anecdotal innuendo of Dr. Eschbach. I have had access to the multicenter data from the Boehringer Mannheim subcutaneous studies, of which you have only heard part reported, and the 'anecdotal' data consisted of 7 patients, of which you have heard Dr. Mion refer to 2 who were on maintenance doses of 2.5 U/kg/day. I think I asked you whether you had ever seen as low a dose as this in a hemodialysis patient?

Baldamus: Is the maintenance dose in any way dependent on the hematocrit you start the patients on?

Bergström: Our material is too limited to draw a conclusion.

Mion: I think one can positively answer your question. For a given dose, if the hematocrit is lower the correction time will be longer, or you will have to increase the dose to shorten the correction period.

Gurland HJ, Moran J, Samtleben W, Scigalla P, Wieczorek L (eds): Erythropoietin in
Renal and Non-Renal Anemias. Contrib Nephrol. Basel, Karger, 1991, vol 88, pp 182–189

Stable Renal Function and Benign Course in Azotemic Diabetics Treated with Erythropoietin for One Year[1]

Clinton D. Brown, Eli A. Friedman[2]

Department of Medicine, State University of New York, Health Science Center at
Brooklyn, Brooklyn, N.Y., USA

Perturbations in blood rheology are thought to contribute to the genesis and progression of micro- and macrovascular complications in diabetes mellitus [1, 2]. Hyperviscosity of whole blood, plasma, and serum and reduced erythrocyte deformability have been linked to the pathogenesis and progression of overt nephropathy in diabetic persons [3, 4]. Therapeutic regimens for diabetic management designed to return blood rheology to normal have been proposed and evaluated positively [5, 6].

Recombinant human erythropoietin (rhEPO) has been shown to increase circulating red blood cell mass in uremic patients sustained by maintenance hemodialysis [7–10]. There is concern that raising whole blood viscosity by increasing red cell mass might worsen hypertension and thereby increase risk of vascular complications in rhEPO-treated uremic diabetics undergoing maintenance hemodialysis [11]. A similar threat exists for the rhEPO-treated diabetic not yet begun on maintenance hemodialysis. Brown et al. [12] reported that mean hematocrit rose 38% in 10 rhEPO-treated azotemic adult predialysis patients and that whole blood viscosity rose appropriately to the value expected for higher hematocrits.

During the last half of the previous decade, more than one-quarter of newly treated uremic patients in the United States have been diabetic [13]. It is likely that diabetics will continue to comprise a large subset of rhEPO-treated subjects both prior to and during the course of maintenance dialysis. To

---

[1] This study was supported in part by a grant from Ortho Pharmaceutical Corp.

[2] We thank Micheal Kieran for competent and conscientious assistance in both patient care and data analysis.

Table 1. Demographics of azotemic diabetic patients

Subject	Sex	Age	Weight kg	Hct %	Serum creatinine mg/dl	Diabetic phenotype
1	F	39	51.9	26	3.0	I
2	M	27	67.0	27	3.4	I
3	M	71	94.7	31	4.2	II
4	F	62	61.1	31	3.7	II
5	M	56	109.7	30	3.4	II

ascertain whether rhEPO treatment imposes a risk of accelerated nephropathy in diabetic subjects, we administered sufficient rhEPO to raise mean hematocrit levels by approximately 33% in 5 azotemic diabetics and followed their renal function and general condition for a period of 12 months.

Patients and Methods

Ambulatory, stable, azotemic anemic diabetic individuals attending the outpatient clinics of University Hospital of Brooklyn and Kings County Hospital Center were recruited for study after obtaining informed consent. Of a total of 11 azotemic subjects not requiring dialytic therapy who began a long-term evaluation of rhEPO, 5 were diabetic and the first year of their treatment forms the substance of the present report. Demographics of diabetic subjects are summarized in table 1. The group of 5 diabetics consisted of 2 insulin-dependent subjects (patients 1 and 2) and 3 noninsulin-dependent subjects (patients 3–5). In each patient, renal insufficiency was attributed to diabetic nephropathy. All were proteinuric ($>$1 g/24 h) and had significant diabetic retinopathy. Renal function was monitored at monthly intervals by measuring serum creatinine concentration. Serum creatinine was measured by autoanalyzer. Whole blood viscosity was determined on a Wells-Brookfield cone-plate viscometer (Brookfield Engineering Corp., Stoughton, Mass.) using the technique described by Wells et al. [14]. Briefly, 1.2 ml of heparinized venous blood was transferred to the cup of the viscometer and viscosity was measured at high and low rates of shear (230 and 23 s^{-1}, respectively) at 37°C. Viscosity is equal to the ratio of shear stress to shear rate and is expressed in millipascal-seconds (mPas). Plasma viscosity was also measured (shear rate of 230 s^{-1}) by the same technique using 1.2 ml of freshly separated plasma. Accuracy of viscosity measurements was monitored by daily repeated determinations of the viscosity of distilled water (0.7–0.95 mPas) and a prepared standard (4.2 mPas) (Brookfield Eng. Corp.). The coefficient of variation was less than 3%. Hematocrit was determined in capillary tube after centrifugation (1,500 g for 10 min). Normal values of whole blood viscosity for our laboratory as measured in a group matched for gender and hematocrit (60% normal adult men and 40% normal adult women,

Table 2. Blood rheologic response in 5 diabetic patients to rhEPO treatment

		Hct, %	Whole blood viscosity		Plasma viscosity
			230 s^{-1}	23 s^{-1}	230 s^{-1}
Pretreatment	mean	29.6	3.62	4.96	1.55
	SD	2.0	0.32	0.98	0.16
Posttreatment	mean	39.5*	4.27**	6.99**	1.60
(12 months)	SD	2.4	0.28	0.88	0.07

*p<0.005; **p<0.001 (comparison of pre- and posttreatment means). Unmarked posttreatment indicates no significant difference from pretreatment mean.

n = 36, hematocrit 40.3±2.56%) are: 4.35±0.53 and 6.83±0.79 mPas for high and low rates of shear, respectively, and plasma viscosity (230 s^{-1}) of 1.57±0.11 mPas (table 4). To approximate whole blood viscosity in anemia, we diluted normal blood to a lower hematocrit by adding autologous plasma to attain a hematocrit of approximately 30%. Whole blood viscosity for 'normal' reduced hematocrit of 30% was 3.49±0.27 and 5.05±0.63 mPas for high and low rates of shear, respectively (table 3).

rhEPO prepared by the Amgen Corp. (Thousand Oaks, Calif.) and provided by Ortho Pharmaceutical Corp. (Raritan, N.J.) was administered intravenously in doses of 50–150 U/kg 3 times weekly until the mean hematocrit had risen to approximately 40%. Maintenance doses of rhEPO were continued at intervals to sustain hematocrit above 35%. Neither the diabetic nor normal subjects had a history of smoking cigarettes.

Data were analyzed using Student's t test for paired and unpaired samples and are expressed as mean ± SD.

Results

Rheologic Response

All 5 diabetic subjects demonstrated a significant rise in hematocrit (p<0.005) from a pretreatment mean of 29.6±2.0 (range 26–31%) to a mean of 39.5±2.4% (range 37–43%) after treatment with rhEPO (table 2). As summarized in table 2, whole blood viscosity measured at both high and low rates of shear rose significantly (p = 0.01 and 0.01, respectively) from a pretreatment level of 3.62±0.32 mPas (high shear rate) and 4.96±0.98 mPas (low shear rate) to 4.27±0.28 and 6.99±0.88 mPas, respectively. Plasma viscosity, however, did not change significantly (p = 0.63).

Table 3. Comparison of blood rheology: diabetic patients (pretreatment) versus normals (after hemodilution)

Parameter			Normals (n = 36, 22 M/14 F)	Patients (n = 5, 3 M/2 F)	p
Hematocrit, %		mean	29.9	29.6	NS
		SD	1.4	2.0	
Whole blood	$230\,s^{-1}$	mean	3.49	3.62	NS
viscosity, mPas		SD	0.27	0.32	
	$23\,s^{-1}$	mean	5.05	4.96	NS
		SD	0.63	0.98	
Plasma	$230\,s^{-1}$	mean	1.57	1.55	NS
viscosity, mPas		SD	0.11	0.16	

Table 4. Comparison of blood rheology: diabetic patients after 12 months of rhEPO treatment versus normals

Parameter			Normals (n = 36, 22 M/14 F)	Patients (n = 5, 3 M/2 F)	p
Hematocrit, %		mean	40.3	39.5	NS
		SD	2.6	2.4	
Whole blood	$230\,s^{-1}$	mean	4.35	4.27	NS
viscosity, mPas		SD	0.53	0.28	
	$23\,s^{-1}$	mean	6.83	6.99	NS
		SD	0.79	0.88	
Plasma	$230\,s^{-1}$	mean	1.57	1.60	NS
viscosity, mPas		SD	0.11	0.07	

Comparison of pretreatment blood rheologic parameters (diabetic patients) to those of normal blood (n = 36, matched for hematocrit and gender), diluted with autologous plasma to a mean hematocrit similar to that of diabetic subjects, revealed no significant difference in either whole blood or plasma viscosity (table 3). Similarly, comparison of rheologic parameters after 12 months of rhEPO treatment to those of normal adults (n = 36, matched for hematocrit and gender), again revealed no significant difference in whole blood or plasma viscosity (table 4).

Table 5. Renal function and clinical course in 5 azotemic diabetics treated with rhEPO: 1 year experience

		Blood pressure, mmHg		Weight	Serum glucose	Serum creatinine
		systolic	diastolic	kg	mg/dl	mg/dl
Initial	mean	149.0	87.8	76.9	142.8	3.5
	SD	20.6	6.6	21.7	73.1	0.4
Final	mean	149.0	76.0	76.3	132.4	3.7
	SD	6.6	8.0	19.7	46.9	0.4
p		NS	NS	NS	NS	NS

Clinical Response

All 5 subjects reported having a sense of improved well-being following treatment with rhEPO. Mean systolic and diastolic blood pressures at the start of the study (149±20.6 and 88±6.6 mmHg, respectively) were unchanged during and after 1 year of rhEPO treatment (149±6.6 and 76±8.0 mmHg, respectively). None of the patients were catabolic; mean body weight at the start (76.9±21.7 kg) was unchanged after 1 year (76.3±19.7 kg) (table 5). The mean serum creatinine concentration of 3.7±0.40 mg/dl in diabetic patients at the end of 1 year of rhEPO treatment was unchanged statistically from its level of 3.5±0.40 mg/dl at the start of the study.

Hospitalization was necessitated for only 1 patient during the study; patient 1 had a reversible rise in serum potassium concentration consequent to administration of enalapril for hypertension which resolved after 3 days in hospital. None of the patients sustained a cerebrovascular or cardiovascular incident during the year of study.

Discussion

Several investigators have reviewed the efficacy and safety of rhEPO treatment for the anemia of renal failure. The general consensus is that rhEPO treatment is both remarkably safe and extraordinarily effective [7–9]. Little reported experience, however, has focused on the safety and efficacy of rhEPO treatment for anemic azotemic diabetic individuals. Raine [11] cautions that the use of rhEPO in patients with chronic renal failure results in a dose-dependent rise in hematocrit which, although abolishing symptoms of anemia, may induce risks associated with an increase in blood viscosity. Also, rhEPO-related increases in blood pressure are of particular concern [8]. Since both hypertension and hyperviscosity are thought to be factors which underlie deterioration in renal function in diabetes [1–3] it is important to determine whether rhEPO treatment in the anemic azotemic diabetic is complicated by an rhEPO-induced loss of renal function.

What is evident from our 5 subjects studied for a mean of 1 year is that rhEPO treatment does not uniformly impart either of the hazards which might have been anticipated when raising the red cell mass in diabetic patients with renal macrovasculopathy manifested by azotemia. None of our azotemic diabetic subjects manifested worsened hypertension, cerebrovascular accident, myocardial infarction, clinically symptomatic retinal hemorrhage or discernible loss of kidney function.

As expected, whole blood viscosity rose in parallel to the rhEPO-induced rise in red cell mass; however, the rise in blood viscosity was proportional to and appropriate for the achieved level of hematocrit. Whole blood viscosity in our diabetic subjects during the pretreatment period compared to that of normal blood diluted with autologous plasma to reach an equivalent subnormal hematocrit (29.6 vs. 29.9%) was not significantly different. Mean plasma viscosity, in rhEPO-treated diabetic persons, was equivalent to that of the normal group at the start and end of study. It is evident from these facts that our study group had 'normal' whole blood (for the level of hematocrit) and plasma viscosity before rhEPO treatment began, a finding representing an unappreciated aspect of our selection bias in a subset of diabetic persons with renal disease. A more complete evaluation of the effects of rhEPO treatment in azotemic diabetic individuals is accomplished by studying a larger number of subjects (including those with elevated blood viscosity prior to rhEPO treatment) for a longer period of time. Therefore, from the data presented in this report, we cannot predict a similar benign clinical course and stability of renal function following treatment with rhEPO in anemic azotemic diabetics with underlying disproportionately high whole blood viscosity and/or elevated plasma viscosity.

We recognize that reliance on the serum creatinine concentration to monitor the course of renal functional impairment in diabetes has been faulted [15–17]. On the other hand, many workers over more than a decade of reporting of progressive renal injury have found that serum creatinine concentration is of *practical importance in predicting the time at which end-stage renal failure will develop [18–20], and a useful tool to gauge renal reserve when determined prospectively every 2–3 months in diabetic nephropathy* [21, 22]. Our experience indicates that an unchanging (stable) serum creatinine concentration is invariably associated with a constant glomerular filtration rate.

Conclusion

From the evidence presented in this report we infer that raising the hematocrit and whole blood viscosity to within the normal range by treatment with rhEPO in azotemic anemic diabetics having appropriate blood viscosity (for the level of hematocrit) and normal blood pressure, produces no clinically obvious vascular complication or discernible progression of diabetic nephropathy over a course of 1 year.

References

1	Barnes, A.J.; Locke, P.; Scudder, P.R.; Dormandy, T.L.; Dormandy, J.A.; Slack, J.: Is hyperviscosity a treatable component of diabetic microcirculatory disease? Lancet *ii:* 789–791 (1977).
2	Prentice, C.R.; Lowe, G.D.: Blood viscosity and the complications of diabetes. Adv. Exp. Med. Biol. *164:* 99–103 (1984).
3	Simpson, L.O.: Intrinsic stiffening of red blood cells as the fundamental cause of diabetic nephropathy and microangiopathy: a new hypothesis. Nephron *39:* 344–351 (1985).
4	Vermes, I.; Steimetz, E.T.; Zeyen, L.J.; van der Veen, E.A.: Rheological properties of white blood cells are changed in diabetic patients with microvascular complications. Diabetologia *30:* 434–436 (1987).
5	Solerte, S.B.; Fioravanti, M.; Patti, A.L.; Schifinao, N.; Zanoletti, M.G.; Inglese, V.; Ferrari, E.: Pentoxifylline, total urinary protein excretion rate and arterial blood pressure in long-term insulin-dependent diabetic patients with overt nephropathy. Acta Diabetol. Latinoam. *24:* 229–239 (1987).
6	Donadio, J.V., Jr.; Ilstrup, D.M.; Holley, K.E.; Romero, J.C.: Platelet-inhibitor treatment of diabetic nephropathy: A 10-year prospective study. Mayo Clin. Proc. *63:* 3–15 (1988).
7	Winearls, C.G.; Oliver, D.O.; Pippard, M.J.; Reid, C.; Downing, M.R.; Cotes, P.M.: Effects of human erythropoietin derived from recombinant DNA on the anaemia of patients maintained with chronic haemodialysis. Lancet *i:* 1175–1178 (1986).
8	Eschbach, J.W.; Egrie, J.C.; Downing, M.R.; Browne, J.K.; Adamson, J.W.: Correction of the anemia of end-stage renal disease with recombinant human erythropoietin: results of a phase I and II clinical trial. N. Engl. J. Med. *316:* 73–78 (1987).

9	Eschbach, J. W.; Adamson, J. W.: Recombinant erythropoietin: implications for nephrology. Am. J. Kidney Dis. *11:* 203–209 (1988).

10	Casati, S.; Passerinin, P.; Campise, M. R.; Graziani, G.; Casana, B.; Perisic, M.; Ponticelli, C.: Benefits and risks of protracted treatment with human recombinant erythropoietin in patients having haemodialysis. Br. Med. J. *295:* 1017–1020 (1987).

11	Raine, A. E. G.: Hypertension, blood viscosity, and cardiovascular morbidity in renal failure. Implications of erythropoietin therapy. Lancet *i:* 97–99 (1988).

12	Brown, C. D.; Keiran, M.; Zhao, Z. H.; Larson, R. H.; Friedman, E. A.: Treatment of azotemic anemic patients with human recombinant erythropoietin raises whole blood viscosity proportional to hematocrit. Abstr. Am. Soc. Nephrol., 1987, p. 37A.

13	Health Care Financing Research Report: End-stage renal disease, 1985, HCFA Publ. No. 03274, Sept. 1987 (US Department of Health and Human Services, Baltimore 1987).

14	Wells, R. F., Jr.; Denten, R.; Merrill, E. W.: Measurement of viscosity of biologic fluids by cone plate viscometer. J. Lab. Clin. Med. *57:* 646–656 (1961).

15	Lopez-Montano, E.; Villalpando-Hernandez, S.; Perez-Pasten, E.; Vargas-Rosendo, R.; Fuentes-Castro, C.; Ramos, L.: Overestimation of creatinine due to interference of glucose in vitro. Implications on creatinine clearance in diabetic patients. Arch. Invest. Med. *15:* 331–338 (1984).

16	Aviram, A.; Ben-Ishay, D.; Chowers, I.; Czaczkes, J. W.: Low plasma creatinine in diabetes mellitus. J. Lab. Clin. Med. *67:* 473–476 (1966).

17	Viberti, G. C.; Bilous, R. W.; Mackintosh, D.; Keen, H.: Monitoring glomerular function in diabetic nephropathy. A prospective study. Am. J. Med. *74:* 256–264 (1983).

18	Jones, R. H.; Hayakawa, H.; Mackay, J. D.; Parsons, V.; Watkins, P. J.: Progression of diabetic nephropathy. Lancet *i:* 1105–1106 (1979).

19	Aubia, J.; Hojman, L.; Chine, M.; Lloveras, J.; Masramon, J.; Llorach, I.; Cuevas, X.; Puig, J. M.: Hypertension and nephrotoxicity in the rate of decline in kidney function in diabetic nephropathy. Clin. Nephrol. *27:* 15–20 (1987).

20	Rutherford, W. E.; Blondin, J.; Miller, J. P.; Greenwalt, A. S.; Vavra, J. D.: Chronic progressive renal disease: rate of change of serum creatinine concentration. Kidney Int. *11:* 62–70 (1977).

21	James, G. D.; Sealey, J. E.; Alderman, M.; Ljungman, S.; Mueller, F. B.; Pecker, M. S.; Laragh, J. H.: A longitudinal study of urinary creatinine and creatinine clearance in normal subjects. Race, sex, and age differences. Am. J. Hypertens. *1:* 124–131 (1988).

22	Norden, G.; Bjorck, S.; Granerus, G.; Nyberg, G.: Estimation of renal function in diabetic nephropathy. Nephron *47:* 36–42 (1987).

Clinton D. Brown, MD, Department of Medicine, State University of New York,
Health Science Center at Brooklyn, 450 Clarkson Avenue, Box 52,
Brooklyn, NY 11203 (USA)

Gurland HJ, Moran J, Samtleben W, Scigalla P, Wieczorek L (eds): Erythropoietin in
Renal and Non-Renal Anemias. Contrib Nephrol. Basel, Karger, 1991, vol 88, pp 190–191

Discussion

to the Paper by C. D. Brown and E. A. Friedman

Rich (Ulm): Did you measure the EPO levels in the serum at the beginning of the study?

Brown: The endogenous EPO levels? No.

Koene (Nijmegen): It is surprising that after 1 year there was no increase in the mean serum creatinine values in your patients. Were there large differences between individual patients?

Brown: No, if you look at the individual responses, there were minor changes either way. Two went down, two went up and one just stayed in the middle. So, given the fact there is a small number of patients this might just have been the luck of the draw. We were quite surprised that there was no deterioration in renal function, and I think that one of the things we didn't appreciate was the fact that all these patients had an appropriate viscosity to begin with. There are patients who are diabetic who have an elevated viscosity, and they may have problems when you increase their hematocrit because there may be a disproportional rise in viscosity.

Scigalla (Mannheim): You are using as a target hematocrit 40%, and that is different to the target in patients on maintenance dialysis. My question is, what is the rationale for this higher target hematocrit in your predialytic patients?

Brown: I think now we probably would opt for a target hematocrit of about 37%. We tried to keep the hematocrit above 35 and a lot of the patients were 39, one was 42 or 43. It turned out that even with lowering the dose, there were some patients, one in particular, who had a persistent very good response to EPO.

Scigalla: Do you think that you would have an incremental improvement if you increased the hematocrit from 30 to 37?

Brown: I think so. We had people who started with hematocrits of 31 who subjectively felt better and were able to do more work. So I think – again, it is a small number of people – there is a difference between 30 and 37, but probably more risk than benefit between 37 and 45.

Williams (Cardiff): To go back to the lack of change in creatinine, I noticed on your blood pressure slide that the diastolic pressures were lower after a year's treatment. Do you think that your patients may have had better antihypertensive therapy during this period of treatment and therefore have maintained their renal function?

Brown: No, as I said before, there was some initial change in antihypertensive medicines but there was no significant difference between pre- and post-treatment blood pressure. So I don't think that explains the preservation of renal function.

Samtleben (Munich): How many of your patients received ACE inhibitors?

Brown: Three.

Samtleben: Were they put on these drugs during the study period?

Brown: They started on these drugs.

Gurland HJ, Moran J, Samtleben W, Scigalla P, Wieczorek L (eds): Erythropoietin in Renal and Non-Renal Anemias. Contrib Nephrol. Basel, Karger, 1991, vol 88, pp 192–199

Renal Function of Pre-Dialysis Patients during Treatment with Recombinant Human Erythropoietin

Robert A. P. Koene, Leon A. M. Frenken

Department of Medicine, Division of Nephrology, University Hospital Nijmegen, The Netherlands

The indications for treatment with recombinant human erythropoietin (rhEPO) in predialysis patients with anaemia do not differ from those in patients treated with haemodialysis or peritoneal dialysis. Experience has shown that the response to the treatment and its side effects are also comparable in these patient groups. At least one qualification must be made regarding a possible influence of the rise in haematocrit (Hct) on renal haemodynamics. In dialysis patients changes in renal blood flow and glomerular filtration rate (GFR) are obviously of no special concern, but in predialysis patients these changes might adversely affect renal function and thus accelerate the rate of progression of renal failure. This concern regarding possible harmful effects of treatment with rhEPO on renal function stems from both theoretical considerations and experimental evidence.

Influence of Increased Haematocrit on Blood Pressure and Renal Haemodynamics

The Hct is the most important determinant of whole blood viscosity. An increase in viscosity leads to an increase in systemic peripheral vascular resistance. Furthermore, the rise in haemoglobin values occurring during treatment with rhEPO will improve oxygenation, and as a consequence, hypoxic vasodilatation, which is always present during the anaemic state, will disappear. This will result in an additional rise in peripheral vascular resistance [1]. It is therefore not surprising that a rise in Hct may lead to systemic hypertension. Such a development is very likely when the Hct is raised within a short period of time. At later stages a haemodynamic resetting may occur with restoration of normal blood pressure, especially in individuals in whom blood pressure was previously normal. In patients with pre-existing hypertension, these secondary compensatory changes appear to be less complete or do not occur at all. Accordingly, large increases in blood pressure during rhEPO treatment have most often been observed in patients with pre-existing hypertension [1].

The detrimental effects of systemic hypertension on renal function are well established. However, the rise in Hct has special consequences for the renal vasculature and this might cause renal damage independently of the effects of systemic hypertension. A rise in blood viscosity causes a disproportionate increase in vascular resistance in the efferent arterioles of the glomerulus. First, the Hct and thus blood viscosity are higher in the efferent arteriole as a consequence of fluid removal by glomerular filtration. Secondly, according to Poiseuille's law, an increase in viscosity will cause a greater rise of efferent than of afferent vascular resistance, since the efferent arterioles are smaller in calibre and have a greater length than the afferent arterioles. Thus, the anatomic structure of the glomerulus and the presence of glomerular filtration per se are responsible for a rise in glomerular intracapillary pressure when the anaemia is corrected. It is important to note that these changes would also be expected to occur even if systemic blood pressure were to remain unaltered. In addition, it has been reported that plasma renin activity may rise with increasing Hct. This may result in an additional rise in efferent vascular resistance via angiotensin-mediated vasoconstriction of the efferent arteriole [2].

Results of Experimental Studies

Studies in experimental animals and in man are generally in keeping with the theoretical considerations discussed above. In human individuals with chronic polycythaemia and increased blood viscosity, renal haemodynamic studies showed an increased filtration fraction (FF), suggesting the presence of an increased glomerular capillary pressure [3, 4]. These changes were attenuated by phlebotomy or isovolemic erythropheresis. The FF also rose in dogs when the Hct was increased by subjecting the animals to low barometric pressure for 6 h daily over 6–10 weeks [5]. Nashat and Portal [6] observed similar increases in FF in dogs when the Hct was raised by isovolemic exchange transfusions. They demonstrated a direct relationship between the rise in Hct and FF, which led them to speculate that a purely passive alteration of the efferent arteriolar resistance accounted for the changes in FF during these acute experiments.

More direct evidence for a rise in glomerular capillary hydraulic pressure has been provided by Myers et al. [7] in experiments in rats in which micropuncture techniques were used. The Hct was artificially raised from a mean normal level of 0.51 to 0.62 l/l with isovolemic exchange of recipient blood by high Hct donor blood. The investigators observed an acute decline in single nephron glomerular filtration rate (SNGFR) but an even larger decline in glomerular plasma flow, resulting in a marked rise in single nephron FF. This was caused by a large rise in glomerular capillary pressure as a result of a highly significant increase in efferent arteriolar resistance.

The detrimental effects of a constantly raised glomerular capillary pressure on renal function have been demonstrated in experiments in rats with partial renal ablation [8]. Sustained glomerular hypertension caused injury to the renal structures resulting in focal glomerulosclerosis and progressive renal insufficiency. All interventions that prevented the development of glomerular hypertension also retarded the rate of progression of the renal disease [9].

The above-mentioned experiments of Myers et al. were performed in polycythaemic animals. One might argue that changes observed in polycythaemic states do not necessarily occur in the clinical situation during treatment with rhEPO when low Hct levels are corrected to normal or, more often, to subnormal values. However, the results of experiments in anaemic rats treated with rhEPO have suggested a detrimental effect on renal function. Gretz et al. [10] were the first to show that five-sixths nephrectomized rats treated with rhEPO had died from acute renal failure at a time when all control animals were still alive. These findings were confirmed by Garcia et al. [11], who performed additional renal haemodynamic studies in a similar remnant kidney model. When the anaemia that developed in these rats after five-sixths nephrectomy was prevented by the administration of rhEPO, the animals exhibited increased proteinuria and more extensive signs of glomerulosclerosis compared to control animal not receiving rhEPO. On the other hand, in animals in which the anaemia was made more severe by feeding an iron-deficient diet, less renal damage developed than in the controls. Micropuncture studies of the kidneys of rhEPO-treated animals showed significantly lower SNGFR and renal plasma flow. In particular, efferent arteriolar resistance was higher. Glomerular capillary hydraulic pressure was highest in the rhEPO-treated animals, whereas anaemia prevented the development of glomerular capillary hypertension.

Table 1. Renal function during the correction phase of rhEPO treatment

Ref.	Patients, n	Duration weeks	Mean serum creatinine, μmol/l[1]	
			before	after
12	11	8	473	518
13	24	8	738	755
14	7	4	469	451

[1] None of the changes is significant.

These observations raised serious concern about the safety of treating predialysis patients with rhEPO. However, it should be understood that there was also a considerable increase in systemic blood pressure during rhEPO treatment in the rat experiments. Systolic blood pressure measured by the tail cuff method rose in control animals from basal levels of 130 mm Hg to a maximum of 185 mm Hg at 6 weeks after the partial nephrectomy. In rhEPO-treated rats, blood pressure was even higher at each time point of the study, and reached a maximum value as high as 210 mm Hg. A significant rise in systemic blood pressure did not occur in the iron-deficient, anaemic animals. In the absence of experiments in which the development of hypertension in rhEPO-treated animals was prevented by the administration of antihypertensive drugs, it remains difficult to decide whether the accelerated renal damage was caused by the systemic hypertension, the glomerular capillary hypertension, or by both factors in concert. Since we know that systemic hypertension per se has a detrimental effect on the kidney, it seems likely that it was at least a significant factor.

Results of Clinical Studies during the Correction Phase

In studies with rhEPO in predialysis patients, almost all investigators have tried to monitor blood pressure meticulously and to adjust antihypertensive treatment when necessary. So far, the experience suggests, that under these conditions, detrimental effects on renal function as observed in rats do not occur. Table 1 summarizes the available data on changes of serum creatinine levels after 8 weeks of rhEPO treatment. In none of the studies, comprising a total of 42 patients, was there a significant increase in the mean

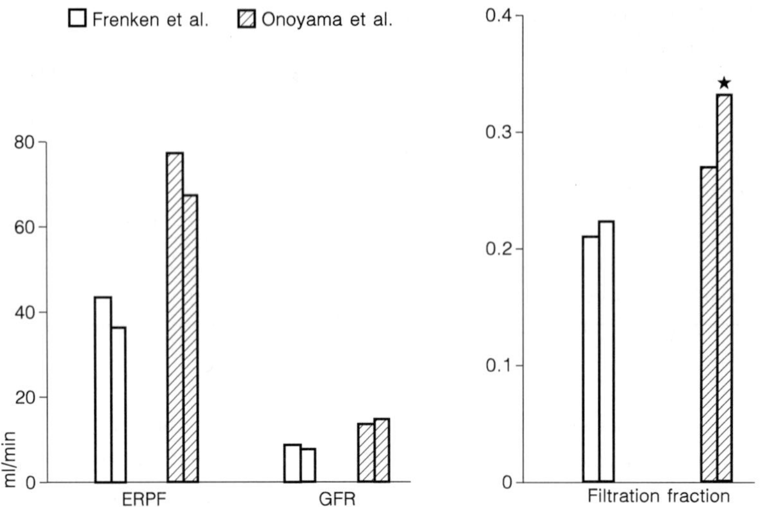

Fig. 1. Renal haemodynamic studies during rhEPO treatment. The first bar in each cluster represents the determinations before the start of the treatment. Values depicted in each second bar were obtained after 12 weeks of treatment (Frenken et al. [15]) or after 4 weeks (Onoyama et al. [14]). Results are means of observations in 8 and 7 patients respectively. The asterisk denotes a statistically significant difference.

serum creatinine value during the correction phase. Therefore, it can be safely concluded that a relatively rapid correction of the anaemia in 4–8 weeks does not have acute detrimental effects on renal function.

In a limited number of patients, data from additional renal haemodynamic studies during treatment with rhEPO are available. Frenken et al. [15] studied *p*-aminohippurate and inulin clearances, as measures of effective renal plasma flow (ERPF) and glomerular filtration rate (GFR) respectively, before and after 12 weeks of treatment. During the period of observation the mean Hct rose from 0.24 to 0.39 l/l. The results of these studies, as depicted in figure 1, demonstrated small and nonsignificant decreases in the mean values of both ERPF and GFR after the correction of the anaemia at 12 weeks. FF also remained unchanged. Onoyama et al. [14], using the same technique, studied 7 patients after 4 weeks of treatment when mean Hct had increased from 0.21 to 0.27. They observed a nonsignificant decrease in ERPF accompanied by a small nonsignificant increase in GFR. As a result there was a significant rise in FF (fig. 1). There was however an important difference between the groups of patients in the two clinical studies. In the first study, patients in whom hypertension developed received additional antihypertensive treatment, whereas in the study of Onoyama et al. no attempt was made to control blood pressure. As a consequence, blood pressure in this latter study rose significantly from a mean value of 171/93 mm Hg before treatment to 190/105 mm Hg. By contrast, mean blood pressure values in Frenken's study were 150/92 mm Hg before treatment and had remained stable after 12 weeks of treatment (148/91 mm Hg). These results show striking similarities to the observations made by Garcia et al. [11] in the rhEPO-treated rats with remnant kidneys. In the rat experiments, a rise in blood pressure was accompanied by an increased glomerular pressure and by a rise of FF. Such a rise in FF also occurred in the clinical situation, unless the development of systemic hypertension was prevented by effective antihypertensive treatment. If the events occurring in man are analogous to those observed in the micropuncture studies in rats, an increase of FF during rhEPO treatment will also reflect a rise in glomerular pressure. Careful control of blood pressure seems therefore of the utmost importance when predialysis patients are treated with rhEPO.

Results of Clinical Studies during the Maintenance Phase

With regard to the effects of long-term correction of the anaemia on renal function, the available data do not yet permit definitive conclusions. Eschbach et al. [16] compared the slopes of the reciprocal serum creatinine values versus time curves during rhEPO therapy with the pretreatment slopes in 17 patients, and found no significant change. This was confirmed in two subsequent studies suggesting that there was no significant change in the rate of progression of renal failure (table 2). However, small changes in progression rate will be difficult to detect. A placebo-controlled trial with a prolonged observation period in a large group of predialysis patients would be necessary to exclude any possible damage. However, it is highly questionable whether a placebo-treated control group can be recruited. A possible alternative would be to study a large group of predialysis patients in whom pretreatment follow-up is long enough to permit calculations of the rates of progression of their renal failure and compare these with the progression rates during one or several years of rhEPO treatment. Ideally, glomerular filtration in these patients should be determined, both before and during rhEPO treatment, by clearance methods which give more reliable information than slopes of reciprocal serum creatinines or creatinine clearances.

Table 2. Progression of renal failure during maintenance therapy with rhEPO: slopes of the regression lines of mean reciprocal serum creatinine values vs. time

Ref.	Patients, n	Mean follow-up months	Mean slope[1]	
			before	end
16	17	7	no change	
13	14	9	–0.036	–0.031
12	10	12	–0.0058	–0.0054

[1] None of the changes is significant.

Conclusion

On the basis of current information, it can be expected that any detrimental effect on renal function will not be very large. Moreover, the benefits of treatment with rhEPO will probably outweigh a possible adverse effect on renal function. Therefore, predialysis patients seem to be eligible for treatment with rhEPO, provided that blood pressure is carefully monitored and controlled.

References

1 Raine, A. E. G.: Hypertension, blood viscosity, and cardiovascular morbidity in renal failure: Implications of erythropoietin therapy. Lancet *i:* 97–99 (1988).
2 Simchon, S.; Chen, R. Y.; Carlin, R. D.; Fan, F. C.; Jan, K. M.; Chien, S.: Effect of blood viscosity on plasma renin activity and renal hemodynamics. Am. J. Physiol. *250:* F40–46 (1986).
3 Scott, H. W.; Elliott, S. R.: Renal haemodynamics in congenital cyanotic heart disease. Johns Hopkins Hosp. Bull. *86:* 58–71 (1950).
4 De Wardener, H. E.; McSwiney, R. R.; Portal, R. W.: Renal haemodynamics in primary polycythaemia. Lancet *ii:* 204–206 (1951).
5 Marshall, L. H.; Hanna, C. H.; Specht, H.: Renal function in the dog during increased blood viscosity produced by simulated altitude exposure. Am. J. Physiol. *171:* 499–505 (1952).
6 Nashat, F. S.; Portal, R. W.: The effects of changes in haematocrit on renal function. J. Physiol. (Lond.) *193:* 513–522 (1967).
7 Myers, B. D.; Deen, W.; Robertson, C. R.; Brenner, B. M.: Dynamics of glomerular ultrafiltration in the rat. VIII. Effects of hematocrit. Circ. Res. *36:* 425–435 (1975).

8   Meyer, T. W.; Rennke, H. G.: Progressive glomerular injury after limited renal infarction in the rat. Am. J. Physiol. *254:* F856–862 (1988).

9   Brenner, B. M.; Meyer, T.; Hostetter, T.: Dietary protein intake and the progressive nature of kidney disease. The role of hemodynamically mediated glomerular injury in the pathogenesis of progressive glomerular sclerosis in aging, renal ablation, and intrinsic renal disease. N. Engl. J. Med. *307:* 652–659 (1982).

10 Gretz, N.; Lasserre, J. J.; Meisinger, E.; Strauch, M.; Waldherr, R.; Kraft, K.; Weidler, A.: Potential side-effects of erythropoietin. Lancet *i:* 46 (1987).

11 Garcia, D. L.; Anderson, S.; Rennke, H. G.; Brenner, B. M.: Anemia lessens and its prevention with recombinant erythropoietin worsens glomerular injury and hypertension in rats with reduced renal mass. Proc. Natl. Acad. Sci. USA *85:* 6142–6146 (1988).

12 Lim, V. S.; DeGowin, R. L.; Zavala, D.; Kirchner, P. T.; Abels, R.; Perry, P.; Fangman, J.: Recombinant human erythropoietin treatment in pre-dialysis patients. Ann. Intern. Med. *110:* 108–114 (1989).

13 Frenken, L. A. M.; Verberckmoes, R.; Michielsen, P.; Koene, R. A. P.: Efficacy and tolerance of treatment with recombinant-human erythropoietin in chronic renal failure (pre-dialysis) patients. Nephrol. Dial. Transplant. *4:* 782–786 (1989).

14 Onoyama, K.; Kumagai, H.; Shimamatsu, K.; Fujishima M.: Effects of human recombinant erythropoietin on anaemia, systemic haemodynamics and renal function in predialysis renal failure patients. Nephrol. Dial. Transplant. *4:* 966–970 (1989).

15 Frenken, L. A. M.; Wetzels, J. F. M.; Sluiter, H. E.; Schrijver, G.; Koene, R. A. P.: Renal haemodynamics and effects of captopril in pre-dialysis patients treated with recombinant human erythropoietin (abstract). Kidney Int. *37:* 551 (1990).

16 Eschbach, J. W.; Kelley, M. R.; Haley, R. N.; Abels, R. I.; Adamson, J. W.: Treatment on the anemia of progressive renal failure with recombinant human erythropoietin. N. Engl. J. Med. *321:* 158–163 (1989).

Robert A. P. Koene, MD, Department of Medicine, Division of Nephrology, University Hospital Nijmegen, PO Box 9101, NL–6500 HB Nijmegen (The Netherlands)

Gurland HJ, Moran J, Samtleben W, Scigalla P, Wieczorek L (eds): Erythropoietin in Renal and Non-Renal Anemias. Contrib Nephrol. Basel, Karger, 1991, vol 88, p 200

Discussion

to the Paper by R. A. P. Koene and L. A. M. Frenken

Koch (Hannover): I doubt the validity of the Garcia data for the purposes of comparison. You have already criticized them for not treating the blood pressure, but we also have to realize that they injected rhEPO into rats. As far as I recall data presented by Dr. Kurtz, he saw interstitial and peritubular morphological changes in rats treated with rhEPO. So I think this is a situation which cannot be used for comparison with your human data, where there was no species difference in the EPO given.

Koene: Has blood pressure been measured in the experiment you refer to? It might be that histological changes occurred due to a rise in blood pressure in these animals. The fact that an increased filtration fraction is observed in rats and man when the blood pressure is not controlled suggests in my view that the rise in systemic blood pressure indeed might play a dominant role in causing renal damage in pre-dialysis patients treated with rhEPO.

Shaldon (Montpellier): I made this point from the Japanese data. One would conclude that if you do not treat the blood pressure you'll get a rise in blood pressure. Do you consider that it is justified to increase hypertensive therapy in order to raise the hematocrit of the preterminal renal failure patient, or did I misunderstand you?

Koene: The Japanese investigators did not treat the patients for hypertension. Their paper does not state whether the patients were treated before rhEPO was started.

Shaldon: My question should be rephrased: Did you have to increase or start antihypertensive therapy in any of these patients in order to maintain normotension during EPO therapy?

Koene: Of 24 predialysis patients we had 9 in whom we had to increase antihypertensive drugs to keep blood pressure stable. That is also the experience in other studies reported in the literature, that in some patients antihypertensive therapy has to be increased to keep the blood pressure stable.

Shaldon: So I will rephrase my question again: If you were not hypertensive and you became hypertensive on EPO therapy would the trade off justify the therapy?

Koene: You have to ask the patient, I think. I believe he or she would say yes, and would take additional antihypertensive drugs in exchange for an improved well-being.

Experience with Recombinant Human Erythropoietin in Children with Renal Anemia

Gurland HJ, Moran J, Samtleben W, Scigalla P, Wieczorek L (eds): Erythropoietin in Renal and Non-Renal Anemias. Contrib Nephrol. Basel, Karger, 1991, vol 88, pp 201–211

Effect of Recombinant Human Erythropoietin Treatment on Renal Anemia and Body Growth of Children with End-Stage Renal Disease

P. Scigalla

On behalf of the European Multicenter Study Group

Although progress in dialysis and transplantation has greatly improved the survival rate of children with end-stage renal disease (ESRD), growth retardation could until recently not be influenced greatly. Only the recent results of clinical studies with recombinant human growth hormone promise a solution to this problem in pediatric nephrology [1]. The EDTA data for 376 pediatric patients who were aged 21 years or older at the time of assessment give a mean ultimate height between 1 and 2 standard deviations (SD) below the mean for females (n = 186) and 2 SD below the mean for males [2].

The earlier chronic renal insufficiency starts and the longer it lasts, the more severe is the growth retardation [3]. Small children are particularly affected because they undergo a period of extremely rapid growth. During the first 2 years, the body size increases by more than 50% and the calorie and protein intake is 2–8 times that of an adult [4].

The growth retardation of uremic children is a multifactorial phenomenon in which the importance of the individual factors varies from patient to patient [5]. The most important pathogenetic factors have been postulated to be as follows [6]: low protein and energy intake; renal osteodystrophy; abnormal endocrine function; acidosis; water/electrolyte disturbances; uremic toxicity, and anemia.

As demonstrated by many authors, renal anemia can be corrected with recombinant human erythropoietin (rhEPO) [7–10]. It was still unknown, however, whether the correction of renal anemia also improves the body growth of uremic children and whether a catch-up growth sets in, as may occur after kidney transplantations. For this reason, we have investigated the effect of the correction of renal anemia with rhEPO on the body growth of children with ESRD.

Table 1. Pediatric nephrologic centers participating in the European Multicenter Study (n = 29)

Clinical center	Responsible trialist	Clinical center	Responsible trialist
Germany		*Switzerland*	
Hanover	PD Dr. Offner	Zürich	Prof. Leumann
Hamburg	Dr. Schwarke		
Berlin	Prof. Zoellner	*Belgium*	
Essen/Essen-Moers	PD Dr. Bonzel/	Brussels	Dr. Janssen
	Prof. Dr. Pistor	Antwerp	Dr. Roodhooft
Cologne	PD Dr. v. Lilien	Liege	Dr. Voz
Marburg	Dr. Gordjani	Leuven	Dr. van Damme
Frankfurt/Main	Prof. Dr. Dippell	*The Netherlands*	
Heidelberg	Prof. Müller-Wiefel	Nijmegen	Dr. Schröder
Freiburg	PD Dr. Leititis	*Austria*	
Münster	Prof. Bulla	Vienna	Dr. Balzar
France			
Strasbourg	Prof. Geisert/Dr. Fischbach		
Lille	Dr. Foulard		
Reims	Dr. Roussel		
Nancy	Dr. André		
Paris	Prof. Bensmann		
Paris	Prof. Loirat/Dr. Maisin		
Paris	Prof. Broyer/Dr. Niaudet		
Nantes	Prof. Guyot		
Rouen	Dr. Landthaler		
Toulouse	Prof. Barthe/Dr. Bouissou		
Clermont-Ferrand	Dr. Palcoux		

Patients and Methods

One hundred and twenty children with ESRD were treated with rhEPO for an average of 41 weeks (range 6–115 weeks) until October 31, 1989, in 29 pediatric nephrology centers. Table 1 lists the clinical centers with the responsible trialists.

Of the 120 ESRD children treated with rhEPO (Boehringer Mannheim GmbH, FRG), 65 were boys (54%) and 55 were girls (46%) with an average age of 13 years (range 2–21 years). The mean duration of dialysis upon entering the trial was 23 months (range 3–14 months). 108 children were treated with hemodialysis (3 × 4–5 h/week) and 12 children were on continuous ambulatory peritoneal dialysis (CAPD).

Before the institution of rhEPO therapy, all children suffered from marked normochromic hypoproliferative anemia. The mean hemoglobin value was 6.5 g/dl, the mean hematocrit was 19.5 vol% and the mean MCHC was 34.2 g/dl. The mean corrected reticulocytes

Table 2. Hematological baseline values (n = 120) in children with ESRD at the onset of RhEPO treatment (median, 25th and 75th interquartiles)

Hematological values	Median	Interquartile range
Hemoglobin, g/dl	6.5	5.9– 7.3
Hematocrit, vol %	19.5	17.4–21.4
MCHC, g/dl	34.2	33.0–35.1
Corrected reticulocytes, %	0.42	0.27– 0.63
Transfusion dependency, n		103
%		86
Serum ferritin, ng/ml	650	222–1,397

were 0.42. Of the 120 ESRD children treated with rhEPO, 103 (86%) were transfusion-dependent until the start of the trial. Most of the polytransfused children suffered from iron overload with mean serum ferritin levels of 650 ng/ml (table 2).

In order to be able to compare the growth of children of different sex and age, the growth data have to be standardized [11, 12]. For this purpose, the SD score for the body height is used which is calculated according to the following formula [13]:

$$\text{Height score} = \frac{\text{Height} - \text{Mean height for age}}{\text{SD of height for age}}$$

In the normal population the SD score ranges between -2 and $+2$ with a mean of zero [14]. In contrast to centile scores, there are no limitations to the values – a very short child has increasingly negative values and a tall child has increasingly positive values. Because of the lack of upper and lower limits, SDs are very easy to use for further statistical analysis.

Most of the children included in the trial (75.5%) were growth-retarded, i.e. their height was below the -2 SD score at the start of the trial.

The median SD score for height was particularly reduced in the group of children with an age up to 5 years. The median SD score in this group is -4.3 (range -5.6 to -1.1). In the other groups of ages the median SD score is approximately -3 (age 5 to $\leq$10 years; range -4.5 to -0.4; $>$10 to $\leq$15 years; range -7.5 to 0.8; $>$15 years; range -7.2 to -0.8). Further, the growth retardation was particularly distinct in children having hereditary nephropathies as primary diseases. In this group the growth retardation was most pronounced in children with cystinosis; the median SD score here was -4.3. On the other hand, there was no difference in the degree of growth retardation between the children with congenital and acquired nephropathies (median SD score of children with congenital nephropathies [-2.79] and with acquired nephropathies [-2.75]).

Study Protocol

After a 14-day run-in period in which the pretreatment values for the individuals safety and efficacy parameters were repeatedly determined, rhEPO therapy was started in 120 anemic and growth-retarded children with ESRD. The children in the chronic hemodialysis

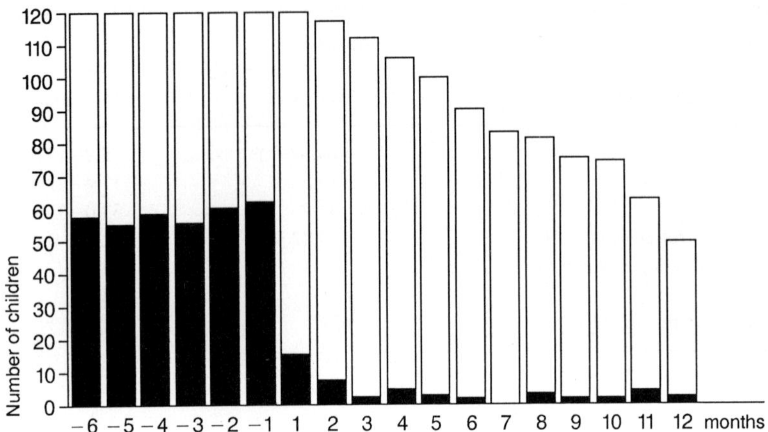

Fig. 1. Number of children with transfusions before and during the first 12 months of rhEPO treatment in children with ESRD. ■ = Blood transfusion; □ = no blood transfusion.

program were intravenously administered an initial dose of 40–100 U/kg b.w. 3 ×/week at the end of hemodialysis. The 12 children in the CAPD program initially received 300 U/kg b.w. once a week. If the target hematocrit of approximately 30 vol% was reached, in the following maintenance period the rhEPO dose was adjusted according to the curve of hematocrit.

Results

Effect of rhEPO Treatment on Renal Anemia

Transfusion dependency was eliminated and renal anemia corrected in all children. As shown in figure 1, immediately after the onset of rhEPO therapy a marked reduction in transfusion rate occurred. Any transfusions performed after the second month of rhEPO therapy were always necessitated by acute indications, e.g. gastrointestinal bleeding or epistaxis, infections such as pneumonia, CMV infection or pyelonephritis or shunt thromboses and shunt revisions.

The hematocrit rose under rhEPO treatment; the weekly increment of hematocrit varied between 0.36 and 1.27 vol% (25th and 75th interquartiles;

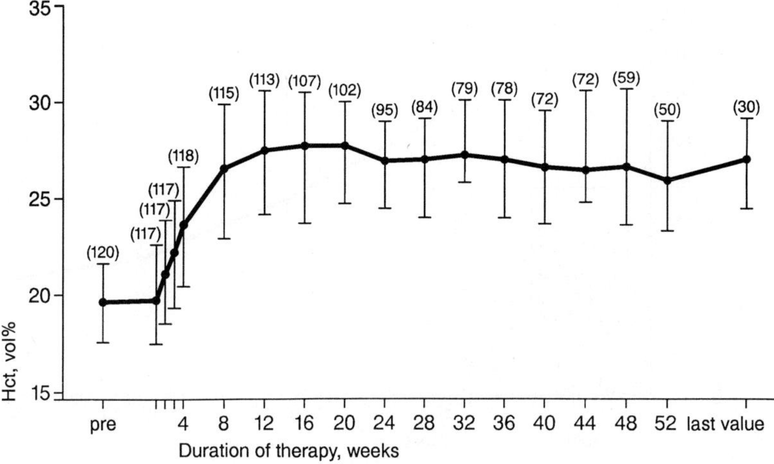

Fig. 2. Course of hematocrit in children with ESRD on rhEPO therapy (median, 25th and 75th interquartile range). Number of patients at each time point in parentheses.

mean 0.9 vol%). The mean target hematocrit of 30 vol% was reached after approximately 3 months. Thereafter the rhEPO dose was adjusted to maintain the corrected hematocrit (fig. 2).

After 12 months, the median rhEPO dose administered was 138 U/kg b.w./week. It is interesting to note that the rhEPO maintenance dose is age-dependent. In the group of children with an age up to 5 years the median weekly rhEPO maintenance dose (rhEPO-MD) was 321 U/kg b.w. (25th and 75th interquartile range: 115 and 441 U/kg b.w., respectively). The weekly rhEPO maintenance dose was lower the older the children were. The median rhEPO-MD in the group of children with an age >5–10 years was 230 U/kg b.w. (25th and 75th interquartile range: 185 and 377 U/kg b.w., respectively) and in the group of children with an age >10–15 years 158 U/kg b.w. (25th and 75th interquartile range: 118 and 219 U/kg b.w., respectively). The lowest rhEPO-MD was in the group of adolescents with an age >15 years, the median rhEPO-MD was 136 U/kg b.w. (25th and 75th interquartile range: 82 and 222 U/kg b.w., respectively), These results show that the younger the children, the more rhEPO is required to keep the hematocrit at a level of 28–30 vol% (fig. 3).

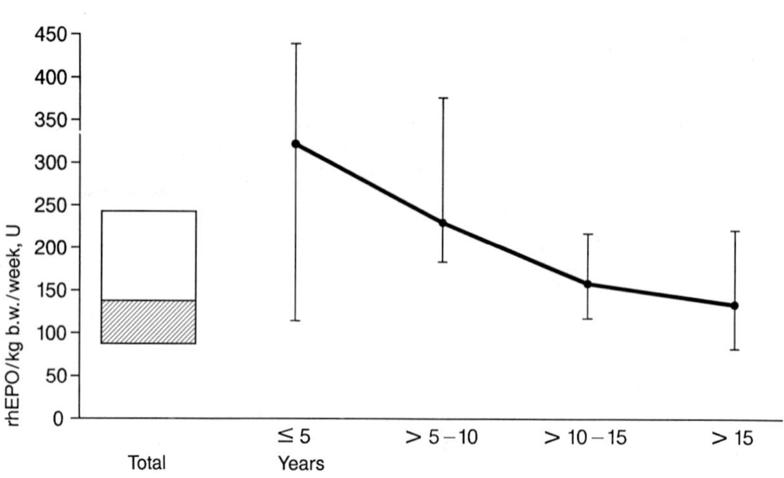

Fig. 3. Weekly rhEPO maintenance dose in children with ESRD after 1 year rhEPO treatment in relation to the chronological age.

Effect of rhEPO on Growth

First of all, the SD scores determined before the start of therapy were compared to those obtained after a minimum of 150 or 300 days of rhEPO therapy. The 76 children who had been treated with rhEPO for over 150 days (average: 351 days) showed no significant changes in the SD score. Even when the children (n = 54) were treated with rhEPO for a minimum of 300 days (average: 409 days), no significant changes were determined in the SD score (table 3).

Further, we looked for a relationship between the changes in SD height scores and the chronological age of the children. Therefore, the children were assigned according to their age to 4 groups (group 1, ≤5 years; group 2, >5 to ≤10 years; group 3, >10 to ≤15 years; group 4, >15 years). The respective courses of the SD height scores were analyzed (fig. 4a–d) and the corresponding statistical values were calculated (table 4).

The analysis of the individual SD height scores for the children in groups 1 and 2 did not reveal any significant changes (fig. 4a, b). In contrast in the >10- to 15-year age group a slight drop in the SD scores is apparent (fig. 4c). However, this drop is not the result of the rhEPO therapy but is due to the fact

Table 3. Changes in SD height scores in children with ESRD on rhEPO treatment

Time rhEPO treatment	n	Δ SD scores of height		
		> +0.25	−0.25 to +0.25	<−0.25
>150 days	76	13	36	27
>300 days	54	10	23	21

Table 4. Changes in SD height scores in children with ESRD on rhEPO treatment (>150 days) in relation to the chronological age

Age group, years	Δ SD scores of height		
	> +0.25	−0.25 to +0.25	<−0.25
≤5	0	2	1
> 5−≤10	3	7	7
>10−≤15	3	16	18
>15	7	11	1

that puberty and growth episodes are normally delayed in uremic children. The drop is thus accounted for by the fact that the SD scores were calculated according to the chronological age of healthy children without making allowance for the stage of puberty or the bone age. Children over 15 years of age show no changes in the SD score (fig. 4d).

Further, it should be investigated whether there is a relationship between the primary diseases leading to uremia and the changes in SD height scores under rhEPO treatment. It is possible that in congenital nephropathies, for example in kidney hypoplasia or dysplasia, not only the growth potential of the kidneys, but of the child as a whole may be impaired. If this phenomenon is significant it may be that the correction of renal anemia is less effective in stimulating growth in children with congenital nephropathies than in patients with hereditary or acquired diseases. To clarify this question, the children were assigned to different groups according to the primary disease leading to uremia. Table 4 shows the SD scores for the body heights determined before

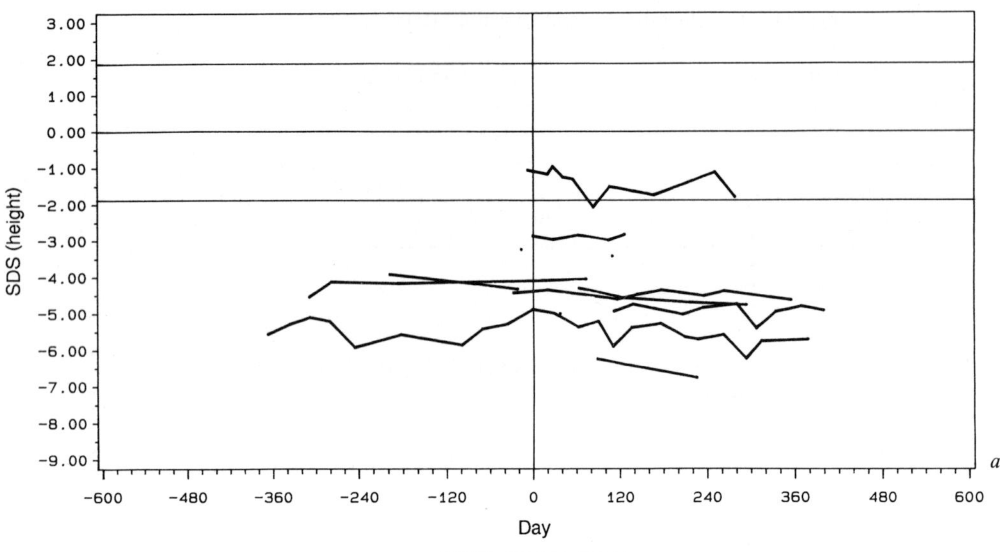

Stratified to age groups

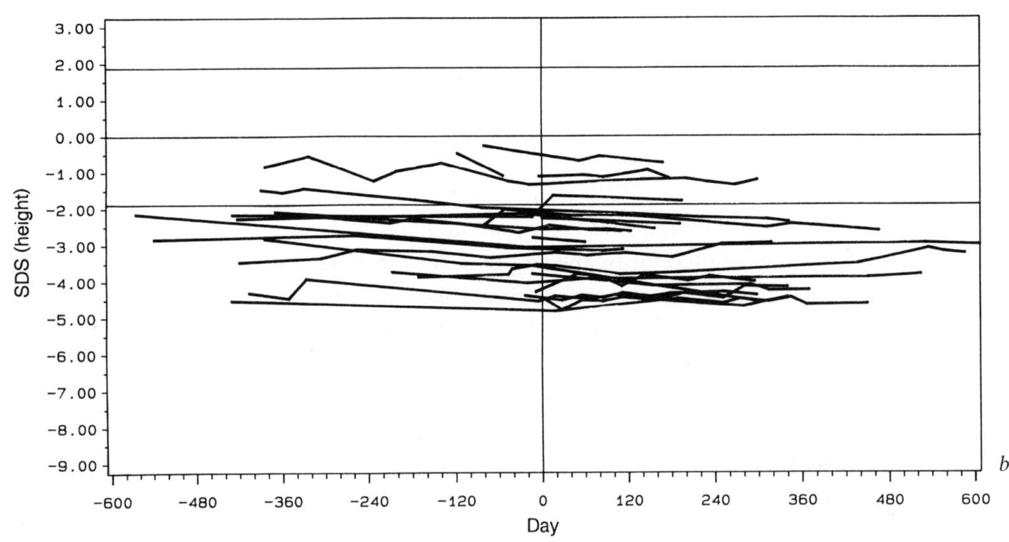

Stratified to age groups

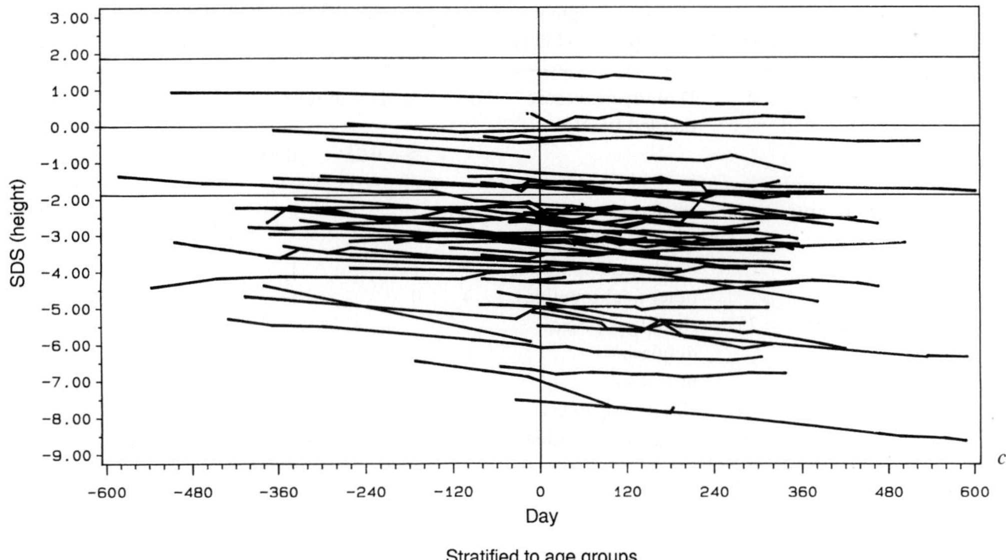

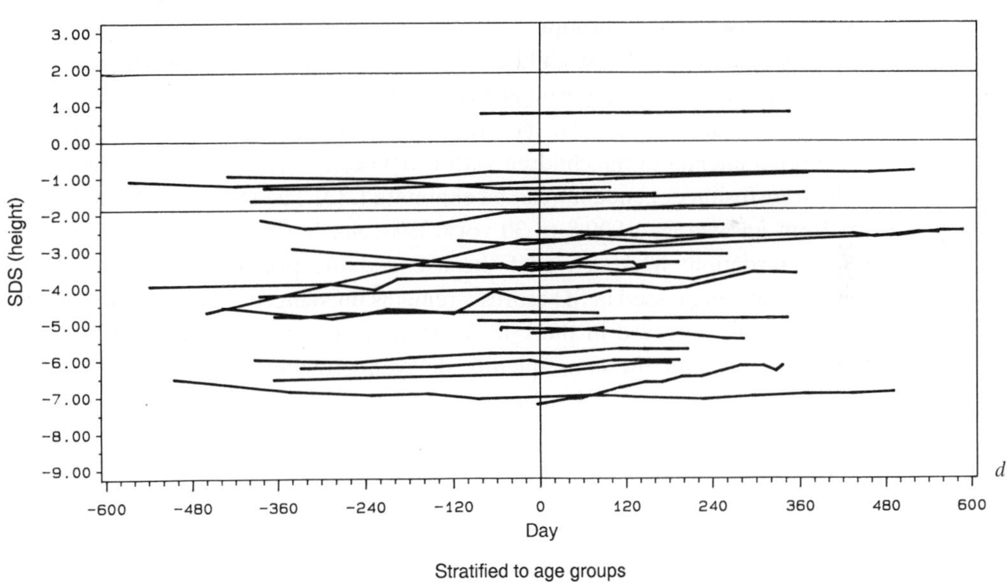

Fig. 4. Individual height scores in relation to chronological age in children with ESRD on rhEPO therapy. Reference lines represent the 3rd, 50th and 97th percentiles of the normal population [15]. Age groups: (*a*) <5 years, (*b*) 6–10 years, (*c*) >10–15 years, (*d*) >15 years.

Table 5. Changes in SD scores of height in relation to the underlying nephropathies in children with ESRD on rhEPO therapy (>150 days)

Type of disease	n	Underlying disease that led ESRD	n	Δ SD scores of height		
				>+0.25	−0.25 to +0.25	<−0.25
Hereditary	15	cystinosis	6	2	3	1
		nephronophtisis/ oligomeganephronia	5	1	1	3
		other nephropathies	4	0	1	3
Congenital	25	renal hypoplasia/ dysplasia	8	1	5	2
		uropathies	17	4	8	5
Acquired	36	glomerulopathies	31	4	17	10
		other nephropathies	5	1	1	3

and after the correction of renal anemia, classified according to hereditary, congenital and acquired diseases. It is obvious that there are no significant differences between these groups.

To summarize: (1) Most children with ESRD who are in the chronic dialysis program show a significant growth retardation. The younger the child and the longer uremia persists, the more severe is the growth retardation. (2) The renal anemia of the children with ESRD can be treated with rhEPO and the transfusion dependency can be eliminated. (3) The increase in hematocrit from an average of 19.8 to 30 vol% does *not* have any effect on the growth retardation; irrespective of the age and the primary disease, the growth deficit – expressed in SD scores – remains unchanged. The slight drop in the SD score observed in the >10- to 15-year age group is the result of delayed puberty and the consequently delayed growth episodes of these children.

References

1   Mehls O, Ritz E, Honzinger EB, et al: Improvement of growth and food utilization by recombinant growth hormone in uraemia. Kidney Int 1988;33:45–52.
2   Combined report on regular dialysis and transplantation of children in Europe. EDTA 1985;82–88.
3   Rizzoni G, Basso T, Setari M: Growth in children with chronic renal failure on conservative treatment. Kidney Int 1984;26:52–58.

4   Holliday MA: Calorie intake and growth in uraemia. Kidney Int 1975;7(suppl 2):73–78.
5   Mehls O, Ritz E, Gilli G, et al: Growth in renal failure. Nephron 1987;21:237–247.
6   Rees L, Rigden SPA, Chantler C, Maycock GB: Growth and methods of improving growth in chronic renal failure managed conservatively. Pediatr Adolesc Endocrinol. Basel, Karger, 1989, vol 20, pp 15–26.
7   Eschbach JW, Egrie JC, Downing MR, Browne JK, Adamson JW: Correction of the anemia of end-stage renal disease with recombinant human erythropoietin. N Engl J Med 1987;316:73–78.
8   Winearls CG, Oliver DO, Pippard MJ, Reid C, Downing MR, Cotes PM: Correction of the anemia of end-stage renal disease with recombinant human erythropoietin. N Engl J Med 1987;316:73–78.
9   Bommer J, Kugel M, Schoeppe W, Brunkhorst R, Samtleben W, Bramsiepe P, Scigalla P: Dose-related effects of recombinant human erythropoietin on erythropoiesis. Results of a multicenter trial in patients with end-stage renal disease. Contrib Nephrol. Basel, Karger, 1988, vol 66, pp 85–93.
10 Schaefer R, Buerner B, Zech M, Denninger G, Borneff C, Heidland A: Treatment of the anemia of hemodialysis patients with recombinant human erythropoietin. Int J Artif Organs 1988;11:249–254.
11 Preece MA: Methodological problems in the assessment of growth and interpretation of growth changes in children with renal disease. Pediatr Adolesc Endocrinol. Basel, Karger, 1989, vol 20, pp 4–14.
12 Barrat T, Broyer M, Chantler C, et al: Assessment of growth. Am J Kidney Dis 1986;7:340–346.
13 Gilli G, Mehls O, Wallstein B, Schärer K: Prediction of adult height in children with chronic renal insufficiency. Kidney Int 1983;24(Suppl 15):48–52.
14 Prader A, Largo RH, Molinari L, Issler C: Physical growth of Swiss Children from birth to 20 years of age. Acta Helv Paediatr 1989:suppl 52.

PD Dr. med. P. Scigalla, Department of Clinical Research,
Boehringer Mannheim GmbH, Sandhoferstrasse 116,
D–6800 Mannheim 31 (FRG)

Gurland HJ, Moran J, Samtleben W, Scigalla P, Wieczorek L (eds): Erythropoietin in
Renal and Non-Renal Anemias. Contrib Nephrol. Basel, Karger, 1991, vol 88, pp 212–214

Discussion

to the Paper by P. Scigalla

Eschbach (Seattle): You made the observation that the longer the duration of uremia
the more the retardation in the growth of uremic children. What would you think about
treating children before they go on dialysis; in other words trying to prevent them from
becoming anemic before they require dialysis? Do you think that they would grow if you could
prevent them from becoming severely anemic? Are there any data on that point?

Scigalla: No. These results show that the hypothesis that renal anemia is responsible for
the growth retardation, or at least is one of the important pathogenetic factors, cannot be
confirmed. On the other hand, the renal anemia is a very important factor in the reduced
well-being and physical working capacity of these children, and therefore it would be advantageous to correct the renal anemia before starting dialysis. Furthermore, we have known for 1
or 2 years that it is possible to correct the growth retardation with recombinant growth
hormone. We know that the concentration of growth hormone in uremic children is increased,
and that the growth retardation is caused by the accumulation of inhibitors of the action of
growth hormone such as IGF1 or IGF2. The first clinical results showed that with growth
hormone the inhibition of growth can be overcome.

Koch (Hannover): In your population the transfusion dependency was 86%, and you
also showed that the older children needed less erythropoietin than the younger ones. What is
the current explanation for these differences from the adult population, the higher transfusion
dependency and the age-related need for erythropoietin?

Scigalla: Transfusion dependency was one of the inclusion criteria, so that the frequency
of transfusion dependency in our study population may well be biased. But, nevertheless, it is
well known that the frequency of transfusion dependency is higher in uremic children than in
uremic adults.

Koch: What is the percentage in the total uremic pediatric population?

Scigalla: I would say it has changed in the last few years, because now many small
children are treated by CAPD from the beginning, and therefore I don't know exactly. I think
nowadays CAPD is the first-choice treatment for children up to the age of 7 years. Formerly
50–60% of children had to be treated with transfusion.

Koch: And why?

Scigalla: Well, I think one of the reasons is blood loss. There is a relatively higher blood
loss in the children than in adults – if an adult loses 10 or 20 ml/day that is much less important
than in a child with a body weight of 10 or 20 kg.

Goldberg (Boston): I am not a pharmacologist, but by giving chemotherapy one thing you quickly learn is that toxicity and efficacy correspond much better to dose per m^2 rather than to dose per kg. Unfortunately, all the EPO studies were done by giving EPO per kg. With adults it doesn't make much difference, but if you look at young children (who have a higher body surface area per kilogram than adults) and recalculate your dose on a basis of per m^2, I think you will find there is no difference in the dose per m^2, although you see what appears to be a difference in dose per kg. I'd like to see the data recalculated in that fashion to see if there is still a difference.

Scigalla: We have already calculated the doses not only on the basis of kg body weight but also on the basis of per m^2. In fact, the difference becomes more distinct. On the basis of body weight the factor was about 2 and if you calculate per m^2 then the factor was 3 or 3.5

Winearls (Oxford): I wonder whether you have really settled this question. You are careful to say in your conclusion that at a hematocrit of 30 there had been no obvious change in growth. But a hematocrit of 30% is very far from correction of anemia. I suggest a better experiment would be to take a group of patients, to correct their anemia fully, and than to look at their growth velocity for the year prior to the correction and for the year afterwards. Then you will get an idea of whether anemia per se made a difference to growth. Do you know in other anemias, for example thalassemia, whether correction of anemia with transfusions makes a difference to growth velocity?

Scigalla: We didn't perform this investigation in other anemias but we also calculated the height velocity, that is, the growth in cm per year, for a period of at least 1 year before starting treatment with erythropoietin and then compared these data with the height velocity during the first year of treatment. We didn't show any differences.

Wardrop (Cardiff): I would like to echo the questions asked by Drs. Winearls and Goldberg. Perhaps your very interesting observation of the higher doses of EPO needed to maintain a given hematocrit in children than in adults reflects increased needs imposed by absolute increases in circulating red cell mass in patients whose bodies are growing. Their increased surface area may also be important and, if they are relatively lean, this would also be associated with a high red cell mass when expressed per kilogram body weight. Moreover, circulating red cell mass and blood volume are quite relevant to oxygen transport by the blood, and are important parameters additional to hematocrit in that regard.

Shaldon (Montpellier): In your long list of causes of retardation of growth in uremic children you included anemia. Is this a sort of dogma or is there any evidence to show that anemia per se really effects growth in children?

Scigalla: No, there are some data for the influence of anemia on growth. Most of these data were derived from animal experiments.

Shaldon: In pediatric medicine you have retarded growth in children who have anemia without other metabolic derangements.

Scigalla: That is very difficult to say. Of course there is thalassemia and other chronic diseases with anemia. However, most of these require a high frequency of transfusion and are therefore associated with iron overload and toxicity, with consequent effects on endocrine function. It is well known, e.g. from children with thalassemia, that iron overload can lead to delayed puberty with growth retardation. Hence, it is difficult to distinguish the effects of the anemia itself from those of iron toxicity. I don't know of any severe chronic anemia without other metabolic disorders and therefore I cannot answer the question directly.

Niemeyer (Hannover): Two comments as a pediatric hematologist. Firstly, I think it has been clearly shown in patients with thalassemia or hypoplastic anemia that children do grow better if you keep the hematocrit up. The second concerns the m^2 versus kg question. Small children have a very high surface area, therefore when we treat them per m^2 we usually overtreat them, especially with chemotherapy. So I think using body weight is a better way of assessing doses than surface area in these patients.

Panel Discussion

Gurland HJ, Moran J, Samtleben W, Scigalla P, Wieczorek L (eds): Erythropoietin in
Renal and Non-Renal Anemias. Contrib Nephrol. Basel, Karger, 1991, vol 88, pp 215–235

Does Exogenous Erythropoietin Down-Regulate Endogenous Erythropoietin?

Chairman: *S. Shaldon,* Montpellier

Panelists: *M. Cotes, E. Goldwasser, D. Kampf, K.M. Koch,
M.A. Goldberg, W. Schaumann*

Shaldon (Montpellier): Good morning ladies and gentlemen. This morning's session is perhaps an unusual one in a scientific setting in that it has had the audacity to have a title which challenges dogma, but does have the humility to put a question mark after the title. Insofar as the audacity is personal, I do not anticipate confirmation of intuitive personal fantasy in the absence of hard data by the panel. Nevertheless, it really has been a pleasure to ask my colleagues to participate in this, some of them with hesitancy and some of them with willingness, but nevertheless they are all here and I'm sure their faces are all familiar to you. On my right I have Dr. Eugene Goldwasser without whose work none of us would probably be here today, then Dr. Cotes on my left-hand side who has been associated with measurements and understanding of erythropoietin (EPO) since the 50s. We have Dr. Goldberg, representative of the new generation of clinicians and molecular biologists, and then we have the pharmacokinetic experts, Dr. Kampf from Berlin and Dr. Schaumann from Boehringer Mannheim, and finally, as my anchorman, we have Prof. Koch, who has considerable clinical as well as scientific experience in this field for the last 20 years.

My own interest in the relationship between EPO and end-stage renal disease (ESRD) was stimulated some 25 years ago when for totally practical reasons, we decided to stop transfusing haemodialysis patients (fig. 1) [1]. This data was derived from 17 patients who had started their dialysis treatment before 1965. We arbitrarily decided to stop all blood transfusions. The duration of previous haemodialysis treatment was 12–41 months with a transfusion requirement of 1–3 units of packed red cells per month. Following cessation of transfusion, the haematocrit fell in all patients to a mean of 17.5 ± 4.5 (range

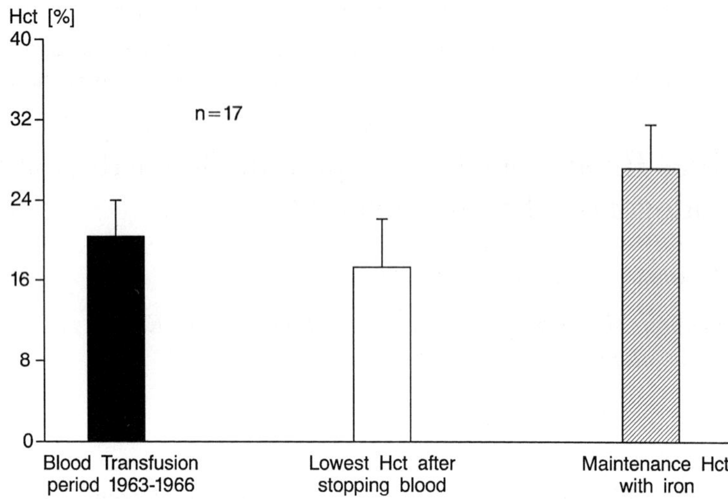

Fig. 1. The effect of stopping blood transfusions in 17 patients on haemodialysis. Derived from data in *Lancet* [1] (see text).

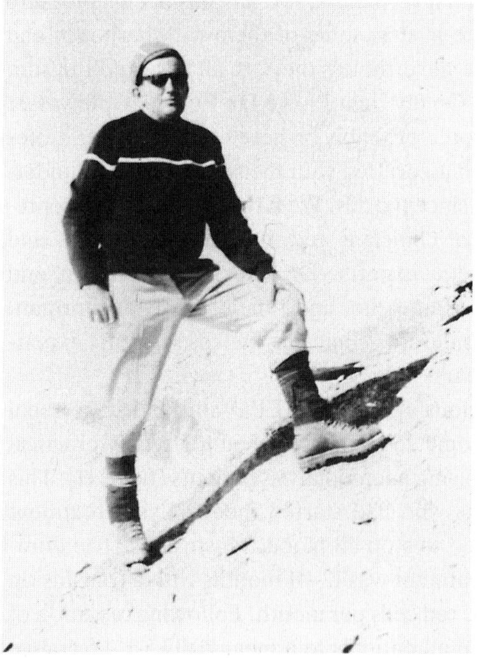

Fig. 2. Haemodialysis patient climbing Mönch in the Jungfrauregion in 1966 (see text).

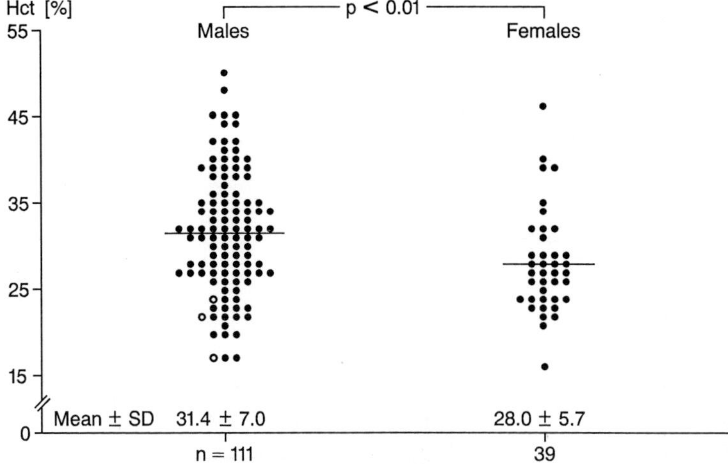

Fig. 3. Haematocrit values of nontransfused haemodialysis patients on treatment at the University Hospital, Frankfurt/Main, December 1978. ○ = Bilaterally nephrectomized patients (data provided by K. Koch).

12–25) vol%. Following the haematocrit through there was a slow but persistent rise in the haematocrit reaching 26.5 ± 6.2 (range 17–39) vol% at 5–18 months following stopping transfusion. In addition, 8 patients developed iron deficiency and required intravenous iron supplements. EPO was detectable in the serum of 50% of these patients after cessation of transfusion [2]. What was even more interesting was that when one of these patients went from sea level in London to live in Lauterbrunnen (Bernese Oberland, approx. 1,200 m altitude), his haematocrit increased from 21 to 34 vol% without exogenous EPO and just on replacement iron. He was an alpinist and was able to climb the Mönch in the Jungfrauregion (fig. 2). With this background, data supplied by Prof. Koch (fig. 3) shows what you could achieve in 1978 in a large dialysis population in terms of mean haematocrit including bilaterally nephrectomized patients with iron replacement and without blood transfusions, androgens or exogenous EPO. (You will note that the mean haematocrit is very close to the target level that many today consider the object of EPO therapy. However, the endogenous EPO response as judged by serum levels measured by RIA (fig. 4) (data of Dr. K.U. Eckardt) in the ESRD patient is inappropriate for the degree of anaemia as compared to anaemic patients with normal renal function. Thus these background data suggest that ESRD patients without poly-

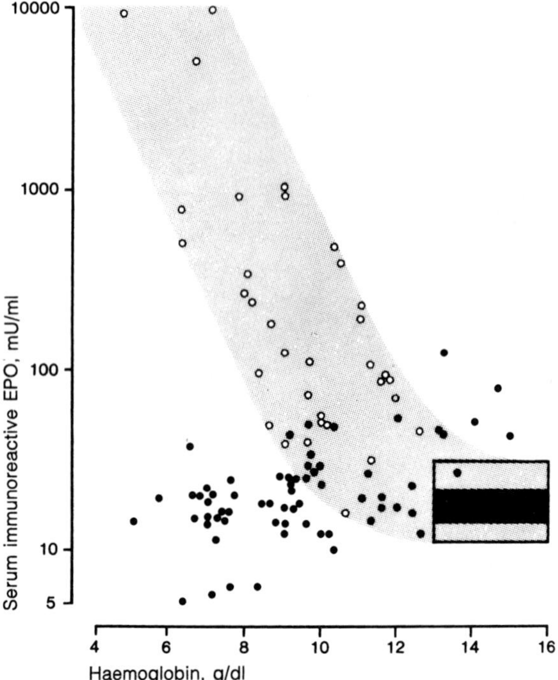

Fig. 4. Serum immunoreactive EPO in renal (filled symbols) and nonrenal (open symbols) anaemias. For comparison, interquartile range of serum immunoreactive EPO in healthy adults (from K.-U. Eckhardt).

cystic kidneys make EPO, but inadequately to completely correct their anaemia, that blood transfusion depresses this response but that altitude hypoxia may stimulate the response.

Finally, the case history which I have asked the panel to comment on has some paradoxical elements to its (fig. 5). The patient, a 57-year-old female, was on haemodialysis for 8 years prior to starting CAPD. She was not transfused and maintained a stable haematocrit of 23 vol% on replacement iron for a number of years. She had an undetermined cause of ESRD (possibly glomerulonephritis) and was anuric. She had no history of liver disease or any evidence of hepatitis during the study. She had a single control EPO serum level of 23 mU/ml at time 0 weeks (measured by RIA by Dr. Eckardt) and I should say that all the serum EPO concentrations measured up to week 30

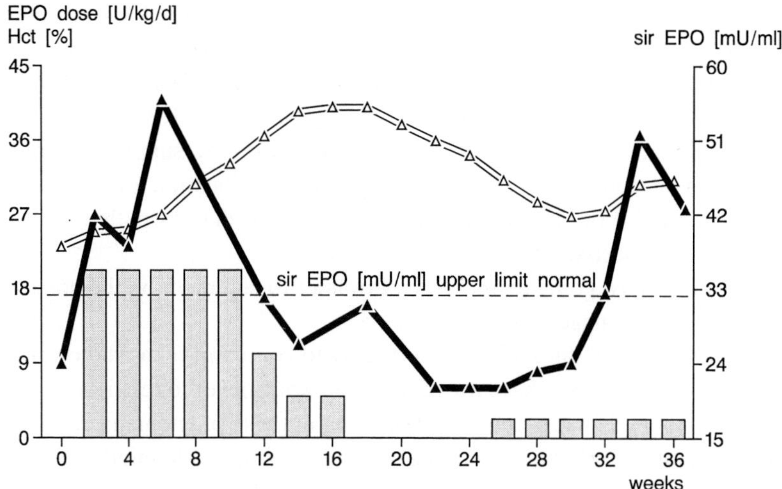

Fig. 5. Case history: patient receiving self-administered daily subcutaneous EPO whilst on CAPD therapy. The patient is on 2.5 IU/kg body weight/day of EPO following 2 months of cessation of EPO therapy (see text). $\triangle$ = Hct; $\blacktriangle$ = serum immunoreactive (sir) EPO. Columns represent daily EPO dose.

were performed within one series of assays. The last three points were done within a second series. The doses of EPO were administered into the thigh subcutaneously every day in the morning. The blood samples were always drawn at 24 h interval from the last dose.

The haematocrit rose from 23 to 41 vol% in the first 16 weeks as the daily EPO dose was diminished from 20 to 5 U/kg body weight/day. During this time, the EPO serum level rose to 57 mU/ml and then fell to 21 mU/ml after EPO was stopped at week 16. The haematocrit then fell slowly until week 30, when it reached 27 vol% and EPO was restarted at 2.5 U/kg body weight/day. The haematocrit then rose to a new steady state at 33 vol% where it has been stabilized. However, there was a significant rise in serum EPO level during weeks 32–36 when it reached 52 mU/ml. I have some difficulty in interpreting this data, and the difficulty is in understanding the mechanism by which this second rise in serum EPO has occurred.

With this background, namely that EPO is produced endogenously in the ESRD patient, that it is inappropriately produced for the degree of anaemia and that the current dogma suggests that the sole mechanism for determining

EPO production in the kidney is hypoxia, we have assembled this panel of experts to discuss the following two questions: (1) Are there other mechanisms which may influence the endogenous production of EPO and/or its effectiveness on the target stem cells such as down-regulation of EPO-producing cells by exogenous EPO or target cell desensitization by suppression of EPO receptors on stem cells? (2) Is there any further justification for continuing the current practice of intravenous EPO 3× week for dialysis patients given the adverse pharmacokinetics?

So I am now going to ask Dr. Goldwasser to comment on the possibilities that have been suggested.

Goldwasser (Chicago): It is very easy to comment on a whole variety of subjects here because I have no information whatsoever to restrict me. Quite a large number of factors could be operating in these phenomena and I will be somewhat non-diplomatic and start with one that comes to mind immediately. Those of us who have been working on EPO assays whether they are bioassays or culture assays or RIAs have to walk around with a burden of suspicion about any single assay point. Looking at these data (fig. 5) and seeing a switch in assay for those last three points, I would like to see a repetition in order to see whether this little burst at the end is reproducible or did something go wrong with that assay? At least in my assay things go wrong all the time and I never would rely on a single point or a single assay for any kind of interpretation, even the ones that I like best. There are other factors that need to be considered in the question raised by this assuming for the time being that the assay is okay. It has been shown fairly conclusively, as brought out yesterday in fact by animal experiments that the direct regulation of EPO production by circulating EPO doesn't seem to operate. It isn't a simple-minded kind of feedback that says at a certain level of EPO the synthesizing system shuts off. That doesn't answer the question raised by Dr. Shaldon yesterday (see discussion to papers of Bommer and Granolleras) about the condition in renal disease. We just don't know. We know, in fact, that the liver can produce EPO in animals. Under severe stress the liver can be quite effective to the extent of about one third or so, that of the kidney in producing EPO for maintenance of red cell production. Whether under longer stress, under conditions inherent with renal disease in man the liver might be even more effective, we just don't know. I think that needs to be found out. Lastly it seems to me that in all of the speculations about the EPO level we have neglected one side of the phenomenon: we are looking at production not at degradation and loss. In some of the animal experiments that we did and that other people have also done, it is very clear that we don't know what happens to EPO when it is injected into a person or an animal. In our experiments in the rat, it seemed to get lost. In the anephric patient, it is not going to be excreted in the urine, where is it going? Why with intravenous injection does it disappear so quickly? It must be an active degradation, I would guess something along the lines of desialation in the circulation and rapid uptake by the liver and perhaps other tissues and then break down into unrecognizable pieces. It is entirely possible that a prolonged half-life or a prolonged appearance in the circulation reflects an inhibition of the breakdown pathway rather than any acceleration of production in the liver or the remnant of the kidney or whatever other organ may be making it. Lastly I come back to the assay: the RIA measures something that reacts with an antibody, we don't know exactly all the things that can react with an antibody, and the finding of a peak by RIA tells us something about what reacts with an antibody but doesn't tell us that we are measuring intact EPO. So I think I have managed to muddy up the situation a little more than it was when we started out. But at least there are alternative ways to approach the problem than the one proposed by our chairman.

Shaldon: I think the chairman merely proposed that you discuss the data. Now I'm going to ask Dr. Eckardt to comment on his assay. The assay was done in duplicate and he was completely blinded in relation to the data.

Goldwasser: I have to clearly indicate, I mean no derogatory remarks about Dr. Eckardt's assay. I have notebooks full of marvellous data based on single assays which we can never replicate.

Eckardt (Zürich): I don't think I should add much more confusion to this than I already did by measuring these values. The only thing I can say is that the difference between 20 and 40 mU/ml is certainly outside the normal variation of the assay but I think Dr. Goldwasser is certainly right and I would like to invite you to send us more samples and see if it is really reproducible. But, apart from this I might perhaps draw your attention to the point that although the data (fig. 5) look very impressive in absolute terms, this difference in EPO is a slight one. Irrespective of the cause why there is such an interesting increase in EPO, there is an increase in haematocrit as well which actually means that the increase in EPO may be real. I think the most important observation from the data is that you have a nice increment of haematocrit with peak levels of about 60 mU/ml EPO in the early phase, which points to a considerable sensitivity towards EPO.

Shaldon: Thank you, Dr. Eckardt. I'll now ask my next colleague from America to comment. Dr. Goldberg will tell us his views on this question.

Goldberg (Boston): I think first of all it's a very interesting observation, but I agree with Dr. Eckardt, I would like to see if it is reproducible in other patients. In addition, having done a lot of RIAs we often have problems as well and when we find small differences we would like to see if the results are reproducible. What I would like to do is to assume for a minute that the answer to the question is yes, that there is feedback inhibition of EPO production. If that were the case then certain things must hold. The first thing is that if the EPO-producing cells are recognizing EPO already made they have to have a mechanism for recognizing it, in other words there must be an EPO receptor on the EPO-producing cells, be it in the kidney or in the liver. Secondly, if EPO binds to this receptor it must then transduce a signal to decrease EPO production and I think that would involve decreasing EPO mRNA levels. Now, what's the data for either of those things occurring? First with regard to the receptor, Dr. D'Andrea in his paper in the journal *Cell* [3], where he described the cloning of the mouse EPO receptor, took the EPO receptor cDNA and probed various tissues including the kidney and the liver by Northern blot analysis and was unable to detect any evidence of a particular EPO receptor in any cells in the kidney or the liver. You could argue that sensitivity of the Northern blot wasn't good enough or you could argue that there is a different receptor that is still yet unknown, but there is no data in favor of that. Secondly, what happens to EPO RNA levels? Again, I am very simplistic and I think it's very hard to work in an intact organism, be it an animal or a man, because there are so many feedback loops that could be participating and that could cause the results described in this patient (fig. 5). The Hep 3B cells, which may have many problems of their own as well, are devoid of a lot of these other feedback loops such as the pulmonary function, cardiac function, changes in hemoglobin oxygen affinity, etc. When you expose them to a certain oxygen tension that's the oxygen tension they see. And when we expose Hep 3B cells to hypoxia and look at EPO mRNA levels over a 24-hour period we don't see a rise and then a subsequent fall, we see a rise in EPO mRNA levels and they stay up until you remove the hypoxic stimulus, even though you're accumulating EPO protein in the media that the cells are exposed to. So again this would go against the idea of feedback inhibition. Thirdly, I think that other data from Dr. Eckardt and the group in Zürich in which they have shown that when you take a rat and you put it in a hypoxic chamber, you see an initial increase in immunoreactive EPO in the serum and then it subsequently falls as do the EPO mRNA levels [4]. And they asked, why does this occur? I don't want to speak for them but in their paper they very elegantly show that this is not caused by a down-regulation due to EPO itself. They showed this by injecting rats with very large doses of EPO and then again making them hypoxic and they observed the same rise in EPO, even though they preinjected the animals with high doses of EPO to begin with. So, having large amounts of EPO they didn't affect the induction of the endogenous EPO. So I think all these data argue against, or do not support, the idea that there is a feedback down-regulation of EPO production. Nonetheless, we are left with a very interesting observation in several patients. Several questions come to mind. Were there subtle changes in liver function? It's well known that hepatitis can sometimes result in changes in EPO secretion for unclear reasons. Was there an acidosis or was there some change in haemoglobin oxygen affinity? Was there a change in cardiac output? Was there a change in renal blood flow? Were there new medications added? These are all questions that need to be addressed. In summary, I cannot explain the observation presented by Dr. Shaldon, but I think it's an important observation, similar to the observations of Eckardt et al. [5]. I think that if we could find the answers to these questions then we could learn a lot more about the regulation of EPO. There is a lot that we still don't know and if we could harness this information perhaps we could even avoid giving rhEPO, although some people might not like this.

Shaldon: Well, Dr. Cotes you've been in this field almost as long as Dr. Goldwasser and he made one or two remarks that I know you wish to discuss. Would you like to comment on the background of this debate and how you interpret the data? In addition, I believe you have some interesting data of your own.

Cotes (Harrow): I would like to draw your attention to two particular points in the case presentation made by Dr. Shaldon (fig. 5). The first is that we have seen a patient who appears to respond to treatment with very small doses of exogenous EPO (2.5 IU/kg body weight/day). The second is that, looking at the estimates of serum EPO (fig. 5), until week 26 these seem to be what might be expected for a patient with renal failure treated with daily subcutaneous EPO and sampled 24 h after each EPO dose. However, from week 26, while the haemoglobin is falling, the serum EPO increases to reach values of about 52 and 43 mU/ml at weeks 34 and 36, respectively. To account for these concentrations, there has almost certainly been an increase in endogenous production of EPO and the possibility arises that additional endogenous EPO contributed to the rise in haemoglobin seen from week 32.

Dr. Shaldon asks whether there is down-regulation of endogenous production of EPO in patients with renal failure in whom anaemia is corrected by treatment with EPO. Our evidence is that this does not usually occur [6]. In a series of anaemic patients on haemodialysis treated with intravenous rhEPO, estimates of serum EPO and of endogenous production of EPO were not

Table 1. Renal anaemia treated with rhEPO [data from 6]

	Haemoglobin[1] g/dl	Serum EPO[2] mIU/ml	Endogenous EPO turnover[3] IU/kg/24 h
Pretreatment	6.3 (1.3)	23.0 (14.1–33.0)	7.0 (2.0–14.3)
Treated	12.3 (1.3)	28.7 (14.7–46.7)	6.4 (3.8–9.5)

[1] Mean (SD).
[2] Geometric mean (range). In treated patients samples were collected 72 h (after the last dose of rhEPO given intravenously.
[3] Mean (range).

changed despite correction of anaemia (table 1). This series of patients was typical of those with renal failure without polycystic kidneys or complicating liver disease, and despite anaemia, serum EPO before treatment was in the normal range. If, despite renal failure, serum EPO is increased, before treatment, down-regulation of endogenous production may occur with correction of anaemia. Estimates of the turnover of endogenous serum EPO give a minimum estimate of the daily production of EPO needed to sustain the concentration found in serum. The calculation depends upon the assumption that the pharmacokinetics of intravenous rhEPO and of endogenous EPO turnover (table 1) of some 7 IU EPO/kg body weight/day (approx. 50 IU/kg/week), may be compared with the amounts of exogenous EPO that are given to treat anaemia. A dose of 17 IU/kg/week is less than a 50% increase above endogenous production. Would this sort of amount, if administered in an appropriate way, be sufficient to correct anaemia?

To try to answer this I want to draw attention to two other models which suggest that a very small increment above the normal serum EPO may be sufficient to sustain a secondary polycythaemia. First, in 30–50% of patients with polycythaemia secondary to chronic hypoxic lung disease, serum EPO is in the range for normal subjects (fig. 6) [7]. My second model (fig. 7) is of climbers going up to a high altitude during an expedition to Mt. Kongur in China [8]. Serum samples were collected at sea level, at 1,500, 3,500 and 4,500 m. After about 10 days, although the haematocrit continued to increase, in contrast, serum EPO, after an initial increase, declined to values which were sometimes no greater than the concentration found at sea level before

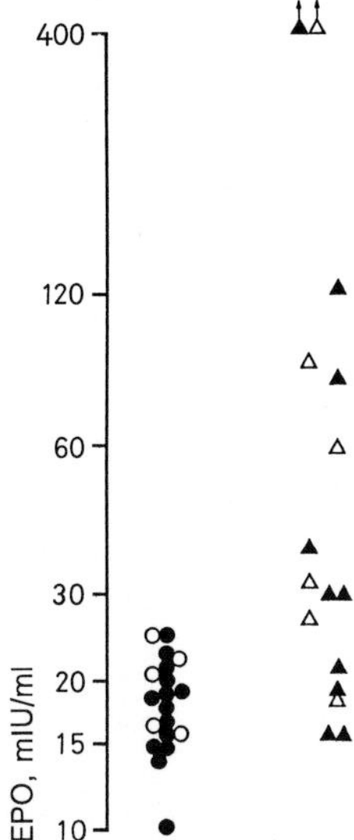

Fig. 6. Estimates of immunoreactive EPO in serum samples from normal healthy men (●) and women (○) and from patients with chronic hypoxic lung disease and secondary polycythaemia (▲ = men; △ = women).

the start of the expedition. Relatively similar results were obtained by Abbrecht and Littell [9] in an earlier study.

Thus, in some instances, polycythaemia was still developing and then maintained although serum EPO was in the range for normal subjects. This data indicates that it may not be necessary to sustain large increases in serum EPO in order to maintain an increase in red cell mass in man. Certainly there is no need for a constant high concentration of serum EPO either for correction of an anaemia or for the maintenance of polycythaemia.

One further point needs to be made in relation to the difficulty of pharmacokinetic studies of rhEPO. Subcutaneous doses of the hormone induce very small increases in the concentration of the hormone in serum and analysis depends upon the assumption that the concentration of endogenous EPO in serum remains constant. This is not always the case as in some subjects there is a diurnal pattern of change [10–12] and it is then difficult to assess the relative contributions of exogenous and endogenous EPO to an estimate of serum EPO, particularly when the exogenous contribution is small.

Shaldon: Very nice, Dr. Cotes, thank your for your excellent presentation. I think the time has come in this panel to shift the emphasis a little bit

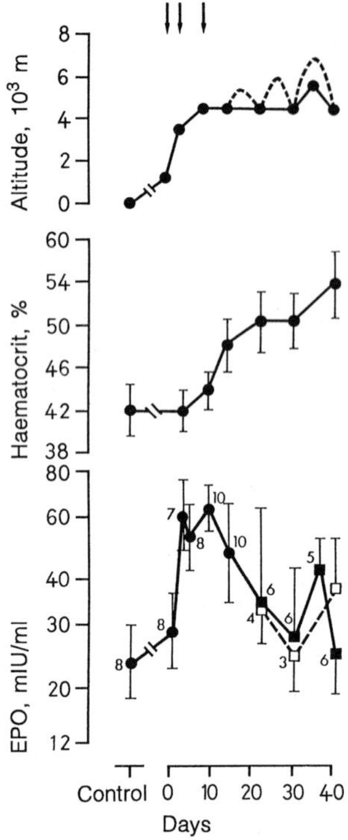

Fig. 7. Mount Kongur expedition: altitude, all subjects (solid line), with additional altitude reached by climbers (dotted line); haematocrit mean for all subjects (± SD); estimates of serum immunoreactive EPO as geometric mean and interquartile range for all subjects (●), for climbers (□), and for scientists (■). Number of subjects are indicated beside each observation. Arrows indicate days of travel.

from speculation and theory and turn more to the practical considerations of the route of administration and perhaps the frequency of administration and in this regard I am going to ask Prof. Schaumann to comment.

Schaumann (Mannheim): Mathematics are supposed to be an exact science but still I'm going to stick with speculations. Starting with your last question, Dr. Shaldon, I will try to explain the relative inefficiency of intravenous EPO.

What we should really study is the effect of EPO and not its serum concentration. Therefore we have tried to translate EPO serum concentrations obtained from pharmacokinetic studies with rhEPO into effect, by using

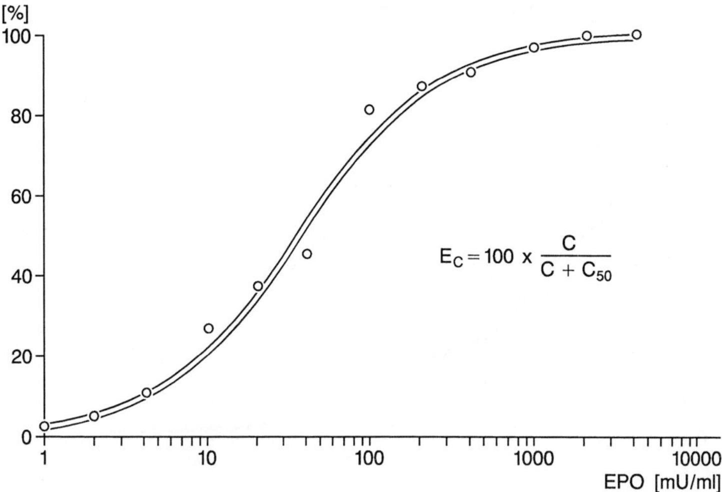

Fig. 8. Concentration-effect curve of EPO in vitro [results from 13]. E_c = Effect in percent of the maximum effect; C = concentration; C_{50} = concentration at half-maximal effect.

data from Todokoro et al. [13]. They showed in vitro a correlation between the concentration of EPO and the increase in hemoglobin-forming cells expressed as percentage (100% being the maximal effect) (fig. 8). The equation derived from the curve shows a correlation coefficient of almost 1 when using a C_{50} (concentration for half-maximal effect) of 35 mU/ml. However, in vivo you very often need different concentrations than in a cell line in vitro to have the same effect. Therefore in our model, in vivo calculation based on Macdougall's [14] pharmacokinetic data of rhEPO, we assumed different C_{50} values of 15, 25 and 50 mU/ml. An equipotent therapeutic effect has been demonstrated between 30 U/kg administered intravenously and 24 U/kg administered subcutaneously to the same patient population (personal communication from Dr. Scigalla). For our model calculation we thus converted the actual serum concentrations – which were obtained from intravenous or subcutaneous administration of 100 U/kg – to 40 U/kg i.v. and 24 U/kg s.c. These converted concentrations were then transformed into percent of maximal effect using the described equation (fig. 9). After intravenous administration, we are close to the maximum for about 24 h. Thereafter, there is a rapid decay due to the half-life of about 6 h. After subcutaneous administration we arrive at about 50–60% of the maximum after 18 h with a slow decay.

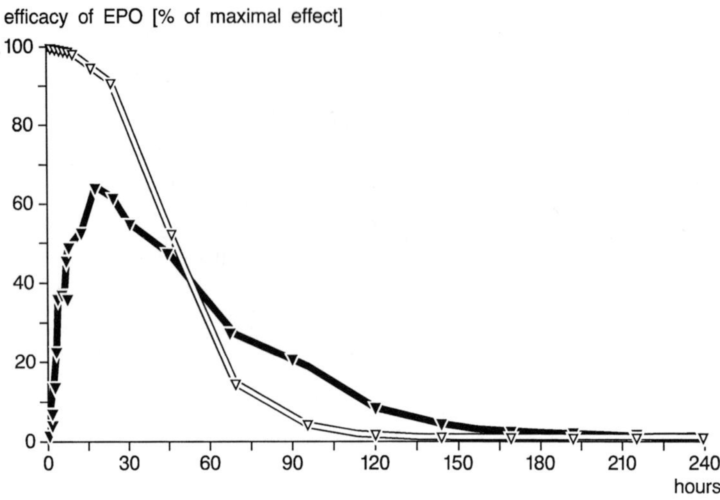

Fig. 9. Efficacy of rhEPO versus time, calculated with $C_{50} = 15$ mU/ml for single doses of 30 U/kg i.v. and 24 U/kg s.c. [data derived from 13].

Table 2. Calculated therapeutic activity of intravenous versus subcutaneous rhEPO

C_{50}, U/l	AUC, % effect × h		i.v.
	30 U/kg i.v.	24 U/kg s.c.	s.c.
Macdougall et al. [14]			
15	4,387	4,370	1.00
25	3,794	3,120	1.22
50	3,012	1,956	1.54
Kampf et al. [15]			
15	3,428	3,978	0.82
25	2,927	2,928	1.00
50	2,267	1,782	1.27

Assuming that the overall therapeutic effect is the product of the effect at a given time versus the duration of action, we calculated the area under the curve (AUC) for intravenous and subcutaneous administration. The results are summarized in table 2. Using a C_{50} value of 15 mU/ml, the AUC for the two administration routes is nearly identical. So how do we explain why the lower dose given subcutaneously is equipotent to the intravenous dose in spite of its low bioavailability of about 20%? The reason is that the excessive concentrations which we find initially, after intravenous injection, don't contribute to the effect. What matters is the long duration of the subcutaneous administration. A similar evaluation was made with the results of Kampf et al. [15]. Here one obtains equipotency between intravenous and subcutaneous therapy with an assumed C_{50} of 25 mU/ml (table 2).

I beg for your indulgence not to put too much emphasis on the actual figures. The hypothesis merely says that you don't need to assume any particular interference with regulation in order to explain the relative inefficacy of intravenous EPO.

Shaldon: Thank you, Dr. Schaumann, I think Dr. Koch has a question for you.

Koch (Hannover): Can you explain with your model the very low doses necessary in daily subcutaneous EPO administration?

Schaumann: We haven't tried yet and actually there we are going to face a difficulty. I discussed the subject with Dr. Macdougall and Dr. Kampf. Please correct me if I'm wrong, what they find is that in many patients the endogenous EPO concentration before treatment, determined by RIA, was not much lower than the average maintenance concentrations during subcutaneous therapy, yet the haematocrit goes up. Applying pure logic to this observation one has to conclude that what was measured initially was not bioactive EPO. The second conclusion is that apparently the biologically inactive (endogenous) EPO goes down during therapy because otherwise the extremely low difference between the concentrations before and during treatment is insufficient to explain the therapeutic effect. This is the dilemma with which we will be left for any model calculation. Should we subtract the endogenous pretreatment value or not? I think we can only obtain an interpretable result if we do not subtract it, which we have done so far.

Shaldon: Nevertheless, it has been reported that significantly lower doses of daily subcutaneous EPO compared to 3× weekly subcutaneous EPO produce the same target haematocrit in the absence of a rise in the serum EPO level. Therefore, are you suggesting that prior to exogenous EPO administration that endogenous EPO has no effect on the stem cell?

Schaumann: The EPO which enters to the stem cell compartment has to pass through the central compartment, and there you do your blood sampling. So, I can only repeat my not very satisfactory speculation, namely that the endogenous EPO measurements do not represent biologically active EPO, and the second is that these values decrease very quickly, as otherwise there is no possibility to correlate the obvious therapeutic success with the serum concentrations.

Cotes: I think that we must acknowledge that haemoglobin would be unlikely to be maintained at the sort of levels we see in patients with renal failure if they did not already have significant amounts of biologically active EPO. There is evidence for this from patients with renal failure and polycystic kidney disease, in whom haemoglobin tends to be higher than in patients with renal disease of other aetiology. The higher haemoglobins are associated with and attributed to the higher concentrations of EPO found in plasma. Plasma EPO was estimated by RIA (the same sort of technique as that used by Dr. Eckardt) and the haemoglobin data in patients with polycystic kidney disease suggests that immunoassay data reflects biological activity. Nonetheless, I don't think that the whole story is yet told in terms of what significant differences occur in the glycosylation patterns of endogenous EPO. There may be differences between molecules of EPO in the duration of biological activity analogous to the sort of differences that are seen within the glycoprotein gonadotrophic hormones. In the case of EPO, it is by no means certain whether changes in glycosylation contribute towards any significant physiological regulatory mechanism.

Schaumann: To my knowledge, glycosylation is probably the only thing that should not interfere with the assay because the deglycosylated EPO is eliminated very rapidly, that is why it shouldn't accumulate in the serum.

Cotes: I don't think we are considering deglycosylated; we are saying that there may be different patterns of glycosylation and there may be some small changes which may alter the properties of some circulating molecules, but we await data on the significance of this and how far it occurs.

Shaldon: Dr. Kampf, as your data has already been partially quoted, would you like to briefly present your observations on peak and trough EPO serum levels?

Kampf (Berlin): From the long-lasting plasma concentration after the subcutaneous administration just shown by Dr. Schaumann, we concluded that it might be possible to reduce the subcutaneous dosage frequency. At the moment, we are treating patients in the maintenance phase with a constant total dose per week reducing the dosage frequency from 3 times to twice to once per week and our very preliminary data in 3 patients show a constant haematocrit value regardless of the frequency of EPO administration. At the same time we measured the trough EPO plasma concentrations 72 h after the subcutaneous administration. The observed trough levels were below the baseline levels obtained at the start of the treatment. But again the differences

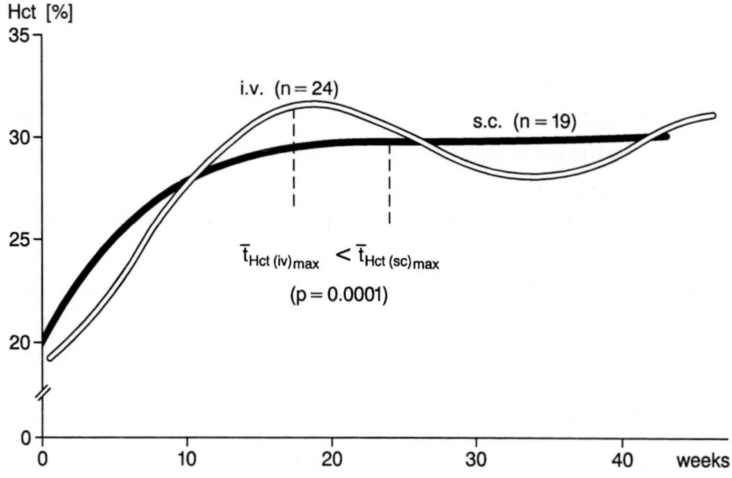

Fig. 10. Time course of haematocrit values in patients treated intravenously and sub-cutaneously with rhEPO. $t_{Hct\,max}$ = Time to reach maximum haematocrit value.

are small, about 30% below baseline levels and the absolute concentrations are low and so the precision of the data is open for discussion. Are these differences only due to the variability in the RIA or are they the consequence of the increase in haematocrit from 22 to 28% or are they indeed a reflection of down-regulation of endogenous EPO by exogenous EPO administration?

Shaldon: Thank you for that provocative data. I think it adds some weight to the discussion, but I think in the remaining period of time it would be appropriate to ask Prof. Koch to put into clinical perspective the potential of subcutaneous EPO, particularly in relationship to avoiding undesirable complications about which we have heard so much.

Koch: Well, as a clinician I have nothing substantial to add to this debate, but my prediction is that in the future we will be only using subcutaneous EPO because first it is cheaper and second it is following a very general principle of pharmacotherapy to use the lowest necessary dose to achieve your therapeutic target and that, I think, increases the safety of treatment. To give you an example, figure 10 shows that when EPO was given intravenously the time to achieve the maximum haematocrit was 18 weeks as compared to 22 weeks in the subcutaneously treated population. And you will note that with the intravenous therapy there is an overshoot of the target haematocrit in the initial phase of treatment and then if you try to correct this you have a backswing. You don't see this using daily subcutaneous EPO, as we are able to adjust the relatively small dose on a daily basis. Our experience in these two groups of patients was that in the intravenous population, 15 out of 24 became hypertensive, whereas in the daily subcutaneous group none had developed hypertension when the target haematocrit was reached. So this is just an example of what I tried to say: there is more safety with daily subcutaneous administration of EPO.

Shaldon: Thank you very much, Dr. Koch. We have still about 10 minutes left and I'm sure that there are people in the audience who would like to pose specific questions to any members of the panel so please don't hesitate to speculate or criticize or add.

Rich (Ulm): Regarding the case history (fig. 5) that has caused all the discussion this morning, could you give us a little bit more information. Were the samples taken at the same time every day?

Shaldon: Yes, these samples were taken in the morning at 24 h after the last dose of EPO. They are part of a study which Boehringer have in hand at the moment. There are several additional cases where data on dose and haematocrit have a similar profile in subcutaneous daily administration.

Baldamus (Köln): I would like to raise the question whether you really need a steady-state EPO concentration to saturate the receptors at the bone marrow or whether it is possible to have small peaks over the day which would do exactly the same?

Shaldon: Dr. D'Andrea, would you like to answer this question?

D'Andrea (Cambridge, Mass.): There has been a lot of reference to the EPO receptor work. Along the lines of EPO production I really cannot make many comments. It appears, as Dr. Goldberg has pointed out, that the EPO receptor is not expressed on the surface of kidney cells which produce EPO. This was done by Northern blot analysis, and this is not a very sensitive technique. So it is still quite conceivable that the cells that produce EPO could respond to EPO. We have not ruled that out. What I think I can respond to is the notion of receptor down-regulation by the target erythroid cells. But again, we do all our experiments in vitro as does Dr. Krantz. We do not do very many in vivo experiments. In vitro it is clear that target cells which have EPO receptors do bind EPO and the EPO is internalized by these cells rapidly. However, EPO in these in vitro studies does not appear to, in any way, increase the degradation of the EPO receptor. That is to say, if one looks at the half-life of the EPO receptor in cells that express it, increasing EPO concentration does not appear to effect the degradation of that receptor. Furthermore, I believe it is naive to think that the EPO receptor is a single receptor that exists as a single state. I think it is very likely that the EPO receptor exists in many different states, in low sensitivity states and high sensitivity states. The EPO receptor, as many groups have already shown, may differ in sensitivity at different times during erythropoiesis. Early red blood cell precursors require very high EPO concentrations whereas later differentiated cells, like CFU-Es, respond to lower concentrations of EPO. We are not dealing with a single EPO receptor population, and its sensitivity may vary as a function of the state of differentiation of the cells.

Shaldon: Dr. Schaumann would like to comment on that.

Schaumann: I have an additional question because I don't think your comments quite answer the question. The question really is how reversible is the binding of the EPO to the receptors because if reversibility is low you may indeed saturate them in a short period of time, then have an effect which lasts much longer than the serum concentrations. So this is the question: What do you know about reversibility of the binding of the EPO to the receptor?

D'Andrea: After EPO binds to the cell surface receptor, the rate of dissociation of EPO from the receptor is extremely slow. It is much slower than the rate of internalization of the EPO by the receptor. The likely molecular events are EPO binding to its receptor at the cell surface followed by rapid internalization and degradation of EPO. So the rate of dissociation is really not a factor.

Goldwasser: I think there is one other factor to consider in response to Dr. Baldamus' question. The best estimates so far indicate that half maximal haemoglobin synthesis can be effected by as few as something like 50 molecules of EPO per target cell. And if your are going to invoke binding and internalization in the kinetics of EPO concentration or the maintenance of EPO concentration you may have to have a room full of cells to reduce a relatively modest concentration in the serum. We are dealing really with small numbers of molecules that are effective and hundreds of millions of molecules in circulation.

Shaldon: Yes, Dr. Eschbach, we have time for a short comment.

Eschbach (Seattle): Stanley, I would like to ask the panel members if they know of any evidence that there is down-regulation in other endocrine feedback mechanisms in the human body.

Shaldon: Well, we don't need to ask the panel, we can ask the total assembled audience about that, the existence of feedback mechanisms on production of hormones by hormones or cytokines by cytokines or paracrines by paracrines?

Cotes: Auto down-regulation of production occurs commonly in other endocrine systems. One example is formation of tri-iodothyronine (T_3), the active form of thyroid hormone thyroxine (T_4). The production of T_4 and indirectly of T_3 is controlled by the pituitary hormone thyrotrophin (TSH). T_3 down-regulates the production of both the hypothalamic thyroid-releasing hormone (TRH) and TSH. Adrenal cortical steroid hormones also exert a similar down-regulatory effect on their own production by reducing production of both hypothalamic corticotrophin-releasing factors and pituitary adrenocorticotrophin.

Shaldon: I think many of the paracrine/endocrine systems either directly or by using prostaglandin synthesis inhibit their own subsequent release. I think this is a well-established regulatory mechanism. Does that answer your question, Dr. Eschbach? The answer would seem to be yes!

Eschbach: I am not convinced.

Shaldon: Well I think we will pass from speculation to facts and hand over the chair to Dr. Scigalla and Dr. Koch for the next session. Thank you very much.

References

1   Shaldon, S.: Chronic dialysis without transfusion. Lancet *i:* 783–784 (1967).
2   Comty, C.M.; Cotes, P.M.; Shaldon, S.: Erythropoietin measurements in patients in end-stage renal failure treated by chronic dialysis therapy. Abstr. 3rd International Congress of Nephrology, Washington 1966.
3   D'Andrea, A.; Lodish, H.; Wong, G.: Expression cloning of the murine erythropoietin receptor. Cell *57:* 277–285 (1989).
4   Eckardt, K.U.; Dittmer, J.; Neumann, R.; Bauer, C.; Kurtz, A.: Decline of erythropoietin formation at continuous hypoxia is not due to feedback inhibition. Am. J. Physiol. *258:* F1432–F1437 (1990).
5   Eckardt, K.U.; Drüeke, T.; Kurtz, A.: Unutilized reserves: The production capacity for erythropoietin appears to be conserved in chronic renal disease. Contrib. Nephrol., vol. 88, pp. 18–31 (Karger, Basel 1991).
6   Cotes, P.M.; Pippard, M.J.; Reid, C.D.L.; Winearls, C.G.; Oliver, D.O.; Royston, J.P.: Characterization of the anaemia of chronic renal failure and the mode of its correction by a preparation of human erythropoietin (r-HuEPO). An investigation of the pharmacokinetics of intravenous erythropoietin and its effect on erythrokinetics. Q. J. Med. *70:* 113–137 (1989).
7   Wedzicha, J.A.; Cotes, P.M.; Empey, D.W.; Newland, A.C.; Royston, J.P.; Tam, P.C.: Serum immunoreactive erythropoietin in hypoxic lung disease with and without polycythaemia. Clin. Sci. *69:* 413–422 (1985).
8   Milledge, J.S.; Cotes, P.M.: Serum erythropoietin in humans at high altitude and its relation to plasma renin. J. Appl. Physiol. *59:* 360–364 (1985).

9   Abbrecht, P.H.; Littell, J.K.: Plasma erythropoietin in men and mice during acclimatization to different altitudes. J. Appl. Physiol. *32:* 54–58 (1972).

10 Miller, M.E.; Garcia, J.F.; Cohen, R.A.; Cronkite, E.P.; Moccia, G.; Acevedo, J.: Diurnal levels of immunoreactive erythropoietin in normal subjects and subjects with chronic lung disease. Br. J. Haematol. *49:* 189–200 (1981).

11 Cotes, P.M.; Brozovic, B.: Diurnal variation of serum immunoreactive erythropoietin in a normal subject. Clin. Endocrinol. (Oxf.) *17:* 419–422 (1982).

12 Wide, L.; Bengtsson, C.; Birgegard, G.: Circadian rhythm of erythropoietin in human serum. Br. J. Haematol. *72:* 85–90 (1989).

13 Todokoro, K.; Kanazawa, S.; Amanuma, H.; Ikawa, Y.: Specific binding of erythropoietin to its receptor on responsive mouse erythroleukemia cells. Proc. Natl. Acad. Sci. USA *84:* 4126–4130 (1987).

14 Macdougall, I.C.; Neubert, P.; Coles, G.A.; Roberts, D.E.; Dharmasena, A.D.; Williams, J.D.: Pharmacokinetics of recombinant human erythropoietin in patients on continuous ambulatory peritoneal dialysis. Lancet *i:* 425–427 (1989).

15 Kampf, D.; Kahl, A., Passlick, J.; Pustelnik, A.; Eckardt, K.-U.; Ehmer, B.; Jacobs, C.; Baumelou, A.; Grabensee, B.; Gahl, G.M.: Single-dose kinetics of recombinant human erythropoietin after intravenous, subcutaneous and intraperitoneal administration. Contrib. Nephrol., vol. 76, pp. 106–111 (Karger, Basel 1989).

Use of Recombinant Human Erythropoietin in Non-Renal Anemia and Surgery

Gurland HJ, Moran J, Samtleben W, Scigalla P, Wieczorek L (eds): Erythropoietin in
Renal and Non-Renal Anemias. Contrib Nephrol. Basel, Karger, 1991, vol 88, pp 238–245

Treatment of Patients with Anemia of Malignancy with Recombinant Human Erythropoietin

F. Herrmann[a], *W. Oster*[b], *R. Mertelsmann*[a,1]

[a]Department of Internal Medicine I, University of Freiburg i. Br., and
[b]Behringwerke AG, Marburg, FRG

Impaired production of erythropoietin (EPO) has been shown to be the major factor contributing to the anemia seen in patients with end-stage renal disease and progressive renal failure [12]. Several clinical trials have shown the efficacy of recombinant human EPO (rhEPO) in the treatment of anemias associated with deficient synthesis of endogenous EPO [4, 7, 15]. EPO treatment has proved to be beneficial for these patients in several aspects, including improvement of quality of life, prevention of transfusion-related risks of infections and of iron overload.

The effects of rhEPO treatment on erythropoiesis in anemic disease states that are not related to renal insufficiency have been, however, controversial. Nevertheless, there are intimations of a role for rhEPO in the treatment of the anemias of rheumatoid arthritis and of the acquired immune deficiency syndrome (AIDS) [1]. In this article we summarize the available data on rhEPO for the treatment of patients with anemia of malignant diseases and for other indications in oncology.

Clinical Experience with rhEPO in Malignancy

The first experiences with rhEPO in malignancy were gathered in a series of patients with anemia due to neoplastic bone marrow involvement by low-grade non-Hodgkin's lymphoma (LG-NHL) and multiple myeloma (MM) [10]. Treatment with the study drug was preceded by a 2-week period of

---

[1] We thank Ms. R. Freitas for the excellent preparation of the manuscript.

placebo administration. rhEPO was started at a comparatively low dose of 150 U/kg body weight (BW) twice weekly, given as an intravenous (IV) bolus injection. If hemoglobin (Hb) values did not increase by at last 1 g/dl, the rhEPO dose was raised after 4 weeks to 300 U/kg BW. A second escalation step of rhEPO to a dose of 450 U/kg BW followed after another 4 weeks in the case of inadequate response.

Four of 5 patients with LG-NHL and initial Hb values below 10 g/dl had a significant response to rhEPO, resulting in a mean increase of Hb levels by 2.1 g/dl (range 0.8–3.3 g/dl) during therapy. One patient with severe extensive disease showed only a minor response with a Hb increase of 0.3 g/dl (fig. 1). All responding patients became independent of erythrocyte transfusions. Improvement in Hb levels was associated with a reduction of serum ferritin values, which were initially high in most patients due to previous polytransfusion by more than 50% in most cases. The prestudy EPO serum levels of all patients were found to be increased (range 74–202 mU/ml).

Two patients in the accelerated phase of chronic myelogenous leukemia (CML) and anemia (Hb<10 g/dl) were also included in the protocol. Using the same route and schedule of rhEPO administration, a significant reduction of ferritin was observed in both as well as an increase in Hb and hematocrit (Hct) with, however, a slope lower than that in the patients with LG-NHL (fig. 2). The EPO serum levels in these 2 CML patients were initially found to be within the normal range (<35 mU/ml).

Recently it has been reported that EPO production by patients with anemia of malignancy is considerably lower when compared to EPO levels seen in patients with a similar degree of anemia caused by iron deficiency [9]. These findings are supported by the EPO serum levels found in our study. The degree of anemia observed, however, does not seem to correlate with the response to exogenous EPO in these patients, even though all laboratory parameters of renal function were within normal limits.

Patients with anemia associated with MM showed responses to rhEPO treatment very similar to those observed in the patients with LG-NHL. Most importantly, the patients also developed increases in platelet (PLT) counts with rhEPO by more than 75%. This might significantly increase therapeutic success in this disease state, which is often complicated by thrombocytopenia. The recent observation of EPO-inducible expansion of megakaryocytic progenitor cells (CFU-Meg) in vitro [2] and the identification of EPO receptors on megakaryocytes, fits well with this in vivo observation.

Most of the patients showed a response to rhEPO in the late phase of the second dose level and most prominently on the highest dose level. Since

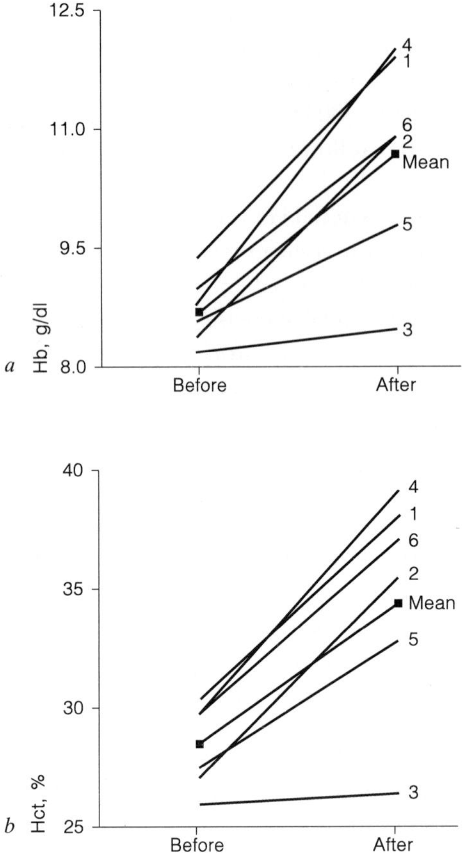

Fig. 1. a Changes in Hb values in 6 patients (indicated by numbers) as measured before and after rhEPO therapy. The line marked by closed squares shows the means of 6 patients. *b* The same information on Hct.

clinical experience with other hematopoietic growth factors in cancer patients [6] has demonstrated that constant drug delivery by continuous IV or subcutaneous (SC) infusion is more effective than IV bolus injection, we have recently changed our treatment protocol. A daily single SC dose of 10,000 U, 5 days/week, was introduced.

For LG-NHL and MM this new treatment modality was clearly associated with a faster increase of Hb and Hct. Figure 3 shows the slopes of Hb increase

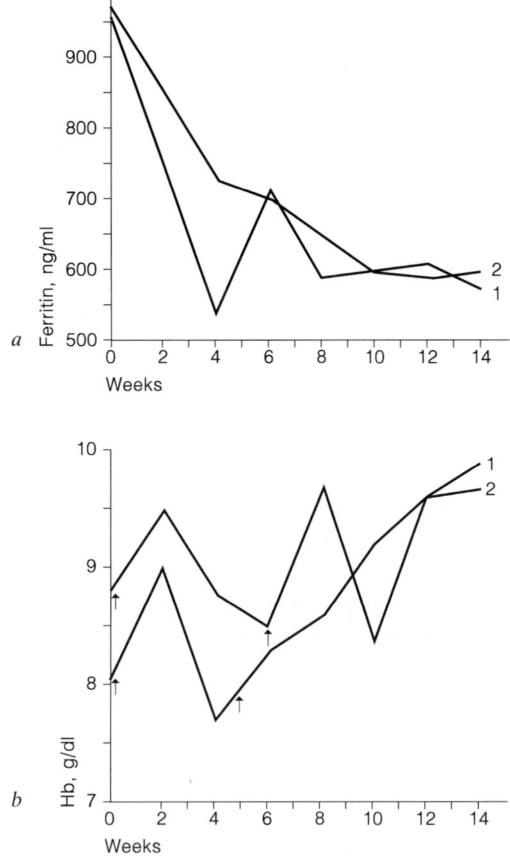

Fig. 2. Courses of serum ferritin *(a)* and Hb *(b)* in 2 patients (indicated by numbers) with CML under rhEPO treatment. The frequency of erythrocyte transfusions (500 ml washed erythrocytes) per 4 weeks is given for each patient. Arrows indicate erythrocyte transfusions during rhEPO treatment.

in 2 patients with LG-NHL and MM with comparable degrees of anemia and disease stage, each of whom was treated by either SC or IV bolus injection. Both SC-treated patients had a more rapid response and rhEPO treatment could be discontinued earlier.

Ten patients with myelodysplastic syndromes (MDS) including RAEB and RAEB-T were also included in our IV bolus injection protocol and are evaluable for the efficacy of rhEPO treatment. There was only a minor or no

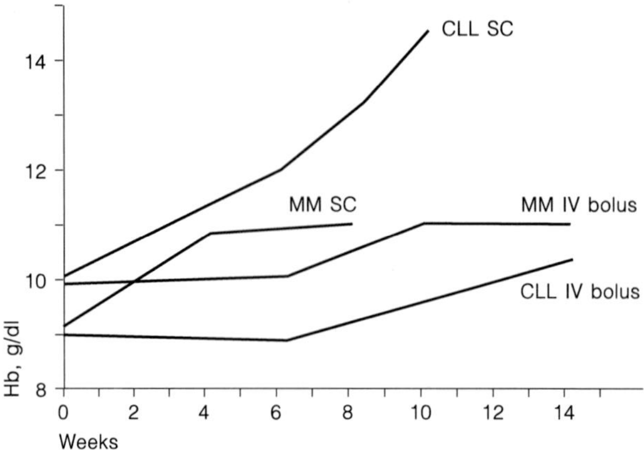

Fig. 3. Courses of Hb with different routes (SC and IV bolus) of rhEPO administration. Doses are indicated in the lower panel. Both patients with MM or CLL had similar stages of disease and equivalent degree of anemia prior to rhEPO therapy. Response of both patients on the SC schedule allowed the earlier discontinuation of rhEPO treatment.

increase in Hb, Hct and erythrocyte counts. However, 4 patients showed a reduction in their erythrocyte transfusion requirements (>50%). In vivo stimulation of erythropoiesis was also reflected by the reduction of serum ferritin values in some of these patients. Two patients also experienced a significantly reduced need for platelet transfusions (>50%), which was maintained for several weeks after rhEPO had been discontinued. However, overall response was less remarkable as compared to patients with LG-NHL and MM. This discrepancy may relate to EPO serum levels which were found to be much higher (range ca. 400–1,200 mU/ml) in our MDS patients, indicating that the mechanism causing anemia in this disorder is dyserythropoiesis rather than EPO deficiency.

Initial experience with rhEPO, given as a SC injection at the dose and duration mentioned above, in anemic patients with osteomyelofibrosis (who usually show high endogenous EPO serum levels similar to those in patients with MDS), suggest that this mode of administration may further enhance its effects on erythropoiesis. However, this question needs to be further investigated.

Preliminary data from other investigators confirm our findings [8]. Patients with anemias due to bone marrow infiltrating NHL and MM tend to show the most impressive responses, whereas the results in patients with MDS remain variable. Several investigators in Europe, Japan and North America

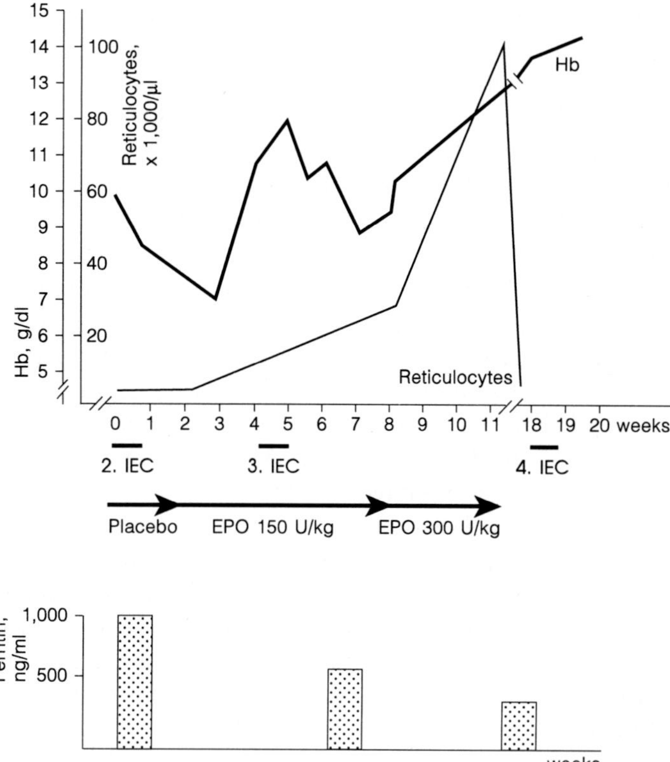

Fig. 4. Course of Hb, reticulocytes and ferritin under rhEPO treatment of a patient receiving anticancer chemotherapy (IEC) with ifosfamide (1,500 mg/m² IV, days 1–5), etoposide (120 mg/m² IV, days 1–3), cisplatinum (30 mg/m² IV, days 4–5).

are currently examining the potential benefit of rhEPO in MDS. Possibly stratification for the various subtypes of MDS (RA, RAEB, RAEB-T) may shed light on the heterogeneous response patterns reported.

Another hope for oncologists relating to anemia is to obtain the means to avoid transfusion therapy when an anemic period can be foreseen, e.g. following chemotherapy. In one well-documented case we showed that rhEPO has the potential to correct the anemia induced by cisplatinum-based treatment [10] (fig. 4). Moreover, we found that the in vivo stimulation of erythropoiesis continued under rhEPO even though further chemotherapy was administered, and the subsequent nadir counts of Hb and PLT were clearly higher as compared to prior nadir counts after identical chemotherapy without rhEPO (Hb 7.0 vs. 8.9 g/dl; PLT 9×10^3 vs. $59 \times 10^3/\mu l$). Again a more than 60% reduction in serum ferritin values was associated with the increase of Hb. The potential for rhEPO to act on erythropoiesis while chemotherapy is continued has also been recently confirmed in a preliminary report by others [5].

Patients with a variety of malignant disease states associated with anemia unrelated to bone marrow infiltration by neoplastic cells or previous chemotherapy have been enrolled in rhEPO trials as well. Data are, however, not yet available. In some cases, rhEPO has been shown to be of potential benefit in pure red cell anemia [3]. Other data show a failure of rhEPO to correct anemia in Fanconi syndrome [14] and Blackfan-Diamond syndrome [Herrmann et al., unpubl. results]. rhEPO is currently also being studied in patients after autologous and allogeneic bone marrow transplantation. A first preliminary report shows the efficacy of rhEPO in hastening the increase of reticulocyte counts and Hct in the phase of transplant recovery [3].

In contrast to adverse events of rhEPO treatment seen in patients with renal disease, cancer patients seem to tolerate rhEPO extremely well. No serious side effects have been reported so far in more than 100 patient treated with rhEPO. The lack of side effects of rhEPO treatment in cancer patients may relate to their shorter history of anemia and the absence of vascular disease, which may represent the major contributing factor to the complications of rhEPO treatment in patients with renal disease.

Although rhEPO has just entered the arena of oncology, this hematopoietic growth factor, with a history going back almost a century [12], seems already to be a promising agent which will improve the treatment of cancer patients.

References

1   Adamson, J.W.; Eschbach, J.W.: Use of recombinant human erythropoietin in humans; in Mertelsmann, R.; Herrmann, F. (eds): Hematopoietic Growth factors in Clinical Applications, pp.129–140 (Marcel Dekker, New York 1990).
2   Dessypris, E.N.; Graber, S.E.; Krantz, D.B.; Stone, W.J.: Effects of recombinant erythropoietin on the concentration and cycling status of human hematopoietic progenitor cells in vivo. Blood *72:* 2060–2065 (1988).
3   Ebell, W.; Bucsky, P.; Diedrich, H.; Seidel, J.; Stoll, M.; Freund, M.; Sens, B.; Tischler, J.; Brune, T.; Riehm,, H.; Poliwoda, H.; Link, H.: Use of recombinant human erythropoietin after bone marrow transplantation (abstract). Mol Biother *1:* 53 (1989).
4   Eschbach, J.W.; Kelly, M.R.; Haley, N.R.; Abels, R.I.; Adamson, J.W.: The treatment of the anemia of progressive renal failure with recombinant human erythropoietin. N. Engl. J. Med. *321:* 158–163 (1989).

5   Henry, D.H.; Rudnick, S.A.; Bryant, E.; Abels, R.I.; Danna, R.P.; Staddon, A.P.;
    Mason, B.A.: Preliminary report of two double-blind, placebo-controlled studies using
    human recombinant erythropoietin in the anemia associated with cancer (abstract).
    Blood *74:* suppl. 1, p. 6 (1988).

6   Herrmann, F.; Schulz, G.; Lindemann, A.; Meyenburg, W.; Oster, W.; Krumwieh, D.;
    Mertelsmann, R.: Hematopoietic responses in patients with advanced malignancy treat-
    ed with recombinant human granulocyte-macrophage colony-stimulating factor. J. Clin.
    Oncol. *7:* 159–167 (1989).

7   Lim, V.S.; DeGowin, R.L.; Zavala, D.; Kirchner, P.T.; Abels, R.; Perry, P.; Fangman,
    J.: Recombinant human erythropoietin treatment in pre-dialysis patients. Ann. intern.
    Med. *110:* 108–114 (1989).

8   Ludwig, H.; Fritz, E.; Kotzmann, H.; Höcker, P.; Gisslinger, H.; Barnas, U.: Erythro-
    poietin treatment for chronic anemia of malignancy (abstract). Blood *74:* suppl. 1, p. 16
    (1989).

9   Miller, C.; Jones, R.; Piantadosi, S.; Abeloff, M.; Spivak, J.: Decreased erythropoietin
    (EPO) response associated with the anemia of malignancy (abstract). Proc. ASCO *8:*
    709 (1989).

10 Oster, W.; Herrmann, F.; Cicco, A.; Gamm, H.; Zeile, G.; Brune, T.; Lindemann, A.;
    Schulz, G.; Mertelsmann, R.: Erythropoietin prevents chemotherapy-induced anemia:
    Case report. Blut *60:* 88–92 (1990).

11 Oster, W.; Herrmann, F.; Gamm, H.; Zeile, G.; Lindemann, A.; Müller, H.-G.; Brune,
    T.; Kraemer, H.-P.; Mertelsmann, R.: Erythropoietin (EPO) for the treatment of
    anemia of malignancy associated with neoplastic bone marrow infiltration. J. Clin.
    Oncol. *8:* 956–962 (1990).

12 Oster, W.; Herrmann, F.; Lindemann, A.; Mertelsmann, R.: Experimental and clinical
    evaluation of erythropoietin ; in Habenicht, A. (ed.): Growth Factors, Differentiation
    Factors, and Cytokines, pp. 232–242 (Springer, Stuttgart 1990).

13 Tischler, H.J.; Leblanc, S.; Brune, H.; Welte, K.; Poliwoda, H.; Link, H.: Recombi-
    nant human erythropoietin in treatment of pure red cell anemia (abstract). Blut *59:* 340
    (1989).

14 Vellenga, E.; de Wolf, J.T.M.; Halie, M.R.: Recombinant erythropoietin failed to
    correct anemia in Fanconi syndrome (abstract). Leukemia *5:* 858 (1989).

15 Winearls, C.G.; Oliver, D.O.; Pippard, M.J.; Reid, C.; Downing, M.R.; Cotes, P.M.:
    Effect of human erythropoietin derived from recombinant DNA on the anemia of
    patients maintained by chronic hemodialysis. Lancet *ii:* 1175–1178 (1986).

Prof. Dr. F. Herrmann, Department of Internal Medicine I, University of Freiburg,
Hugstetter Strasse 55, D–7800 Freiburg i. Br. (FRG)

Gurland HJ, Moran J, Samtleben W, Scigalla P, Wieczorek L (eds): Erythropoietin in
Renal and Non-Renal Anemias. Contrib Nephrol. Basel, Karger, 1991, vol 88, pp 246–247

Discussion

to the Paper by F. Herrmann et al.

Krantz (Nashville): In the myelodysplasia patients that have so far been reported to
respond to EPO, I haven't found a case that had a karyotypic abnormality. I wonder if any of
your 4 cases had such abnormalities.

Herrmann: We have not routinely done karyotypic studies. As far as I know, one of the
patients had 5q– syndrome and another had an isochromosome 17.

Wardrop (Cardiff): Did you get any impression as to whether this potent stimulation of
erythropoiesis led to any reduction in neutrophil production?

Herrmann: We have not observed any effect on the white cell count.

Jacobs (Cardiff): Could Dr. Herrmann clarify whether the patients with non-Hodgkin's
lymphoma and CLL myeloma were pre-chemotherapy, post-chemotherapy, or at what stage?

Herrmann: A requirement for entrance into the study was that the patient had received
no chemotherapy in the previous 4 weeks. Most of them, however, had had chemotherapy
prior to this. Patients with chronic myelogenous leukemia had concomitant therapy with
hydroxyurea.

Erslev (Philadelphia): You mentioned that in your patients with chronic myelogenous
leukemia, the endogenous EPO production was normal. How low did the hemoglobin fall
without any EPO response?

Herrmann: Below 8 g/dl.

Essers (Aachen): Did you look at the blast population in the myelodysplastic syndrome?

Herrmann: Yes. The blasts did not respond to EPO, at least not proliferatively.

Goldberg (Boston): With regard to the myelodysplasia patients, even the ones that had
endogenous EPO levels of 1,000 mU/ml responded?

Herrmann: No.

Goldberg: Did the ones that responded have low levels?

Herrmann: Yes, although there was no obvious correlation between endogenous EPO
levels and response. In general, only patients with an EPO level below 500 responded.

Krantz: We are also treating myelodysplasia patients, and 2 of our patients had EPO
levels of 1,000 and I think Dr. Hirashima has also seen that. So the response doesn't seem to
relate necessarily to the EPO level, as long as it isn't too high. All our patients with more than
1,000 U have not responded.

Niemeyer (Hannover): In the myelodysplastic patients who responded to EPO, did you then stop therapy?

Herrmann: No.

Eschbach (Seattle): This is for Dr. Herrmann and Dr. Krantz. You mentioned that your patients had serum EPO levels as high as 5,000 mU/ml. If you give subcutaneous EPO in the doses you used I doubt whether you're going to get levels as high as that. So how do you explain why they responded?

Herrmann: I don't know for sure, but it might well be that we are measuring in the RIA biologically less active EPO.

Krantz: Dr. Eschbach, I believe you're thinking of uremic patients who have very low EPO levels when you say that a given amount of EPO will raise the EPO level only so much. In these patients, where you already have high endogenous levels, you are going to build upon that high endogenous level that much more, since we now know that there is no down-regulation of EPO production.

Goldberg: Did the patients who had previously received chemotherapy and might have had a recovering bone marrow continue to have the same elevated hematocrits when they had been off EPO for several months, or did they fall back down?

Herrmann: No. The hematocrit continued to be elevated for at least 6 weeks.

Goldberg: Is another possibility that these patients are recovering from chemotherapy and that you were seeing a recovering bone marrow?

Herrmann: I don't think our patients had anemia caused by previous chemotherapy.

Hellström (Stockholm): Did you see any changes in the bone marrow in the patients responding to therapy?

Herrmann: We have not routinely investigated the bone marrow in the myelodysplastic patients.

Gurland HJ, Moran J, Samtleben W, Scigalla P, Wieczorek L (eds): Erythropoietin in
Renal and Non-Renal Anemias. Contrib Nephrol. Basel, Karger, 1991, vol 88, pp 248–251

Chemotherapy-Induced Anemia

Carole B. Miller

The Johns Hopkins Oncology Center, Baltimore, Md., USA

Anemia is a common cause of morbidity in patients with cancer. While
mild anemia is present in cancer patients prior to treatment with cytotoxic
chemotherapy, the anemia often worsens with treatment. The anemia associated with cancer and chemotherapy is normochromic, normocytic with an
inappropriately low reticulocyte count. Serum iron and iron-binding capacity
are low and morphologic examination of the bone marrow reveals normal
erythroid precursors and normal or increased stainable iron [1]. Erythroid
progenitors (BFU-E and CFU-E) size, number, and degree of hemoglobiniza-
tion are normal in the marrows of patients with cancer and maintain normal
sensitivity to erythropoietin (EPO) in vitro [2]. The anemia of cancer and
chemotherapy is morphologically similar to the anemia of other chronic diseases (renal failure, rheumatoid arthritis, HIV infection).

Transfusion is not without significant morbidity in patients receiving
chemotherapy [3,4]. Acute side effects (transfusion reactions and alloimmuni-
zation) are not uncommon. As the long-term remission and cure rate in
patients with some cancers increases, long-term complications of blood transfusion such as hepatitis, with the potential for development of hepatoma and
cirrhosis [5, 6], become increasingly important issues for the oncologist. Methods of treatment of the anemia associated with chemotherapy without the use
of red blood cell transfusions could lessen the morbidity associated with
chemotherapy and improve the quality of life in patients with cancer.

An inappropriately low EPO response to anemia is seen in anemias associated with renal failure [7] and other chronic diseases (HIV infection [8], rheumatoid arthritis [9]). Treatment of the anemia of chronic renal failure with
rhEPO has been highly successful [10, 11], suggesting that EPO deficiency may
be the etiology of the anemia of renal failure. It is possible that the anemia of
cancer and chemotherapy may also be partially due to inappropriately low EPO
response to anemia, and therefore may also respond to therapy with rhEPO.

Methods and Results

In order to determine if the anemia of cancer and chemotherapy was associated with inadequate EPO production, EPO levels were analyzed in 74 nonhypoxemic anemic patients [12] with cancer using a sensitive commercially available radioimmunoassay [13]. Twenty-four patients with iron deficiency anemia were used as controls, as they have a normal EPO response to anemia [14]. Compared to the controls, where EPO levels increased as hemoglobin decreased, there was no significant correlation between EPO levels and hemoglobin levels in the cancer patients, and EPO levels did not increase as hemoglobin levels decreased. Using analysis of covariance [15], the EPO response to anemia was significantly lower in the cancer patients than in the controls. The EPO response to anemia was decreased in the patients with cancer who had not been previously treated, but was significantly more depressed in the patients receiving chemotherapy. There was no difference in the EPO response to anemia in patients who were treated with cisplatin-containing regimens versus noncisplatin-containing regimens. This effect was not related to clinical nephrotoxicity or severe malnutrition. These data suggest that the anemia of cancer is in part mediated by EPO deficiency.

In order to determine whether the anemia associated with chemotherapy can be improved with treatment with exogenous EPO, we participated in a cooperative phase I/II study of rhEPO [16] (Marogen, provided by Chugai-Upjohn). Patients who were anemic (hemoglobin <11.0 g/dl) as a result of chemotherapy were eligible. Patients were required to have a good performance status and normal renal, liver, and cardiac function. rhEPO was given intravenously 5 times a week for 4 weeks during the course of chemotherapy at escalating dose levels (25–300 IU/kg). Ten patients are treated at each level – 5 on cisplatin chemotherapy and 5 on chemotherapy that did not include cisplatin. The cisplatin arm was terminated after the 200 IU/kg dose level because of slow patient accrual on this arm and evidence of activity at lower dose levels. Patient accrual has recently been completed.

There was no acute toxicity associated with rhEPO administration. Hypertension did not appear to be associated with a response to EPO in this group of patients with cancer as was seen in the patients with renal insufficiency. At the highest dose level (300 IU/kg), two thrombotic episodes were seen at sites of Hickman catheters. Additional patients were accrued at this dose level to determine if this is an EPO-related toxicity (3 patients are still receiving therapy).

Preliminary results from this study demonstrate activity at the 100 and 200

IU/kg dose levels in both the cisplatin and noncisplatin arms of this study. The mean hemoglobin increase in the evaluable patients after 4 weeks of treatment with rhEPO at the 100 and 200 IU/kg dose levels was 1.9 and 3.0 respectively in the cisplatin arm and 1.2 and 1.6 respectively in the noncisplatin arm. This increase in hemoglobin does not appear to be an artifact related to the timing of chemotherapy and the administration of EPO. Four patients (3 noncisplatin, 1 cisplatin) are currently under treatment.

Discussion

These data suggest that the anemia of cancer and chemotherapy is associated with decreased EPO response to anemia. The etiology of the decreased EPO response to anemia in patients who are receiving chemotherapy is unknown but may be due to the direct inhibition of EPO production in the kidney [17]. It therefore appears that the anemia of cancer and chemotherapy may be at least partially due to the inadequate EPO response to anemia seen in these patients. This is further supported by the preliminary results that demonstrate considerable activity of rhEPO in the treatment of the anemia of chemotherapy-induced anemia, as described above. Phase III placebo-controlled studies [18, 19] of rhEPO at a dose of 150 IU/kg given subcutaneously, 3 times a week for 12 weeks, in the anemia associated with chemotherapy have also shown significant increases in hematocrit in the treatment arms when compared to the control arms. Quality of life appears to be improved by treatment with EPO in preliminary analysis as well [19].

In conclusion, treatment of the chemotherapy-induced anemia with EPO appears to be well tolerated in patients who are receiving chemotherapy. Treatment with rhEPO appears to increase the hemoglobin despite continued administration of chemotherapy and thus may improve the quality of life in patients who are receiving chemotherapy, reduce transfusion-related complications, and decrease the need for homologous blood donation.

References

1   Cartwright, G.E.: The anemia of chronic disorders. Semin. Haematol. *3:* 351–355 (1966).
2   Dainiak, N.; Kulkarni, V.; Howard, D.; Kalmant, M.; Dewey, M.; Hoffman, R.: Mechanisms of abnormal erythropoiesis in malignancy. Cancer *51:* 1101–1106 (1983).
3   Phares, J.C.: Hematologic support of the patient with malignancy. Cancer Growth Prog. *10:* 180–188 (1989).

4   Schiffer, C.A.; Wiernik, P.H.: Hematologic considerations in cancer; in Calabresi, P.; Schein, P.S.; Rosenberg, S.A. (eds): Medical Oncology, pp. 1358–1370 (Macmillan, New York 1985).

5   Fukuda, A.; Sugimachi, K.; Tokudome, S.; Ikeda, M.; Koga, S.; Hirohata, T.: Blood transfusion as a risk factor for cirrhosis and liver cancer: A matched case-control study. J. Natl. Cancer Inst. *81:* 1189–1190 (1989).

6   Beasley, R.P.; Hwang, L.Y.; Lin, C.C.: Hepatocellular carcinoma and hepatitis B virus. Lancet *ii:* 1129–1133 (1981).

7   Spivak, J.L.: Erythropoietin. Blood Rev. *3:* 130–135 (1989).

8   Spivak, J.L.; Barnes, D.C.; Fuchs, E.; Quinn, T.C.: Serum immunoreactive erythropoietin in HIV-infected patients. JAMA *2612:* 3104–3107 (1989).

9   Hochberg, M.C.; Arnold, C.M.; Hogans, B.B.; Spivak, J.L.: Serum immunoreactive erythropoietin in rheumatoid arthritis: Impaired response to anemia. Arthritis Rheum. *31:* 1318–1321 (1988).

10 Eschbach, J.W.; Egrie, J.C.; Downing, M.R.; Browne, J.K.; Adamson, J.W.: Correction of the anemia of end-stage renal disease with recombinant human erythropoietin: Results of the phase I and II clinical trial. N. Engl. J. Med. *316:* 73–88 (1987).

11 Casati, S.; Passerini, P.; Campise, M.R.; Graziani, G.; Cesana, B.; Perisic, M.; Ponticelli, C.: Benefits and risks of protracted treatment with recombinant erythropoietin in patients having haemodialysis. Br. Med. J. *295:* 1017–1020 (1987).

12 Miller, C.B.; Jones, R.J.; Piantadosi, S.; Abeloff, M.D.; Spivak, J.L.: Decreased erythropoietin response in patients with the anemia of cancer. N. Engl. J. Med., *322:* 1689–1693, 1990.

13 Egrie, J.C.; Cotes, P.M.; Lane, J.; Gaines Das, R.E.; Tam, R.C.: Development of a radioimmunoassay for human erythropoietin using recombinant erythropoietin as a tracer and immunogen. J. Immunol. Methods *99:* 235–241 (1987).

14 Ward, H.P.; Kurnick, J.E.; Pisarczyk, M.J.: Serum level of erythropoietin in anemias associated with chronic infection, malignancy and primary hematopoietic disease. J. Clin. Invest. *50:* 332–335 (1971).

15 Snedecor, G.W.; Cochran, W.G.: Statistical Methods; 7th ed., pp. 365–388. (Iowa State University Press, Ames 1967).

16 Miller, C.B.; Platanias, L.C.; Ratain, M.J.; Hart, R.D.; Ettinger, D.S.; Mills, S.R.; Jones, R.J.: A phase I/II trial of erythropoietin in the treatment of chemotherapy-induced anemia in patients with cancer (abstract). Proc. ASCO *9:* 194 (1990).

17 Fisher, J.W.; Roh, B.L.: Influence of alkylating agents on kidney erythropoietin production. Cancer Res *24:* 983–988 (1964).

18 Henry, D.H.; Rudnick, S.A.; Bryant, E.; Abels, R.; Danna, R.; Staddon, A.; Mason, B.: Preliminary report of two double-blind, placebo-controlled studies using recombinant human erythropoietin in the anemia associated with cancer (abstract). Blood *73:* suppl. 8 (1989).

19 Henry, D.; Keller, A.; Kugler, J.; Silver, R.; Danna, R.; Staddon, A.; Mason, B.; Abels, R.: Treatment of anemia in cancer patients on cisplatin chemotherapy with recombinant human erythropoietin. Proc. ASCO *9:* 182 (1990).

Carole B. Miller, MD, The Johns Hopkins Oncology Center, Oncology 2–127, 600 North Wolfe Street, Baltimore, MD 21205 (USA)

Gurland HJ, Moran J, Samtleben W, Scigalla P, Wieczorek L (eds): Erythropoietin in Renal and Non-Renal Anemias. Contrib Nephrol. Basel, Karger, 1991, vol 88, pp 252–253

Discussion

to the Paper by C. B. Miller

Herrmann (Berlin): I am not sure whether you can answer this question because this was not a controlled study, but did you look at the white count and platelet recovery? Was there any compromise?

Miller: There did not appear to be any compromise in either. In our preliminary analysis of the cycles before and after treatment with EPO there did not appear to be any change in the white count nadir. However, the study is still in progress and the formal analysis has not been done. We also have not seen any changes in platelets. It did not appear that we had to delay courses of chemotherapy because of lowered white cell counts.

Baldamus: (Cologne): I would like to make a comment concerning serum EPO levels during chemotherapy. In using various regimens we only found a rise in serum EPO levels during treatment of seminomas with a combination of bleomycin, cis-platinum and etoposid. Serum EPO levels rose beyond the value expected for the degree of anemia. The pathogenetic background so remains unexplained since simultaneous serum biochemistry showed neither hepatic (EPO degradation) nor renal (EPO production) involvement. However, the future follow-up of this unexpected rise of serum EPO as a consequence of specific chemotherapeutic drugs might help to clarify the unknown mechanisms in EPO production and/or degradation.

Miller: Early in the course of chemotherapy with other regimens there have been marked increases in EPO levels, potentially related to the chemotherapy. This has been seen in patients undergoing both bone marrow transplant and treatment for leukemia. Your observation is very interesting.

Essers (Aachen): Was there any change in performance status and weight?

Miller: Anecdotally, yes, the patients whose hematocrit/hemoglobin went up improved. However, this is a phase I/II study and we cannot formally analyse the performance status.

Winearls (Oxford): How did you define normal renal function?

Miller: As a serum creatinine of less than 1.5 mg/dl. We did not do 24-hour urine collections for creatine clearance. We just used an oncologist's view of normal renal function, I am sure, instead of a nephrologist's view.

Winearls: I think this may be relevant. These are very sick patients, who with a creatinine of 1.5 mg, might have really quite depressed renal function. So what you may be in fact seeing is acute renal impairment causing suppression of EPO responses, and that ought to be taken into account in interpreting the responses.

Miller: In looking at the EPO response to anemia in the patients with cancer, we looked for a correlation within the patients who all had 'normal' renal function. We looked for a relationship between the serum creatinine and the EPO response to anemia, and there did not appear to be any correlation. In our patients undergoing treatment we did not look at that question at all.

Winearls: In your graph correlating EPO levels with hematocrit, the line seemed to depend very much on 6 data points. Three iron-deficient patients had relatively higher EPO levels than 3 cancer patients that had 'normal' levels. One would feel more confident if there were more data points in that particular part of the graph.

Miller: There were some data presented at the most recent American Society of Clinical Oncology meeting from the phase III double-blind study an rhEPO in patients receiving chemotherapy. Those data appeared similar to ours, supporting the idea that these patients do have a decreased EPO response.

Gurland HJ, Moran J, Samtleben W, Scigalla P, Wieczorek L (eds): Erythropoietin in
Renal and Non-Renal Anemias. Contrib Nephrol. Basel, Karger, 1991, vol 88, pp 254–265

Improvement in Anemia by Recombinant Human Erythropoietin in Patients with Myelodysplastic Syndrome and Aplastic Anemia

Kunitake Hirashima, Masami Bessho, Ituro Jinnai

First Department of Internal Medicine, Saitama Medical School, Moroyama,
Saitama, Japan

Recently, progress in genetic engineering techniques has allowed the
production of sufficient recombinant human erythropoietin (rhEPO) for clinical trials. Since the reports of Winearls et al. [1] and Eschbach et al. [2], the
clinical importance of rhEPO has been established in the treatment of anemia
with chronic renal failure.

In Japan, we have already treated over 1,000 severely anemic chronic
hemodialysis patients with rhEPO (Epoch; Chugai Pharmaceutical Co. Ltd.,
Tokyo, Japan). A remarkable improvement in anemia was observed in over
95% of these patients without any severe adverse effects [3].

We have now expanded the clinical application of rhEPO with trials in
severe refractory anemias such as aplastic anemia (AA) and myelodysplastic
anemia (MDS), a trial of anemia associated with chronic inflammation such as
rheumatoid arthritis, and a trial designed to reduced the amount of blood used
during operations in association with autotransfusion.

The efficacy of rhEPO in AA and refractory anemia was uncertain because of the very high level of endogenous EPO in the plasma of these
patients. However, we already had experimental evidence of an improvement
in the congenital hypoplastic anemia of the W/W^v strain of mice by rhEPO
administration in large amounts [4]. In the present study, we aimed at the
improvement of the anemic state in AA and refractory anemia by reducing the
requirement of red blood cell transfusion by the administration of a large dose
of rhEPO. Four of 12 such patients responded to rhEPO according to our
evaluating criteria, including an increase in hemoglobin and a decrease in the
transfusion requirement.

Materials and Methods

Subjects

Eight patients with MDS and 4 with AA were studied after giving informed consent as approved by the human subjects review committee at our institution. The etiology of the disease was unknown in all of the patients. The clinical characteristics at enrollment are shown in table 1. The median age was 36 years (range 21–83).

The diagnosis of MDS was made according to the French-American-British (FAB) criteria. Two patients with MDS had been treated previously with bolus methylprednisolone and vitamin D_3. Five patients were dependent on periodical red cell transfusions. Chromosome analysis revealed an abnormal karyotype in 1 patient with RAEB-t (case 7).

In all patients with AA, a pancytopenia in the peripheral blood and a hypocellularity in the bone marrow was present. One of the 4 patients had received previous treatment with methylprednisolone and antilymphocyte globulin (ALG). All patients were dependent on red cell transfusions.

All patients in both groups were ambulatory and had Karnovsky performance scores of >50% with a life expectancy of at least 3 months. Adequate renal and hepatic function were required in all patients. Patients were also required to have no evidence of iron deficiency. None had received chemotherapy or ALG for at least 4 weeks before starting rhEPO.

Test Drug

The rhEPO was provided by Chugai Pharmaceutical Co. Ltd. The specific activity of the test drug corresponds to 180,000 IU/mg polypeptide equivalent of rhEPO.

Dose and Dosing Schedule

Patients received rhEPO by intravenous injection 3 times/week for at least 4 weeks. Doses were 3,000, 6,000 or 12,000 units/day. The body weight of all patients was comparable, and average body weight was 60 kg; therefore, 3,000 units/day was roughly 50 units/kg. Six patients received 3,000 units and the other 6 patients 6,000 units as an initial dose.

Laboratory Tests

All patients were admitted to our hospital and evaluated by a complete history, physical examination and laboratory tests including a complete blood count, a white cell differential reticulocyte count, a serum biochemical profile, urinalysis, prothrombin time and partial thromboplastin time. These tests were monitored periodically during treatment with rhEPO. Detailed morphological studies on the peripheral blood and bone marrow aspirate were also performed periodically. A ferrokinetic study including red cell iron utilization, plasma iron clearance rate and a red cell life span study by ^{51}Cr were performed in each case. For an assay of erythroid progenitors (colony-forming units, erythroid), bone marrow mononuclear cells were cultured following Ficoll-Hypaque separation by the methylcellulose culture technique of Iscove et al [5]. Serum EPO concentration in these patients was measured by radioimmunoassay.

Evaluation

A favorable response to rhEPO was defined as an increase of hemoglobin concentration of 1.5 g/dl or more 8 weeks after the initiation of rhEPO in transfusion-independent patients. In transfusion-dependent patients it was regarded as effective if the requirement for red cell transfusion decreased over 50% compared with the average amount in 4 weeks during the

Table 1. Clinical and laboratory characteristics of patients with MDS or AA

Patient No.	Age	Sex	Dx	Months after Dx	Previous Tx (months)	Hb g/dl	Corrected ret., %	Neutro-phils, 10^9/l	Platelets 10^9/l	CFU-E/10^5 BM cells	BFU-E/10^5 BM cells
1	29	F	RA	18	mPLS (+20) VitD$_3$ (8)	6.3	1.3	1.6	12	88	1.4
2	65	F	RA	11	NT	8.6	1.2	1.0	37	80	9.4
3	73	F	RA	4	NT	5.1	0.6	0.2	34	4	0.6
4	60	F	RARS	8	NT	5.8	0.8	0.8	64	6	0.6
5	83	F	RAEB	17	VitD$_3$ (8)	7.3	1.5	0.9	120	157	14.6
6	63	M	RAEB-t	6	NT	6.8	0.2	2.1	33	0	0
7	57	M	RAEB-t	2	NT	6.2	0.1	0.2	54	0	0
8	53	M	RAEB-t	5	NT	7.4	0.3	0.2	27	ND	ND
9	68	M	AA	7		9.3	0.8	0.7	47	14	3.3
10	21	F	AA	16	mPLS (+16) ALG (+5)	5.9	1.3	0.6	10	118	8.6
11	62	F	AA	5	NT	6.6	0.4	0.5	30	128	4.6
12	73	F	AA	4	NT	7.5	0.1	0.5	49	0.6	0

ND = Not determined; NT = no treatment; RA = refractory anemia; RARS = refractory anemia with ring sideroblast; RAEB = refractory anemia with excess of blasts; RAEB-t = RAEB in transformation; AA = aplastic anemia; mPLS = methylprednisolone; VitD$_3$ = vitamin D$_3$; PSL = prednisolone; ALG = antilymphocyte globulin.

pretreatment period. Patients judged as responsive according to these criteria were eligible for maintenance therapy with rhEPO. Treatment was discontinued in patients who had severe adverse effects or when progression of the disease was documented.

Results

Improvement in Anemia in Transfusion-Independent Cases

Therapeutic efficacy was assessed as an improvement in the hemoglobin concentration, as previously mentioned. This was observed in 1 patient with refractory anemia with an excess of blasts (RAEB, case 5) (table 2).

Decrease in Transfusion Requirement

In the transfused patients, efficacy was evaluated as a decreased requirement. This was observed in 2 patients (cases 1 and 2) with refractory anemia and 1 patient with AA (case 9). Cases 1 and 9, who were dependent on red cell transfusion and responded very well to rhEPO, were commenced on maintenance therapy by rhEPO. They became transfusion-independent because of a continued increase in hemoglobin with rhEPO (table 2).

Increase in Mean Corpuscular Volume (MCV) and in the rhEPO-Responsive Cases

An increase in the MCV and mean corpuscular hemoglobin (MCH) of red cells was observed in several cases (table 3). A marked increase in both values was observed in cases 1, 5, 9 and 11. All except case 11 were responsive according to our evaluation.

Decrease in EPO Concentration after rhEPO Administration

The serum EPO concentration before rhEPO treatment was extremely high in all patients, ranging from 694 to 9,840 mU/ml. Following rhEPO treatment, a decrease in EPO concentration was observed in 3 of the patients (case 1, 5 and 9) who had an increase in hemoglobin concentration. As shown in table 2, no precise correlation between the efficacy of EPO and the titer of serum EPO concentration was observed.

Relationship between the Number of Erythroid Progenitors and the Responsiveness to rhEPO

The number of erythroid progenitor cells was estimated in 11 cases by CFU-E assay before rhEPO treatment (table 1). The number of CFU-E in the marrow was very heterogeneous before the initiation of treatment. The pres-

Table 2. Effect of rhEPO on erythropoiesis of patients with MDS or AA

Patient No.	Doses of rhEPO × 10³ units (weeks)	RBC 10¹²/l		Hb g/dl		Hct %		Corrected ret. %		Serum EPO mU/ml		Transfusion of RBCs ml/month	
		BF	AT	BF	AT	BF	AT	BF	AT	BF	AT	BF	AT
1[1]	6 (4), 12 (+50)	1.92	3.16	6.3	13.9	20.2	42.3	1.3	5.1	919	114	900	0
2	6 (4), 12 (2)	2.46	2.61	8.6	8.6	26.5	27.9	1.2	1.0	1,240	2,000	0	0
3[1]	3 (4), 6 (4), 12 (4)	1.62	1.78	5.1	5.8	15.4	17.2	0.6	0.7	986	956	1,000	400
4	6 (4), 12 (1)	1.81	1.79	5.8	5.7	19.8	19.1	0.8	1.0	1,570	2,100	0	0
5[1]	3 (4)	2.23	3.40	7.3	11.8	24.2	36.5	1.5	0.7	1,040	244	0	0
6	3 (4)	2.32	1.96	6.8	5.9	20.7	18.0	0.2	0.1	694	1,060	600	400
7	3 (4), 6 (4)	2.01	1.85	6.2	5.6	19.2	17.0	0.1	0.1	2,290	7,230	1,200	1,200
8	6 (4)	2.32	2.03	7.4	5.9	21.3	18.3	0.3	0.1	1,240	ND	900	800
9[1]	3 (4), 6 (4), 12 (+86)	2.73	3.16	9.3	12.2	26.7	38.1	0.8	2.6	2,790	394	500	0
10	6 (4), 12 (4)	1.92	1.53	5.9	5.2	18.2	14.9	1.3	0.3	9,840	ND	800	500
11	3 (4), 6 (4), 12 (4)	2.06	1.64	6.6	5.6	19.4	17.5	0.4	0.8	2,280	2,630	800	600
12	6 (4), 12 (4)	1.38	2.63	7.5	7.9	22.1	24.5	0.1	0.1	1,720	ND	1,000	800

[1]Responsive cases evaluated by our criteria.
ND = Not determined; BF = before rhEPO treatment; AT = after rhEPO treatment.

ence of CFU-E in the marrow was verified in all patients who responded to rhEPO, and in some nonresponsive patients, CFU-E were also detectable in the marrow (case 2, 4, 10–12).

Ferrokinetic Study

As shown in table 4, in 2 cases (cases 1 and 9) who responded well, a significant improvement in plasma iron disappearance (PID) and red cell utilization (RCU) of radioiron was observed.

Other Data

rhEPO had no effect on the white cell count, the white cell differential count, and the percentage of blasts in the marrow. A transient increase in platelets was seen in 1 RAEB-t patient (case 6). The cellularity and the fraction of erythroblasts in the marrow both increased in cases 1 and 9.

Adverse Effects

We have seen no adverse effects of rhEPO. No progression of the disease which could be attributed to rhEPO was seen.

Case Reports

The clinical courses of 3 patients who had excellent responses to rhEPO are shown in figures 1–3.

Case 1 (fig. 1): Case 1 was a 29-year-old woman who was referred of our hospital because of anemia in April 1987. She was 24 weeks' pregnant. Laboratory tests showed hemoglobin 3.7 g/dl, WBC 33 × 10^9/l with 73% neutrophils, and platelets 46 × 10^9/l. Bone marrow examination revealed a hypocellular marrow with hypercellular islands. Chromosome analysis of the bone marrow showed a normal karyotype. Blood and marrow smears showed dysplastic changes in neutrophils, erythroblasts, and megakaryocytes. Based on these findings, she was diagnosed as having a refractory anemia. In August 1987 (the 40th week of pregnancy), she gave birth to a normal female weighing 2,890 g. The infant's peripheral blood count was normal. In October 1987, she was treated with bolus methylprednisolone, but no clinical improvement was observed. In November 1988, oral vitamin D$_3$ was started but was not effective. The patient received approximately 900 ml of red cell transfusion per month prior to the initiation of rhEPO treatment. In October 1988, she received 6,000 units of rhEPO 3 times/week for 4 weeks. While a transient increase in reticulocytes was observed, hemoglobin did not change. Over an interval of 2 weeks, she received 50 µg of GM-CSF (provided by Shering-Plough Co.) for 5 days as a part of a phase 1 trial of GM-CSF. A slight and transient increase in leukocytes and reticulocytes was seen. After 2 weeks, she received 12,000 units of rhEPO 3 times/week. The reticulocytes increased consistently and the hemoglobin increased to an almost normal level. When hemoglobin reached 13.9 g/dl in July 1989, rhEPO administration was reduced to twice weekly. Since October 1989, the weekly dose of rhEPO has been

Table 3. Change in MCH and MCV after rhEPO

Patient No.	Dx	MCH, pg		Increase of MCH	MCV, fl		Increase of MCV	Serum EPO mU/ml	BT requirement ml/month
		before	after		before	after			
1[1]	RA	31.6	40.0	+8.4	93.3	130.7	+37.4	349	900→0
2	RA	35.0	34.0	−1.0	107.7	106.9	− 0.8	1,240	0→0
3[1]	RA	31.5	32.6	+1.1	95.1	96.6	+ 1.5	986	1,000→400
4	RARS	32.0	31.9	−0.1	109.4	106.7	− 2.7	1,570	0→0
5[1]	RAEB	33.4	40.1	+6.7	104.2	123.2	+19.0	1,040	0→0
6	RAEB-t	29.3	30.1	+0.8	89.2	91.8	+ 2.6	694	600→400
7	RAEB-t	30.8	30.1	−0.7	95.5	90.1	− 3.6	2,290	1,200→1,200
8	RAEB-t	31.9	29.1	−2.8	91.8	90.1	− 1.7	1,240	900→900
9[1]	AA	34.1	38.2	+4.1	98.1	118.7	+20.6	2,790	500→0
10	AA	30.7	34.0	+3.3	94.8	97.4	+ 2.6	9,870	800→500
11	AA	32.0	34.1	+2.1	94.2	106.7	+12.5	2,280	800→600
12	AA	31.5	30.0	−1.5	92.9	93.1	+ 0.2	1,720	1,000→800

[1] Responsive cases evaluated by our criteria.

Table 4. Detailed hematological data of patients responsive to rhEPO

	Hb g/dl	RBC ×10^{12}/l	Hct %	MCV fl	MCH pg	Ret. 10^9/l	CFU-E 2×10^5	Serum Fe µg/dl	Ferritin ng/ml	PID h	% RCU	Half-life of RBC days
Case 1: refractory anemia												
Before	7.2	227	21.2	93.3	31.6	38.6	176	211	2,730	3.7	30.3	15.2
After	12.6	411	41.1	130.7	40.0	94.5	54	226	3,450	2.0	96.1	15.5
Case 9: aplastic anemia												
Before	9.3	273	26.7	98.1	34.1	38.2	28	189	361	5.0	19.9	23.0
After	13.2	347	41.1	118.7	38.2	97.2	129	165	349	1.8	78.0	33.2

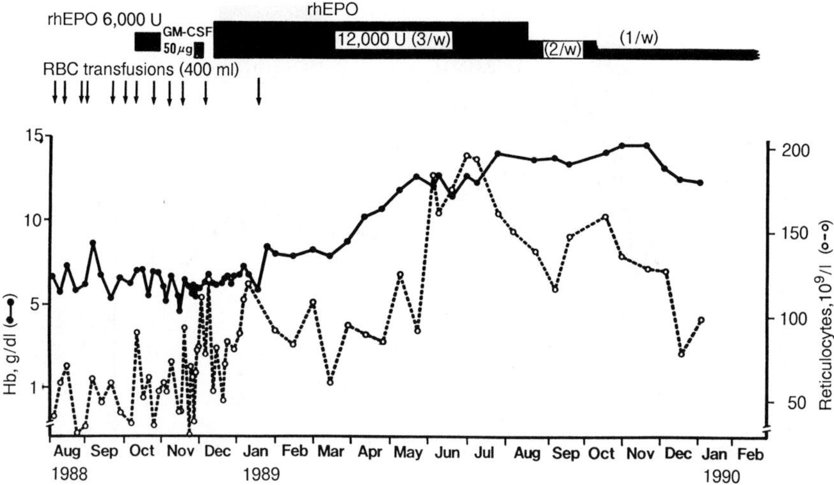

Fig. 1. Clinical course of case 1: M.A., 29, F, RA (MDS). An arrow indicates a 400-ml red cell transfusion. The frequency of rhEPO administration was reduced to twice weekly from July 1989, and then to weekly from October 1989. The reticulocyte count and the hemoglobin concentration decreased slightly, but the parameters have remained stable. The patient became completely transfusion-independent.

continued as maintenance therapy and the patient has no longer required red cell transfusion. The serum EPO concentration decreased following the improvement in the anemia. The ferrokinetic study revealed an improvement in PID and RCU. The red cell life span did not change.

Case 5 (fig. 2): Case 5 was an 83-year-old woman who was referred to our hospital because of anemia in October 1986. Laboratory tests showed hemoglobin 6.4 g/dl, WBC 1.4×10^9/l and platelets 98×10^9/l. The marrow aspirate was normocellular with 13.2% myeloblasts. No chromosomal abnormality was observed. Based on these findings, RAEB was diagnosed. Oral vitamin D_3 administration resulted in no clinical improvement. In March 1988, treatment with 3,000 units rhEPO 3 times/week was started. Following a reticulocytosis, hemoglobin increased from 7.3 to 11.8 g/dl and serum EPO decreased from 1,024 to 244 mU/ml. After 4 weeks of administration, treatment was discontinued. The reticulocytes decreased immediately and the hemoglobin concentration decreased gradually, reaching 6–7 g/dl 4 weeks after the cessation of EPO. Furthermore, the serum EPO concentration again rose, reaching 1,024 mU/ml. In June 1988, the administration of EPO was resumed. However, a significant increase of hemoglobin was not observed because she suffered from severe acute cholecystitis during this period.

Case 9 (fig. 3): Case 9 was a 68-year-old man who was referred to our hospital because of anemia in August 1987. Laboratory tests revealed hemoglobin 5.7 g/dl WBC 2.8×10^9/l with 26.1% of neutrophils and platelets 42×10^9/l. A bone marrow aspirate was moderately hypocellular. No significant dysplasia of hemopoietic cells was observed. He needed approximately

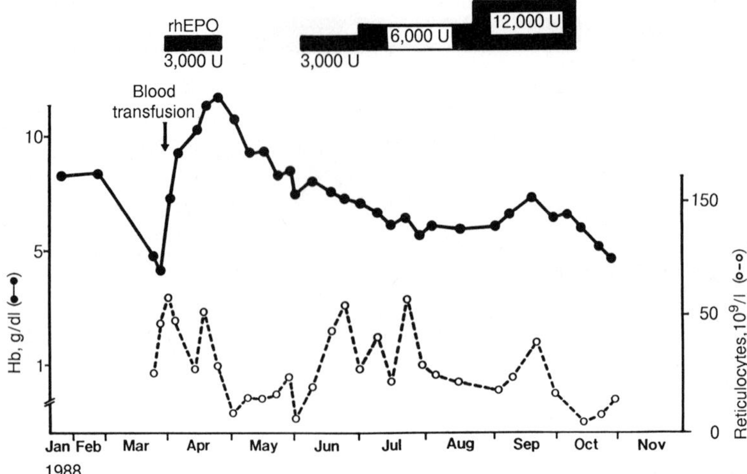

Fig. 2. Clinical course of case 5: K.N., 83, F, RAEB (MDS). After 4 weeks administration of 3,000 units rhEPO 3 times/week, the treatment was stopped. The hemoglobin fell to the pretreatment value 4 weeks after the cessation of rhEPO.

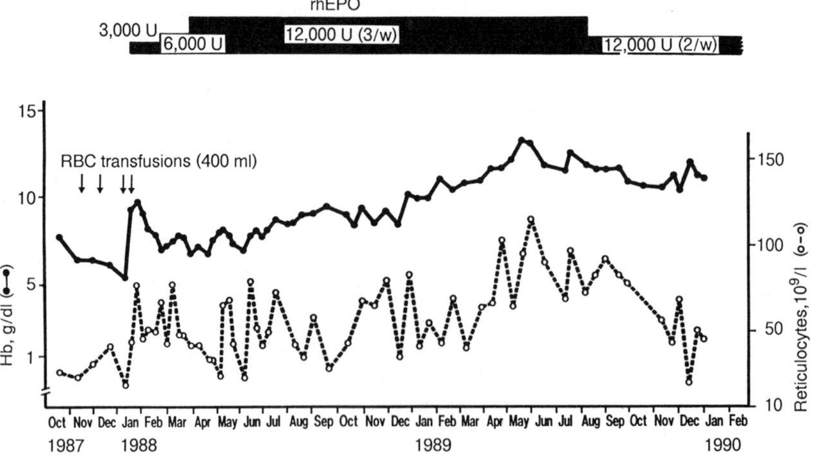

Fig. 3. Clinical course of case 9: T.S., 68, M, AA. The frequency of rhEPO administration was reduced to twice weekly from August 1989. The hemoglobin remains stable, and the patient has remained transfusion-independent.

500 ml red cell transfusion per month to maintain the hemoglobin concentration at 6–7 g/dl. He received no specific treatment for AA. In January 1988, he received 3,000 units rhEPO 3 times/week for 4 weeks. Although the reticulocytes increased immediately, the hemoglobin concentration increased only gradually. The dose of rhEPO was increased to 6,000 units 3 times/week. After 4 weeks, the dose was further increased to 12,000 units 3 times/week and this dose was continued until August 1989 as maintenance therapy. The hemoglobin concentration increased to 12.2 g/dl and the serum EPO concentration decreased 490 mU/ml. He has been maintained on 12,000 units rhEPO twice weekly, and no longer needs red cell transfusion. The ferrokinetic study revealed marked improvement and the red cell life span was normalized.

Discussion

In our experience of over 1,000 cases of severe anemia associated with chronic renal failure treated with rhEPO, the effect was remarkable and the adverse effects minimal if precise attention and care was paid to controlling hypertension. Moreover, the appearance of antibody to rhEPO has not been observed in over 2 years since the initiation of clinical application. Based on this confirmation of the safety of rhEPO, trials in nonrenal anemias are now in progress. MDS and AA are untreatable except in a few patients who are able to receive bone marrow transplantation from related HLA-matched donors, and a small proportion of patients who respond to immunosuppressive agents. More of these patients are forced to rely on periodic blood transfusion, with the risk of the infection with viral hepatitis, ATL, AIDS and multiorgan failure after transfusion hemosiderosis. If rhEPO were even partially effective in these diseases, it would be worthwhile for such patients. However, because of the high level of the serum EPO concentration in these patients, the efficacy of rhEPO was regarded as questionable. Recently, we have tried treatment with a large dose of rhEPO in congenitally anemic mice and cured the anemia [4]. This strain of W/W^v mice was shown to have severe anemia due to a congenital deficiency of pluripotential hemopoietic stem cells. If a dose of 8,600 units/kg rhEPO was given to these mice every day for a week, the hemoglobin increased from 10.1 to 13.5 g/dl and the number of reticulocytes increased from 43.6 to 91.0 × 10^4/mm^3. Thus a high dose of EPO was effective in curing the anemia of mice having a serum EPO concentration about 150 times higher than normal mice.

A clinical trial of rhEPO in AA and MDS patients was initiated based on this experimental evidence. Four of the 12 patients showed a favorable response without side effects. Especially in 2 patients (cases 1 and 9) the effect of rhEPO was remarkable. In case 1, the hemoglobin concentration increased

Table 5. Multicentre study of rhEPO[1] in MDS and AA (Japan 1990)

	Not transfused cases (increase of Hb > 1.5 g/dl/8 weeks)		Transfused cases (decrease of requirement of BT > 50% compared with pretreatment)		Total cases	
	n	%	n	%	n	%
29 institutes in Japan						
MDS	2/9	22.2	5/21	23.8	7/30	23.3
AA	0/2	0.0	5/13	38.5	5/15	33.3
Saitama Medical School						
MDS	1/3	33.3	2/5	40.0	3/8	37.5
AA	0/0		1/4	25.5	1/4	25.5

[1] Dose of rhEPO 6,000–12,000 units, 3 times/week.

from 6.3 to 13.9 g/dl and she became transfusion-independent during maintenance therapy with rhEPO. Case 9 with AA has received maintenance therapy for more than 100 weeks; he also became transfusion-independent with rhEPO and his hemoglobin remains stable. In these 2 patients, markedly enhanced erythropoiesis was also demonstrated by the ferrokinetic study. It is highly unlikely that the improvement in these cases could be ascribed to a spontaneous remission unrelated to rhEPO administration because the improvement in hematological parameters was limited to the erythroid series. Moreover, in case 5, the response was clearly dependent on EPO administration. Further evidence of the efficacy of EPO includes the increase in MCV and MCH immediately after the administration of rhEPO. According to the previous work of Lajtha and Oliver [6], Stohlman [7] and ourselves [8], the skipped division pathway of erythroblasts is induced by a very high titer of serum EPO, such as with severe bleeding or the hemolytic state, and macrocytosis occurs as a result. With the high dose administration of rhEPO to W/W^v mice, an increase in MCV was also observed after the improvement of anemia. Although further studies are necessary to elucidate the mechanism, a residual normal erythroid clone in these patients may be responding to a high titer of rhEPO and a skipped division may take place.

A remaining important problem is that of how to select patients who will respond to rhEPO. In this study, the pretreatment EPO level in serum was not closely related to the effectiveness. RAEB-t patients and AA patients with very hypocellular bone marrow did not respond, nor did patients with no erythroid colony formation during in vitro culture. Further detailed analysis, including assay of the EPO receptor, remains to be performed.

Although the number of patients was small in this present study, we have proceeded to a multicenter study in Japan, including 29 institutes. Up to now, 30 cases of MDS and 15 cases of AA have been enrolled. The efficacy of EPO following the same criteria as in this study is 23.3 and 33.3%, respectively (table 5). No patients have had any serious adverse side effects, and particularly no episodes of hypertension have occurred. To conclude, rhEPO is a promising therapeutic tool for treating some patients with MDS or AA.

References

1   Winearls, C. G.; Oliver, D. O.; Pippard, M. J., et al.: Effects of human erythropoietin derived from recombinant DNA on the anemia of the patients maintained by chronic hemodialysis. Lancet *ii:* 1175–1177 (1986).
2   Eschbach, J. W.; Egrie, J. C.; Downing, M. R., et al.: Correlation of the anemia of end-stage renal disease with recombinant human erythropoietin. Results of a combined phase I and phase II clinical trial. N. Engl. J. Med. *316:* 73–78 (1987).
3   Suzuki, M., et al.: Dose-finding, double-blind, clinical trial of recombinant human erythropoietin (Chugai) in Japanese patients with end-stage renal disease. Contrib. Nephrol., vol. 76, pp. 179–192 (Karger, Basel 1989).
4   Cynshi, O., et al.: Effects of recombinant human erythropoietin on anaemic W/W^v and Sl/Sl^d mice. Br. J. Haematol., in press.
5   Iscove, N. N.; Sieber, F.; Winterhalter, K. H.: Erythroid colony formation in culture of mouse and human bone marrow: Analysis of the requirement for erythropoietin by gel filtration and affinity chromatography on agarose-concanavalin A. J. Cell Physiol. *83:* 309–320 (1974).
6   Lajtha, L. G.; Oliver, R.: Studies on the kinetics of erythropoiesis: A model of the erythron; in Wolstenholme, G. E. W.; O'Connor, M. (eds): Ciba Foundation Symposium on Haemopoiesis, pp. 289–324 (Churchill, London 1960).
7   Stohlman, F., Jr.: Observation on the kinetics of red cell proliferation; in Sohlman, F., Jr. (ed.): The Kinetics of Cellular Proliferation, pp. 318–331 (Grune & Stratton, New York 1959).
8   Hirashima, K.; Takaku, F.: Regulation of erythropoiesis. Jpn. Nucl. Med. *2:* 69–74 (1963).

Kunitake Hirashima, MD, First Department of Internal Medicine,
Saitama Medical School, 38 Morohongo, Moroyama, Iruma-Gun,
Saitama, 350–04 (Japan)

Gurland HJ, Moran J, Samtleben W, Scigalla P, Wieczorek L (eds): Erythropoietin in
Renal and Non-Renal Anemias. Contrib Nephrol. Basel, Karger, 1991, vol 88, pp 266–270

Erythropoietin and the Myelodysplastic Syndrome

A. Jacobs, D. Culligan, D. Bowen

Department of Haematology, University of Wales College of Medicine, Cardiff, UK

The myelodysplastic syndrome (MDS) represents a clonal abnormality of
haemopoietic stem cells which progresses to a preleukaemic state [1, 2]. It
probably develops as a sequence of events in which the earliest stages may be
difficult to detect by conventional pathological techniques. It seems increasingly likely that the mechanism of progression from a trivial haematological
aberration to overt leukaemia involves sequential genetic changes resulting in
abnormal control of cell proliferation and differentiation. Expansion of an
abnormal clone may be related to independence from normal growth factors,
insensitivity to normal inhibitory factors and suppression of normal haemopoiesis. In many cases, clonal evolution is accompanied by increasing chromosome abnormalities, increasingly malignant characteristics in the bone marrow, and eventually acute myeloblastic leukaemia (AML). Usually neither the
nature of the genetic insult nor the lesion produced is known, though MDS
may follow either chemical or radiation attack on the marrow.

The haematological picture of MDS includes peripheral blood cytopenias
associated with a cellular bone marrow in which the cells appear dysplastic and
have a high premature death rate. There are numerous functional abnormalities in progenitor cells, immature myeloid cells and in the end cells of all
lineages [2, 3]. Recent observations suggest that the early stages of MDS may
be associated with minimal haematological signs [4] and the classical clinical
syndromes have already evolved through several genetic changes, the haemopoietic marrow being composed of a mixed cell population comprising normal
cells and an unknown proportion of abnormal stem cells and their progeny at
different stages of premalignant evolution. The response of these various
populations to haemopoietic growth factors is unknown and may differ from
case to case.

Serum Erythropoietin in Patients with Myelodysplastic Syndromes

While the primary abnormality of haemopoietic cells in MDS and their failure to grow adequately in vitro in the presence of added growth factor suggests a failure of response to cytokines [2, 5, 6], the bone marrow in vivo commonly shows active erythropoiesis and in many cases there is marked erythroid hyperplasia.

Erythropoietin (EPO) promotes differentiation of committed erythroid precursor cells [7, 8] and is synthesized in response to hypoxia [9–11] but the exact mechanisms responsible for EPO production under physiological and many pathological conditions are still not clear. In patients with anaemia, excluding those with renal disease, there is usually an inverse relationship between the circulating level of EPO and the haemoglobin concentration. However, this is not always the case and some anaemic patients have been described in whom the plasma level of EPO is lower than expected [12].

We have previously reported on plasma concentrations of EPO in 46 patients with various clinical manifestations of MDS [13]. The results suggested that although an overall relationship between the degree of anaemia and circulating EPO levels was observed, in some patients the EPO response may not match the degree of anaemia. The highest EPO levels were found in those patients with erythroid hypoplasia in the bone marrow but there was considerable variation in serum EPO levels amongst patients with similar haemoglobin concentrations.

Plasma Clearance of an Intravenous Bolus Dose of rhEPO

We have recently studied the clearance of an intravenous bolus of 150 U/kg of rhEPO (Boehringer Mannheim GmbH) in 10 subjects with myelodysplasia. Basal blood samples were taken immediately preinjection, and at frequent intervals over the first 24 h, at 12-hour intervals on day 2 and daily thereafter for a total of 5 days. Serum was separated and stored at –30 °C until analysis. Serum EPO concentration was measured by Dr. B. Ehmer using a specific radioimmunoassay [14]. Basal serum EPO concentration varied from 210 to 5,984 mU/ml. Plasma half-time clearance ($t_{1/2}$) measured up to 36 h varied considerably from 3.9 to 20.0 h. A significant positive correlation was found between $t_{1/2}$ and basal EPO concentration. The sites of elimination of EPO from serum are uncertain but attention has focused mainly on the liver, kidney, and bone marrow. Experimental animal evidence for the role of the liver in EPO clearance is conflicting [15]. Recent studies rhEPO in the rat suggest that little unmodified ^{125}I-EPO is cleared by the liver, in contrast to the desialated protein which undergoes rapid hepatic clearance [16]. Renal excretion accounts for about 10% of EPO clearance [17, 18], but may in addition represent direct secretion from the production site in the renal tubular cells. The first suggestion that bone marrow consumption of EPO may be significant came from Stohlman and Brecher [19] who demonstrated a slower decline in plasma EPO levels on discontinuation of 16 h exposure to simulated altitude of 23,000 ft, in irradiated rats, compared with controls. They surmised that utilization of serum EPO was reduced due to the diminished bone marrow mass in the irradiated group. Patients with erythroid hypoplasia have higher serum EPO levels for a similar haemoglobin concentration than those with erythroid hyperplasia [20] and if transfused to suppress endogenous EPO production, show a slower rate of decline of serum EPO than expected [21]. There is, however, evidence against the bone marrow playing a major role in EPO clearance from serum. Expansion of the erythron in renal anaemia following recombinant EPO therapy did not alter the $T_{1/2}$ clearance of rhEPO [22], and the $t_{1/2}$ of iodinated rhEPO in rats with erythroid hyperplasia did not differ significantly from rats with erythroid hypoplasia [23]. Reasons for the marked variation in EPO clearance between patients with MDS are entirely unknown.

Treatment of Anaemia in MDS with rhEPO

We have administered subcutaneous rhEPO to 10 patients with MDS in an attempt to improve their anaemia and reduce transfusion requirements. Ten patients, 5 male and 5 female, aged 23–79 years (mean 64 years), were studied. All patients had a steady-state haemoglobin concentration of <10 g/dl or were transfusion dependent. They were treated with rhEPO (Boehringer Mannheim UK) as a single daily subcutaneous injection 6 days/week. The initial dose was 60 units/kg/day rising to 90 units/kg/day if there was no response in the first 6 weeks. A response was defined as a rise in haemoglobin concentration of ≥1.0 g/dl and/or a reduction in the average monthly transfusion requirement during the treatment period compared to the 16 weeks before treatment. Treatment was stopped if the haemoglobin concentration rose to a level >11.0 g/dl for 2 consecutive weeks and at 16 weeks in all other instances.

Eight out of 10 patients showed no change in haemoglobin concentration or transfusion dependency over the 16-week period. Two out of 10 patients had a steady increase in haemoglobin concentration above baseline. One with RAEB had a rise in haemoglobin concentration from 9.5 to 11.4 g/dl at 6 weeks, but failed to maintain this, and thereafter declined steadily to pretreatment levels at 16 weeks, despite rhEPO being increased to the higher dose. The other, with RA, showed a rise in haemoglobin concentration from 9.9 to 11.3 g/dl at week 5 and 11.2 g/dl at week 6 when therapy was stopped. The decline in haemoglobin concentration in the patient with RAEB was associated with a fall in serum ferritin concentration to iron-deficient levels.

Discussion

The haematological data suggest that 2 out of our 10 patients have responded to rhEPO therapy and similar results have been observed in small groups of MDS patients by Dr. Hellstrom (Uppsala), Dr. Hast (Stockholm) and Dr. Merchav (Haifa). We are uncertain how such responses may be predicted, the optimal dose of rhEPO required to produce this effect or the optimum plasma EPO level to be attained. We remain equally uncertain of the nature of the responding cells in the bone marrow or their sensitivity to EPO or other growth factors.

References

1   Jacobs, A.; Clark, R.: Pathogenesis and clinical variations in the myelodysplastic syndrome. Clin. Haematol. *15:* 925–951 (1986).
2   Jacobs, A.: Do we have a model? Br. J. Cancer *55:* 1–5 (1987).
3   May, S. J.; Smith, S. A.; Jacobs, A.; Williams, A.; Baileywood, R.: The myelodysplastic syndrome analysis of laboratory characteristics in relation to the FAB classification. Br. J. Haematol. *59:* 311–351 (1985).
4   Bowen, D. T.; Jacobs, A.: Primary acquired sideroblastic erythropoiesis in non-anaemic and minimally anaemic subjects. J. Clin. Pathol. *42:* 56–58 (1989).
5   Ruutu, T.; Partanen, S.; Lintula, R.; Terenhoui, L.; Knuutila, S.: Erythroid and granulocyte macrophage colony formation in myelodysplastic syndromes. Scand. J. Haematol. *32:* 395–402 (1984).
6   Milner, G. R.; Testa, N. G.; Geary, G. A., et al: Bone marrow culture studies in refractory cytopenia and smouldering leukaemia. Br. J. Haematol. *35:* 251–261 (1977).
7   Erslev, A.: Humoral regulation of red cell production. Blood *8.* 349–357 (1953).
8   Spivak, J. L.: The mechanism of action of erythropoietin. Int. Cell Cloning *4:* 139–166 (1986).
9   Kuratowska, A. Z.; Lewartowski, B.; Michalak, E.: Studies on the production of erythropoietin by isolated perfused organs. Blood *18:* 527–534 (1961).

10   Caro, J.; Schuster, S.; Ramirez, S.; Badiavas, E. V.; Costa-Giomi, P.; Weinmann, R.: Transcriptional activations of the erythropoietin gene in response to hypoxia or cobalt. Blood *72:* 112A (1988).

11   Schooley, J. C.; Mahlmann, L. J.: Evidence for the de novo synthesis of erythropoietin in hypoxic rats. Blood *40:* 662–700 (1972).

12   Sherwood, J. B.; Goldwasser, E.; Chilcote, R.; Carmichael, L. D.; Nagel, R. L.: Sickle cell anaemia patients had low erythropoietin levels for their degree of anaemia. Blood *67:* 46–49 (1986).

13   Jacobs, A.; Janowska-Wieczorek, A.; Caro, J.; Bowen, D. T.; Lewis, T.: Circulating erythropoietin in patients with myelodysplasia. Br. J. Haematol. *73:* 36–39 (1989).

14   Ergie, J. C.; Cotes, P. M.; Lawe, J., et al.: Development of rapid immunoassays for human erythropoietin using recombinant erythropoietin as tracer and immunogen. J. Immunol. Methods *99:* 235–241 (1987).

15   Emmanouel, D. S.; Goldwasser, E.; Katz, A. L.: Metabolism of pure human erythropoietin in the rat. Am. J. Physiol. *247:* F168–F176 (1984).

16   Spivak, J. L.; Hogans, B. B.: The in vivo metabolism of recombinant human erythropoietin in the rat. Blood *73:* 90–99 (1989).

17   Steinberg, S. E.; Garcia, J. F.; Matzke, G. R.; Mladenovic, J.: Erythropoietin kinetics in rats: generation and clearance. Blood *67:* 646–649 (1986).

18   Macdougall, I. C.; Roberts, D. E.; Neubert, A.; Dharmasena, A. D.; Coles, G. A.; Williams, J. D.: Pharmacokinetics of recombinant human erythropoietin in patients on continuous ambulatory peritoneal dialysis. Lancet *i:* 425–427 (1989).

19   Stohlman, F.; Brecher, G.: Humoral regulation of erythropoiesis vs. relationship of plasma erythropoietin level to bone marrow activity. Proc. Soc. Exp. Biol. Med. *100:* 40–43 (1959).

20   de Klerk, G.; Rosengaten, P. C. J.; Det, J. W. M.; Goudsmit, R.: Serum erythropoietin (ESF) titres in anaemia. Blood *58.* 1164–1170 (1981).

21   Hammond, G. D.; Ishikawa, A.: The rate of disappearance of erythropoietin following transfusion of severely anaemic patients; in Jacobson, Doylem (eds): Erythropoiesis, pp. 128–133 (Grune & Stratton, New York 1962).

22   Egrie, J. C.; Eschbach, J. W.; McGuire, T.; Adamson, J. W.: Pharmacokinetics of recombinant human erythropoietin administered to haemodialysis patients. Kidney Int. *33:* 262 (1988).

23   Piroso, E.; Flaherty, K.; Caro, J.; Erslev, A.: Erythropoiesis half-life in rats with hypoplastic and hyperplastic bone marrows. Blood *74:* suppl. 270A (1989).

Prof. A. Jacobs, MD, Department of Haematology, University of Wales College of Medicine, Heath Park, Cardiff CF4 4XN (UK)

Gurland HJ, Moran J, Samtleben W, Scigalla P, Wieczorek L (eds): Erythropoietin in
Renal and Non-Renal Anemias. Contrib Nephrol. Basel, Karger, 1991, vol 88, pp 271–272

Recombinant Human Erythropoietin at High Dose Is Effective for the Treatment of the Anemia of Myelodysplastic Syndromes

J. P. H. Laporte[a], *F. Isnard*[a], *P. Fenaux*[b], *M. Woler*[c], *A. Najman*[a]

[a]Service des Maladies du Sang, Hôpital Saint-Antoine, Paris;
[b]Service d'Hématologie, Lille, France, and
[c]Boehringer Mannheim GmbH, Mannheim, FRG

The myelodysplastic syndromes (MDS) are a heterogeneous group of clonal hematopoietic disorders characterized by bone marrow dysplasia and ineffective hematopoiesis [1]. Most MDS patients are anemic with a normal or low reticulocyte count. The content of erythroblasts in the bone marrow is usually high, with gross dyserythropoietic appearances. Besides very rare cases which are vitamin B_6 responsive, red cell transfusion remains the sole therapy.

In an attempt to improve red cell production we administered recombinant human erythropoietin (rhEPO) to 6 patients with MDS without excess of blasts in the bone marrow [2] as part of a phase I trial. Four patients were followed for refractory anemia (RA) with ringed sideroblasts (RARS), and 2 for RA. One of the latter group presented a deletion of the long arm of chromosome 5. Four of the 6 patients were receiving regular transfusions. The rhEPO was given subcutaneously with a progressive increase in dose from 40 IU/kg 3 times/week up to 300 IU/kg. The induction period lasted 3 months. In patients who responded to the treatment, a decreasing dose protocol allowed us to find the optimal dose to maintain the benefits of the treatment. So far, a beneficial effect was observed in 5 of 6 patients. Two patients regained a normal hemoglobin level (10–14 and 9–13 g/dl). One patient gained 2.5 g/dl of hemoglobin (7.5–10 g/dl), while 2 other patients have had a mild response and gained between 1 and 1.5 g/dl. Among the 4 patients requiring transfusions, 2 are no longer transfusion-dependent (1 with a normal hemoglobin level and 1 has had a decrease of 66% in transfusion requirement). No change in the number of granulocytes or platelets was noted, except in 1 patient whose platelet count increased from 15,000/mm^3 (with platelet transfusions to 55,000/mm^3). The patient who did not respond was the only one with a 5q⁻ syndrome.

These preliminary results indicate that high-dose rhEPO stimulates in vivo erythropoiesis in some cases of RA. A correlation with the in vivo studies cannot be established till now, although patients with a higher number of erythroid progenitors or with the best result in a dose-response evaluation seem to be in the best responders. Notwithstanding its clinical importance, the in vivo sensitivity to rhEPO appears to be a new parameter in the evaluation of the dyserythropoiesis in MDS, the significance of which remains to be explained.

References

1   Jacobs A, Clark RE: Pathogenesis and clinical variations in the myelodysplastic syndromes. Clin Haematol 1986;15:925–951.
2   Bennett JM, Catovsky D, Daniel MT, et al: Proposals for the classification of the myelodysplastic syndromes. Br J Haematol 1982;51:189–199.

Dr. J. Laporte, Department of Hematology, Hôpital Saint-Antoine,
184, rue du Faubourg Saint-Antoine, F–74012 Paris (France)

Gurland HJ, Moran J, Samtleben W, Scigalla P, Wieczorek L (eds): Erythropoietin in
Renal and Non-Renal Anemias. Contrib Nephrol. Basel, Karger, 1991, vol 88, pp 273–275

Discussion

to the Papers by K. Hirashima et al., A. Jacobs et al., and
J. P. H. Laporte et al.

Wardrop (Cardiff): The speakers have all described very different dosage schedules;
they've ranged tremendously from perhaps 100 U three times a week to 1000,000 U a week. As
Dr. Jacobs has said, the MDS and other refractory anemias are extremely heterogeneous
themselves. How does one set about deciding what the correct dosage is in those patients who
are responders? It seems to me that the variety in diagnosis and the discrepancy in treatments
are very impressive.

Jacobs: I think the optimal dose for starting depends basically on how much Boehringer
Mannheim ar going to charge for the drug in the first place. We selected the dose prag-
matically and we obtained some clear responses. If we have a response where the patient's
hemoglobin goes up to 13 g, we then halve the dose, and continue to halve the dose, until we
find the lowest dose that will maintain an optimal hemoglobin. We titrate each patient
individually. It may be that they will show the same pattern, but I don't know yet.

Merchav (Haifa): I'd like to know if you have any idea how GM-CSF induced the EPO
response in your refractory anemia patient, and whether you have gone back to your EPO
non-responders and tried stimulating them with GM-CSF prior to an additional trial of
rhEPO.

Hirashima: We assume that GM-CSF acts on more immature progenitor cells than
CFU-E and BFU-E and so synergistic effects will occur. But the supply of GM-CSF was very
limited and so we only gave 5 μg/day for 5 days in case 1. We have 2 additional patients in
whom we tried this therapy with good results. We also tried combining G-CSF with EPO but
that didn't work.

Herrmann (Freiburg): I would like to know something about the subtypes of the aplastic
anemia in your studies. Were they severe, very severe or moderately severe? I would also like
to know something about the pretreatment status of your patients.

Hirashima: We treated 4 patients with aplastic anemia in this study. We classified the
aplasia as mild, moderate, or severe depending on the number of neutrophils, platelets and
reticulocytes. Two cases were severe and two moderate. The responding patient had moderate aplastic anemia and had had no pretreatment.

Herrmann (Freiburg): You have treated a patient with severe aplastic anemia for 2 years
with EPO alone and had no problems managing the granulocytopenia and thrombocytopenia?

Hirashima: His granulocyte and platelet counts have not changed during two and a half years of rhEPO therapy.

Cavill (Cardiff): Dr. Hirashima, our experience in measuring reticulocyte volumes in several thousand samples makes me sceptical that the extremely high MCH and MCV that you reported in your responding patients could be attributed to reticulocyte counts. Have you any other possible explanation for the remarkably high MCH and MCV that you saw in some of your patients?

Hirashima: As I have already mentioned, a marked increase in MCV and MCH may be related to a skipped division of late erythroblasts under the influence of a high serum EPO concentration.

Hellström (Stockholm): Did any of you observe any changes in the bone marrow regarding the percentage of erythropoiesis or bone marrow fibrosis before and after treatment?

Hirashima: Erythroid cellularity improved in all the responsive cases. Bone marrow fibrosis was not apparent either before or after treatment in any of the cases.

Eschbach (Seattle): May I offer another explanation for the elevation in the MCV? I suspect your patients were iron-overloaded from transfusions. Do you know their serum ferritin levels? Dialysis patients who are iron-overloaded have high MCVs, and in my experience, the MCVs of those patients increase to over 110, even to 120, with rhEPO therapy.

Hirashima: Thank you for a good suggestion. We measured serum ferritin levels in all cases before and after EPO, so I will examine those results with your suggestion in mind. However, one of the responsive patients was not transfusion dependent, so you might suspect that she was not iron-overloaded.

Herrmann (Berlin): Did you supplement with folate?

Hirashima: No, but the levels of folate and of vitamin B_{12} were normal.

Miller (Baltimore): Did you look at CFU-E and BFU-E in your patients, and based on the data from Dr. Hirashima, do you feel that it's indicated to limit patients based on in vitro data? Could you then comment on the potential use of CFU-E and BFU-E to predict which patients would not respond to EPO?

Jacobs: I think it would be very difficult to be dogmatic on the basis of 10 treated patients. We looked at BFU-E and CFU-E before and after EPO and we couldn't see any changes, but of course the majority of these patients have very few colonies and some have none at all. We didn't see any difference in marrow morphology.

Krantz (Nashville): In your patients that received iron, were you treating iron deficiency or an inadequate use of the iron that was on board?

Jacobs: The first patient's serum ferritin was initially 150 and during treatment came down to 40, which is not officially an iron-deficient level, but I guess iron was being utilised and the supply was running out. The other one started out at 45 and came down to an iron-deficient level, so that was certainly iron deficiency.

Wardrop: I think what Dr. Hirashima was describing was stress erythropoiesis. I don't think he meant to imply that he was describing reticulocytosis necessarily, but with these very big doses of rhEPO, I think one would expect stress erythropoiesis for the reasons that Dr. Hirashima described in his diagram. One would also perhaps expect an increase in fetal hemoglobin, and this might be a means of assessing the effect of rhEPO in patients who are responders. I wonder if any of the speakers have looked at fetal hemoglobin levels in patients receiving high doses of rhEPO.

Jacobs: We haven't looked routinely but occasionally you see patients with a high hemoglobin-F level before treatment.

Erslev (Philadelphia): Since we believe that EPO production is a physiological function, I think the rational choice of a specific dose of rhEPO would depend on the endogenous level at the onset of treatment. When you have in mind that endogenous level which is necessary for production to meet destruction, then, if you want to increase the production level, you have to go beyond what endogenously has been produced. It is to me incredible to hear that some of your patients responded to what must be considered homeopathic doses compared to an endogenous EPO production in the thousands.

Jacobs: I think there are two points that we really can't get to grips with. Firstly we don't know the EPO sensitivity of the cells we are looking at. The other point, which I didn't raise, is that one of the features of MDS is that the abnormal clone, by some mechanism we don't understand, is suppressing normal hemopoiesis. So there are suppressive mechanisms going on as well which we also know nothing about. I don't think we understand at all what's happening.

Laporte: In the W/W mouse model which Dr. Hirashima showed us there is anemia and a myelodysplastic bone marrow, and the levels of endogenous EPO are very high. This mouse responds to very high doses of recombinant EPO. Therefore, I don't think that the endogenous EPO level should be a marker for determining dosage.

Gurland HJ, Moran J, Samtleben W, Scigalla P, Wieczorek L (eds): Erythropoietin in
Renal and Non-Renal Anemias. Contrib Nephrol. Basel, Karger, 1991, vol 88, pp 276–280

Treatment Trial with Recombinant Human Erythropoietin in Children with Congenital Hypoplastic Anemia

C. M. Niemeyer[a], *E. Baumgarten*[b], *J. Holldack*[c], *I. Meier*[d], *G. Trenn*[e],
A. Jobke[f], *K.-U. Eckhardt*[g], *A. Reiter*[a], *S. Sauter*[a], *H. Riehm*[a]

[a]Children's Hospital, Medical School of Hannover; [b]Children's Hospital of the Free
University, Berlin; [c]University Children's Hospital, Freiburg i. Br.; [d]Vestsches
Children's Hospital, Datteln; [e]Department of Internal Medicine, University of Essen;
[f]Chnopfsches Children's Hospital, Nürnberg, FRG; [g]Department of Physiology,
University of Zürich, Switzerland

Congenital hypoplastic anemia (Diamond-Blackfan anemia) is a congenital anomaly of erythropoiesis characterized by a normochromic, often macrocytic anemia with reticulocytopenia [1]. The bone marrow shows normal cellularity with markedly decreased erythroid precursor cells but normal myeloid and megakaryocytic maturation [2]. The clinical course of the syndrome is variable and characterized by spontaneous remissions in some patients, while others have a life-long dependency on steroids or erythrocyte transfusions. Although the pathogenesis of the anemia remains obscure, there is a general consensus that the erythroid stem cell may be defective. Some in vitro studies have demonstrated that the proliferation and differentiation of the erythroid progenitor cells could be increased to the normal range by the addition of higher than usual concentrations of erythropoietin (EPO) [3]. In vivo, patients with Diamond-Blackfan anemia are known to have increased serum EPO levels. We have previously shown that in patients with myelodysplastic syndrome, recombinant human EPO (rhEPO) can stimulate erythropoiesis despite high endogenous serum EPO levels [4]. In this study, we therefore wished to investigate whether the administration of rhEPO could improve erythropoiesis in patients with congenital hypoplastic anemia.

[1] We thank Boehringer Mannheim GmbH (FRG) for continuing support and for the
provision of rhEPO.

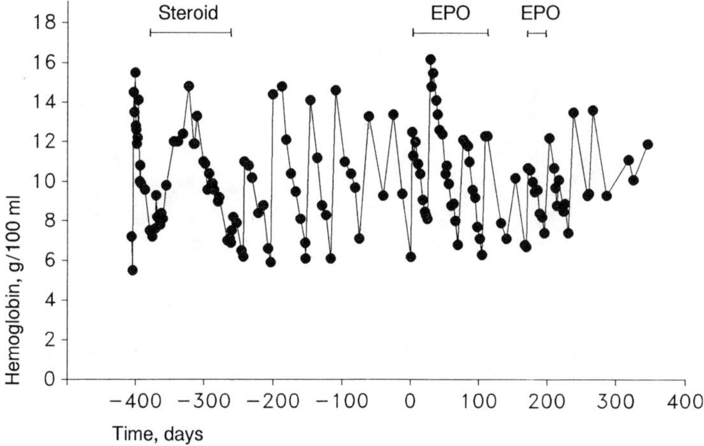

Fig. 1. Hemoglobin concentrations of patient 1. The patient is a 15-month-old boy who had failed steroid therapy and was red cell transfusion dependent.

Patients, Material and Methods

Nine patients with congenital hypoplastic anemia entered the trial. Their ages ranged from 2.5 months to 24 years (2.5 months, 3.5 months, 15 months, 2 years, 2 years, 4 years, 5 years, 9 years, 24 years). Six patients had been unresponsive to steroid treatment and were red cell transfusion dependent. In 3 patients erythropoiesis was dependent on high dose steroid therapy. Two patients received iron chelation therapy with daily desferrioxamine. Prior to rhEPO treatment all medications including steroids were discontinued.

rhEPO was administered subcutaneously at increasing dosages, each dose being given for 4 weeks. The initial starting dose was 10, 30 or 90 U/kg/dose. After 4 weeks the dosages were tripled to 30, 90, or 270 U/kg/dose and subsequently doubled to 540 U/kg/dose. In a second part of the trial, 3 patients received a daily dose of 500 U/kg. In 2 of the 3 patients this dose was increased to 2,000 U/kg/day. The duration of rhEPO treatment was as long as 5 months.

Physical examinations were performed weekly. Complete blood counts, including reticulocytes (corrected for the anemia), serum chemistries and iron parameters were done serially throughout the study. EPO concentrations in serum or plasma were determined by radioimmunoassay [5]. Samples for these measurements were collected about 4 h after the subcutaneous administration of the drug. Bone marrow aspirates for morphology were performed prior to the beginning of the study and at least once during the study period.

Results

During rhEPO administration none of the patients showed a rise in reticulocytes or hemoglobin concentration. All patients remained red cell transfusion dependent. Figures 1–3 illustrate the course in 2 patients. In 1 pa-

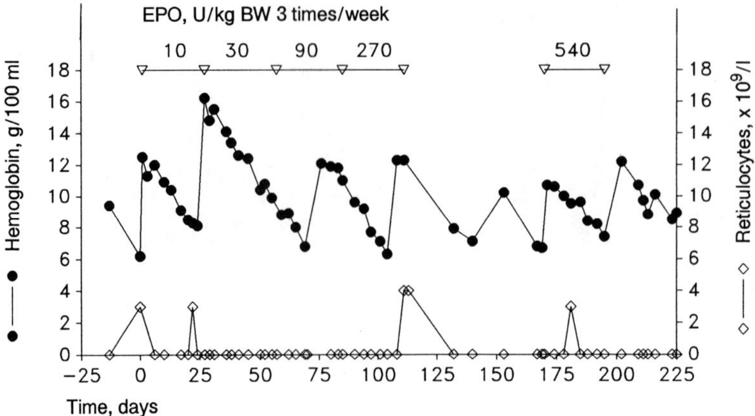

Fig. 2. Hemoglobin concentrations and absolute reticulocyte counts of patient 1 during rhEPO administration.

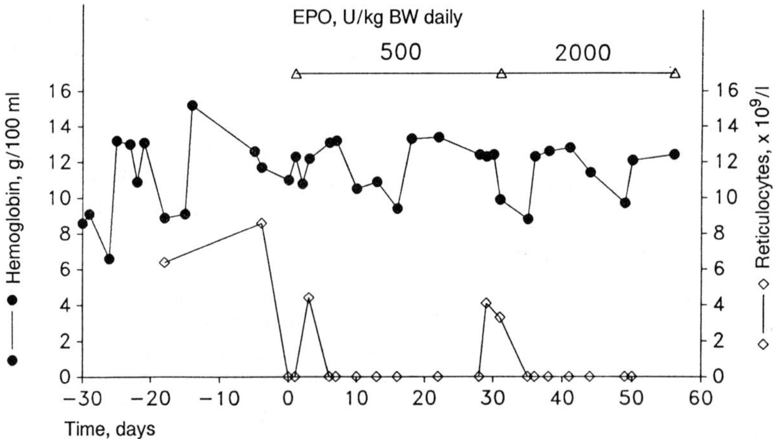

Fig. 3. Hemoglobin concentrations and absolute reticulocyte count of patient 7 (2.5-month-old girl) during rhEPO administration.

tient the discontinuation of steroid therapy prior to rhEPO administration was followed by a decrease in platelet count. This prompted the cessation of rhEPO administration in this patient. All other patients did not show any significant changes in platelet, leukocyte or differential counts during the rhEPO trial.

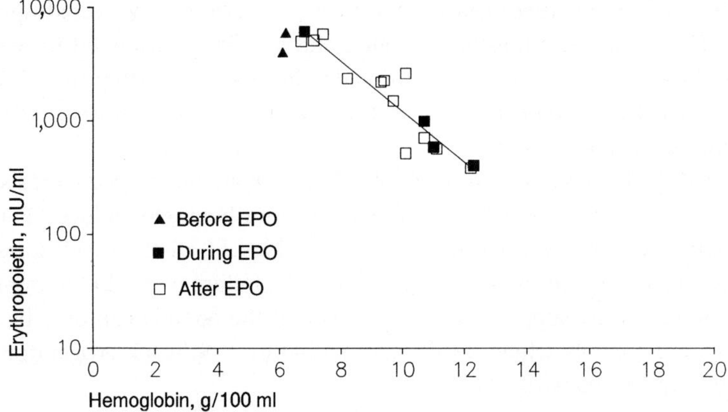

Fig. 4. Relationship of EPO serum/plasma levels to hemoglobin concentrations in patient 1.

rhEPO was tolerated extremely well. Physical examinations remained unchanged. None of the patients developed evidence of increased blood pressure. Blood chemistries remained within the normal range, with the exception of patient 1. This patient showed a tenfold increase in serum alkaline phosphatase during the administration of rhEPO at 270 U/kg/dose 3 times/ week. After the discontinuation of rhEPO treatment the enzyme level normalized, and remained within the normal range despite re-introduction of rhEPO at a higher dose level of 540 U/kg/dose.

Serum/plasma EPO concentrations and hemoglobin levels were inversely correlated. They showed a linear regression when plotted on a semilogarithmic scale (fig. 4). rhEPO administration up to 500 U/kg/day did not result in increased serum EPO concentrations.

Discussion

We have previously shown that the presence of high endogenous serum EPO levels does not preclude the responsiveness to rhEPO therapy. Following rhEPO administration, patients with myelodysplasia can correct their red cell transfusion dependency, although serum EPO levels during therapy are not significantly increased above pretreatment values [4]. In Diamond-Blackfan anemia hematopoiesis is characterized by erythroid aplasia rather than by dysplasia of red cell precursors. Similar to our observations in myelodysplasia, serum EPO concentrations are elevated and inversely correlated to the hemoglobin level. This study was performed to investigate whether the administration of rhEPO could improve erythropoiesis in patients with congenital hypoplastic anemia.

None of the patients with Diamond-Blackfan anemia showed a response to rhEPO therapy with increase in reticulocytes or hemoglobin level. Peripheral blood counts and bone marrow morphology of all three cell lines remained unchanged during the study period. The failure of rhEPO to improve erythropoiesis may support the hypothesis that the anemia can only be corrected by cytokines which render the immature erythroid progenitor cell BFU-E more responsive to EPO [6].

While it was not efficacious, rhEPO therapy was tolerated extremely well. There were no side effects even at doses as high as 14,000 U/kg/week. The excellent tolerance in our young patient population may facilitate studies on the clinical efficacy of rhEPO in other anemias of childhood.

References

1 Diamond LK, Blackfan KD: Hypoplastic anemia. Am J Dis Child 1938;56:464–467.
2 Alter, BP: Childhood red cell aplasia. Am J Pediatr Hematol Oncol 1980;2:121–139.
3 Lipton JM, Kudisch M, Gross R, Nathan DG: Defective erythroid progenitor differentiation system in congenital hypoplastic (Diamond-Blackfan) anemia. Blood 1986;67:962–968.
4 Niemeyer CM, Eckhardt KU, Sauter S, Reiter S, Riehm H: Recombinant human erythropoietin has unique functional capacity (abstract). Pediatr Res (in press).
5 Eckhardt KU, Kurtz A, Hirth P, Scigalla P, Wieczorek L, Bauer C: Evaluation of the stability of human erythropoietin in samples for radio immuno assay. Klin Wochenschr 1988;66:241–245.
6 Halperin DS, Estrov Z, Freedman MH: Diamond-Blackfan anemia: promotion of marrow erythropoiesis in vitro by recombinant interleukin-3. Blood 1989;73:1168–1174.

Dr. Charlotte Niemeyer, Klinikum der Albert-Ludwigs-Universität Freiburg, Universitäts-Kinderklinik, Mathildenstrasse 1, D–7800 Freiburg i. Br. (FRG)

Gurland HJ, Moran J, Samtleben W, Scigalla P, Wieczorek L (eds): Erythropoietin in Renal and Non-Renal Anemias. Contrib Nephrol. Basel, Karger, 1991, vol 88, p 281

Discussion

to the Paper by C. M. Niemeyer et al.

Herrmann (Freiburg): Have you had a chance to use IL-3 in your patients with Blackfan-Diamond disease?

Niemeyer: No, we haven't used IL-3 yet. I know it is the obvious next thing to do, but we have been hesitant. We have treated 2 children with aplastic anemia with IL-3 and both got quite sick, with fevers. Children with Blackfan-Diamond anemia do well, they go to school and have normal activity. They just come in every 4 weeks for a transfusion. So we were not willing to use IL-3 in this patient population.

D'Andrea (Boston): Have you looked at bone marrow from patients before and after treatment with EPO? Was there a change in bone marrow morphology during treatment?

Niemeyer: We have looked, and there was no change in bone marrow morphology. We also performed cultures for BFU-E and CFU-E and there was no change in progenitor growth either.

D'Andrea: What is the normal bone marrow response during the first year of life to EPO? Is the response normal compared to that of older children?

Niemeyer: We are currently looking at that. We are looking at cord blood and the sensitivity towards EPO compared to that of normal adult bone marrow. So far we have not seen any differences in either serum-containing or serum-free culture systems.

Gurland HJ, Moran J, Samtleben W, Scigalla P, Wieczorek L (eds): Erythropoietin in Renal and Non-Renal Anemias. Contrib Nephrol. Basel, Karger, 1991, vol 88, pp 282–292

The Role of Recombinant Human Erythropoietin in the Management of Anemia Associated with Acquired Immunodeficiency Syndrome

Marc B. Garnick[a], *Robert Abels*[b], *Seth A. Rudnick*[b]

[a] Genetics Institute, Inc., Cambridge, and Harvard Medical School, Boston, Mass.;
[b] The R. W. Johnson Pharmaceutical Research Institute, Raritan, N.J., USA

The recent introduction of recombinant human erythropoietin (rhEPO), available through recombinant DNA technology, has allowed its use in a multitude of clinical settings [1–6]. Myelosuppression and anemia are the major hematological toxicities of patients who are infected with human immunodeficiency virus (HIV), or in individuals receiving antiviral therapy with zidovudine, formerly azidothymidine (AZT) [7, 8]. Recent studies have indicated that individuals receiving zidovudine may have their anemia ameliorated by the concomitant administration of rhEPO. Both the correction of hemoglobin and hematocrit levels, and a decrease in the necessity for transfusions have been achieved with the use of rhEPO. Side effect profiles have been minimal. Moreover, long-term (greater than 1 year) administration of rhEPO may allow patients to avoid chronic transfusions. The administration of rhEPO to patients with AIDS may help decrease the necessity for blood transfusions [9, 10].

The epidemic of HIV infection and resulting AIDS is one of the greatest public health problems of modern times. It is estimated that approximately 1–1.5 million Americans are believed to be carriers of HIV. Reports from 1988 state that greater than 80,000 cases of AIDS have been reported to the Center for Disease Control, with a resultant 45,000 deaths. It is anticipated that approximately 285,000 cases of AIDS will be expected by the end of 1991. A recent interim analysis of AIDS cases around the world suggests substantial underreporting of the disease. As of May 20, 1990, there have been greater than 250,000 reported cases of AIDS worldwide; however, due to the substantial underreporting, it is estimated that greater than 600,000 total cases actually exist [*USA Today,* May 23, 1990]. The countries with the greatest incidence include the United States, Uganda, Zaire, Brazil and France, with the United States having a substantially greater incidence than the other countries.

Hematological toxicity accounts for much of the morbidity and mortality associated with AIDS treatment. Recent estimates suggest that in the early 1990s, 40% of patients infected with AIDS will be red blood cell (RBC) transfusion dependent. In one estimate, 2 units of blood per patient per month has been calculated; in the United States alone this would mean an incremental increase in the blood supply by approximately 1 million units per year. This would be a substantial burden on a health care system already perplexed by rising health care costs. Moreover, the detrimental aspects of blood transfusions in terms of immunosuppression should be avoided in the already immunocompromised AIDS patient [11]. It thus becomes important to establish the role of therapies to reduce the anemia and transfusion requirements in patients either with AIDS alone, or in AIDS patients receiving zidovudine.

Several studies have demonstrated that untreated patients with AIDS or AIDS patients treated with zidovudine have a significant incidence of leukopenia, thrombocytopenia, and anemia. In one study [12], serum-immunoreactive erythropoietin (siEPO) and hemoglobin levels were measured in 152 patients infected with HIV. Elevated levels in siEPO were seen in HIV-infected patients. Anemia was present in 18% of these HIV-infected patients and in 75% of patients with clinical AIDS. In a subpopulation of patients who were treated with zidovudine, hemoglobin levels fell to <10 g/l in approximately half the patients; however, the siEPO levels in these patients rose nearly 10-fold compared to untreated patients for any given level of anemia (fig. 1, 2). For HIV-infected patients there was an inappropriately low level of EPO compared to patients with uncomplicated iron deficiency anemia. However, the ability of patients to produce EPO is definitely intact and can be exaggerated following zidovudine therapy. Despite this, even high circulating levels of siEPO fail to stimulate erythropoiesis adequately.

More recent studies have demonstrated that the number of burst forming units erythroid (BFU-E) in a normal bone marrow exposed to an antiviral such as zidovudine caused a substantial diminution in the number of BFU-Es at relatively low levels of exposure [13].

A recent study assessing the severity of anemia caused by zidovudine in patients with AIDS demonstrated that a substantially and significantly higher number of patients treated with zidovudine required transfusions. In one study of greater than 150 patients, 46% of 83 patients required transfusions

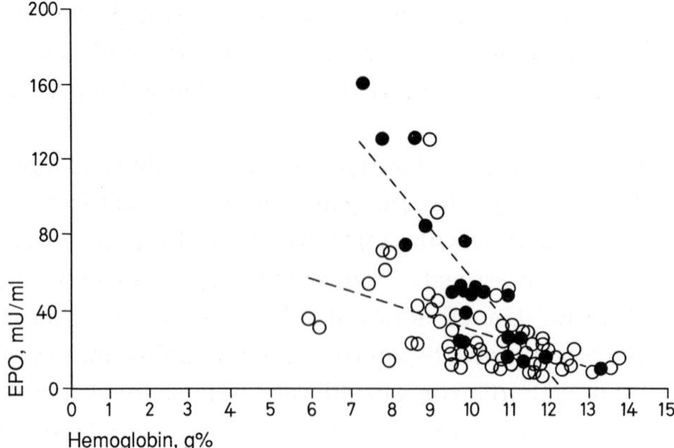

Fig. 1. Relationship between hemoglobin and siEPO in 55 anemic, untreated patients with AIDS (○) and 23 patients with iron deficiency anemia (●). For the AIDS patients the equation for the regression line was y = –6.6× + 91.9 (r = 0.05; p < 0.01). From [6].

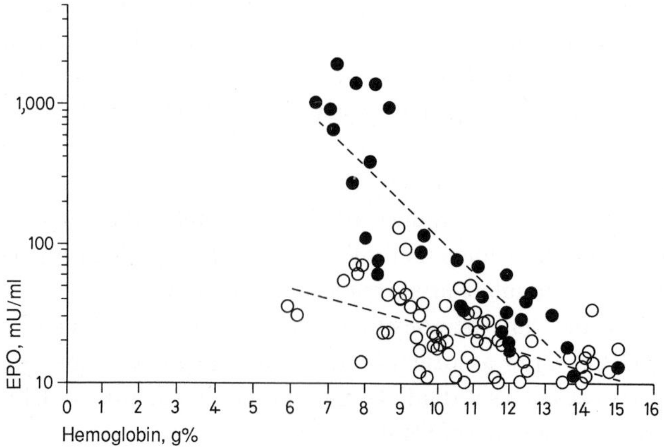

Fig. 2. Relationship between hemoglobin and siEPO in untreated patients with AIDS (○) and 31 AIDS patients treated with zidovudine (●). The equation for the regression line for the zidovudine-treated patients was y = –127.7× + 1,561 (r = 0.63; p < 0.001). The difference between the slopes was significant (p < 0.01). Data from [6].

during zidovudine therapy compared to only 15% of 74 patients in the placebo population [7, 8]. Thirty-two percent of zidovudine patients versus 3% of placebo-treated patients required multiple transfusions. Hemoglobins of <7.5 g/dl developed in 31% of patients receiving zidovudine compared to only 3% in placebo patients. An additional 18% of patients developed hemoglobins of <6.5 g/dl compared to no patients in the placebo population.

Materials and Methods

The currently available published studies evaluating the use of rhEPO in patients with AIDS receiving zidovudine were reviewed. This is predominantly composed of a study sponsored by the R. W. Johnson Pharmaceutical Research Institute, done in conjunction with investigators from the University of Miami, Fla.; The Porton Medical Group, Sherman Oaks, Calif.; New England Deaconess Hospital, Boston, Mass.; Graduate Hospital, Philadelphia, Pa.; Los Angeles Oncologic Institute, Los Angeles, Calif.; UCLA School of Medicine, Los Angeles, Calif.; Orlando, Flo.; Community Research Initiative, N.Y., and Beth Israel Medical Center, N.Y. [10].

This study was a multicenter investigation in which the role of rhEPO to treat the anemia of patients with AIDS receiving zidovudine was investigated. This was a double-blind placebo-controlled study. Patients received rhEPO at doses of 100 U/kg or placebo intravenously 3 times weekly. The design of this study included 12 weeks of rhEPO therapy or until a hematocrit of 38–40% was achieved. The objective of this study was to determine the safety and efficacy of rhEPO; the major end point was an assessment of transfusion requirements. Nonprimary end points included assessment of hemoglobin, hematocrit, and quality of life.

Sixty-three patients were entered into the study, and entry characteristics are seen in tables 1–3. The age of patients was 18–75 and individuals needed to have a documentation of AIDS who were receiving zidovudine. The diagnosis of AIDS was established by demonstrated lymphocytopenia of $<1 \times 10^9$ cells/l and, when possible, a CD4 count of $<0.4 \times 10^9$ cells/l. Individuals had to demonstrate antibody to HIV and have had a documented history of opportunistic infection. Individuals were required to have a performance status of 0–2 and the hematocrit of ≤30%. Individuals had to be either transfusion dependent or have demonstrated a diminution in the hematocrit of 15% since initiation of zidovudine therapy.

Individuals were excluded if they had evidence of other hematological disorders or non-AIDS/non-zidovudine related anemia, uncontrolled hypertension, seizures, history of substance abuse, iron deficiency, recent androgen or cancer chemotherapy administration, or the presence of an active opportunistic infection which required active therapy.

In addition to routine monitoring with typical laboratory values, individuals also had a baseline serum (siEPO) obtained using a radioimmunoassay (Smith-Kline Bioscientific Laboratory, Van Nuys, Calif.). In this study, individuals were stratified for analysis based upon endogenous levels. Low endogenous EPO levels were defined ≤500 IU/l. Individuals with >500 IU/l were considered as having high levels. In this study, the number of patients having high EPO levels was 21%, with 79% of patients having low EPO levels. These data were identical for both patients treated with EPO and placebo. Figure 3 demonstrates the baseline endogenous EPO levels.

Table 1. Characteristics of the patient population [data from 2, p. 203]

	rhEPO	Placebo
Sex		
Male	29	33
Female	0	1
Race distribution		
Caucasian	27	31
Other	2	3
Age		
Median	37	38
Maximum	51	64
Minimum	24	24

Table 2. rhEPO + zidovudine (AZT) in AIDS

Age 18–75
AIDS on AZT
Lymphocytopenia ($<1 \times 10^9$/liter; CD4$<0.4 \times 10^9$/liter)
Antibody to HIV
Documented Hx of OI
PS = 0–2
Hct $\leq$ 30
Tx-dependent
Decrease in Hct up 15% since AZT

Table 3. rhEPO/AZT exclusions

Other hematologic disorders
Uncontrolled hypertension
Seizures
Substance abuse
Fe deficiency
Recent androgen/cancer chemotherapy
Active OI
Non-AIDS/AZT anemia

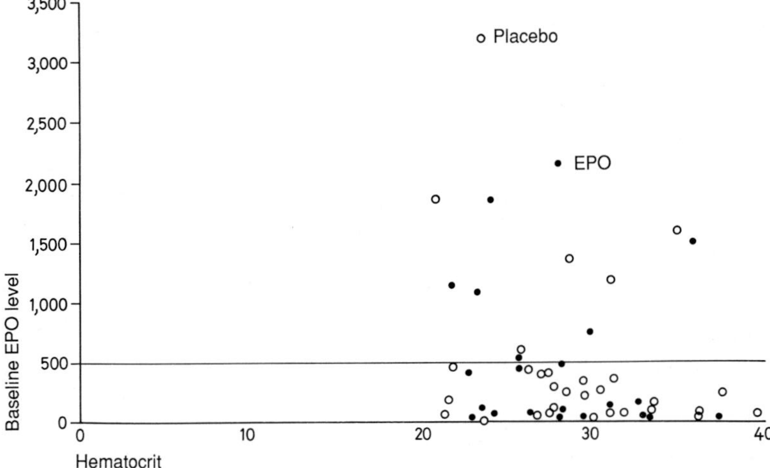

Fig. 3. RWJ-PRI rhEPO study (protocol No. H87–037), treatment of anemia in AIDS patients also receiving zidovudine: baseline endogenous EPO levels. From [6].

Results

The main end point in this study was the dependency and number of transfusions required during the double-blind phase. As mentioned, hemoglobin and hematocrit were secondary and not primary end points because patients could receive transfusions at the discretion on their physician. Table 4 demonstrates the number of patients who received transfusions at baseline, months 1, 2, and 3, and at end point during the last month of study.

The number of patients in this study demonstrated that 23 rhEPO and 27 placebo patients respectively were actively being transfused at the initiation of the study. At the end of the study, only 11 patients in the rhEPO group compared to 21 patients in the placebo group required transfusions. If one stratifies these transfusion requirement data according to the endogenous level of EPO, there were 16 individuals in the low EPO group receiving rhEPO and 21 patients in the placebo group. At the study end point the number of patients requiring transfusions fell to 5 and 17 respectively.

These results were less striking in individuals who had high EPO levels. In this population there were 7 patients assigned to rhEPO who were transfused, compared to 6 at the study end point. In the placebo group, 6 patients at baseline were transfused compared to 4 patients at the end point. Likewise, if

Table 4. Patients receiving transfusion (number in study in parentheses) of packed red cells or whole blood, according to serum level of endogenous EPO [data from 10]

Level of endogenous EPO	Receiving transfusion[1]				
	baseline	month 1	month 2	month 3	month 4
≤500 IU/l					
EPO group	16 (22)	10 (22)	7[2] (21)	5[2] (20)	5[2] (22)
Placebo group	21 (26)	13 (25)	16 (24)	15 (23)	17 (25)
>500 IU/l					
EPO group	7 (7)	7 (7)	7 (7)	6 (7)	6 (7)
Placebo group	6 (6)	5 (6)	5 (6)	3 (5)	4 (6)
All					
EPO group	23 (29)	17 (29)	14 (28)	11 (27)	11 (29)
Placebo group[3]	27 (34)	18 (33)	21 (31)	18 (29)	21 (33)

[1] Baseline refers to the 3 months before beginning the study medication, and end point to the last month of participation.
[2] Significantly fewer than placebo ($p \leq 0.05$).
[3] Data on endogenous EPO levels were not available for 2 patients in the placebo group, and information on transfusions was not available after the first dose in 1 patient.

the data were evaluated relating to number of units of blood transfused per patient in the entire group, 29 patients required 1.7 units/patient at baseline in the individuals assigned to rhEPO. At the end of the study this had fallen to 1.48 units/patients. In the placebo group, 1.87 units/patient were transfused at baseline compared to 2.58 units/patient at the end of the study (table 5).

Stratification according to low EPO levels demonstrated that in the rhEPO-treated patients, the baseline and end point values were 2.3 and 0.84 units respectively. In the placebo-treated patients, the values were 1.68 units at baseline compared to 2.74 units at end point. Both of these numbers are very highly statistically significant.

In the high rhEPO patients, the number of units transfused at baseline were 3.1 units/patient compared to 2.5 at end point. In the placebo-treated patients this was 3.32 units at baseline compared to 2.78 at end point. These numbers were not statistically significant.

An additional aspect of this study was the demonstration of well-being in terms of energy level, work ability, and a global assessment of quality of life.

Table 5. Units of packed red cells or whole blood transfused (number of patients in parentheses), according to serum level of endogenous EPO [data from 10]

Level of endogenous EPO	Units transfused[1]				
	baseline	month 1	month 2	month 3	end point
≤500 IU/l					
EPO group	1.31 (22)	1.18 (22)	1.23^2 (21)	0.92^2 (20)	0.84^2 (22)
Placebo group	1.68 (26)	2.15 (25)	2.80 (24)	2.17 (23)	2.74 (25)
>500 IU/l					
EPO group	3.10 (7)	4.86 (7)	3.29 (7)	3.50 (7)	3.50 (7)
Placebo group	3.32 (6)	3.19 (6)	3.35 (6)	2.43 (6)	2.78 (6)
All					
EPO group	1.74 (29)	2.07 (29)	1.74 (28)	1.59 (27)	1.48 (29)
Placebo group[3]	1.87 (34)	2.21 (33)	2.81 (31)	2.14 (29)	2.58 (33)

[1] Units at baseline refer to the mean number of units per month in the 3 months before treatment with the study medication began, and units at end point to the mean number of units during the last month of participation.
[2] Significantly fewer than placebo ($p \leq 0.05$).
[3] Data on endogenous EPO levels were not available for 2 patients in the placebo group, and information on transfusions was not available after the first dose in 1 patient.

Using a visual analogue scale at baseline and then again at the end of the study, it was demonstrated that energy level and quality of life parameters were improved and approached statistical significance (table 6). This was mainly seen for the comparison of the low EPO patients versus the placebo-treated patients. There was no improvement in well-being assessments with rhEPO in the high endogenous EPO patients compared to placebo.

The side effect profiles most frequently reported in this double-blind study included pyrexia, fatigue, rash, headaches and diarrhea. None of these were more frequent in the rhEPO versus placebo-treated patients. Individual patients ended up going off study both in the rhEPO group and the placebo group. The main reasons for this were either discontinuation of zidovudine or the development of a rash in the rhEPO population. In the placebo population, individuals were discontinued because of pancytopenia, rash, discontinuation of zidovudine, the development of plasmacytoma, and opportunistic

Table 6. Well-being assessments[1]: change from baseline to end point treatment [data from 6]

Assessment	rhEPO (100 U/kg)		Placebo	
	n	median change	n	median change
Energy level				
Low EPO	20	8.5[2]	22	–1.0
High EPO	7	–4.0	6	10
All patients	27	8.0	29	0
Work capacity				
Low EPO	20	8.0	22	–7.5
High EPO	7	–5.0	6	–7.0
All patients	27	7.0	29	–6.0
Quality of life				
Low EPO	20	13.5[3]	22	–9.5
High EPO	7	–9.0	6	–0.5
All patients	27	10.0	29	–7.0

[1] A higher score indicates improvement.
[2] $p = 0.064$ for between-treatment-group comparison.
[3] $p = 0.084$ for between-treatment-group comparison.

infection. Many of these were secondary to the natural history of AIDS infection. Serious adverse drug reactions that occurred were relatively limited. There was no difference in the development of opportunistic infections in either the rhEPO versus placebo-treated patients.

Discussion

This cardinal and landmark study evaluating the use of rhEPO versus placebo in patients infected with HIV who are receiving zidovudine demonstrated that individuals could be selected for response to rhEPO based upon endogenous serum EPO levels. Individuals with ≤500 IU/l of EPO could have a reduction in transfusion requirements and an improvement in quality of life and increases in hemoglobin in hematocrit. This was accomplished without any increase in overall side effects. The implications of this study are profound. The likelihood of decreasing the overall burden on the health care system as relates to blood transfusion may indeed be ameliorated by the use of rhEPO. Longer term studies currently underway may demonstrate chronic benefit in transfusion requirements for AIDS patients treated with zidovudine.

Addendum

On March 15, 1990, the FDA Advisory Committee recommended that erythropoietin be approved for patients with HIV infections receiving zidovudine (AZT) in a dose of 40–100 mg per week or less with an endogenous erythropoietin level of less than or equal to 500 IU/liter.

References

1   Scigalla, P.; Wieczorek, L.; Bicker, U.: Treatment of renal anemia with recombinant human erythropoietin: European experience; in Garnick, M. B. (ed.): Erythropoietin in Clinical Applications; An International Perspective, p.141 (Dekker, New York 1990).

2   Sobota, J.: Erythropoietin treatment of end-stage renal disease: North American and Japanese experience; in Garnick, M. B. (ed.): Erythropoietin in Clinical Applications; An International Perspective, p.183 (Dekker, New York 1990).

3   Koene, R. A. P.; Frenken, L. A. M.: The use of erythropoietin in predialysis patients; in Garnick, M. B. (ed.): Erythropoietin in Clinical Applications; An International Perspective, p. 221 (Dekker, New York 1990).

4   Jabs, K.; Harmon, W. E.: Potential use of erythropoietin in the pediatric population; in Garnick, M. B. (ed.): Erythropoietin in Clinical Applications; An International Perspective, p. 255 (Dekker, New York 1990).

5   Goodnough, L. T.: Erythropoietin in the surgical setting; Garnick, M. B. (ed.): Erythropoietin in Clinical Applications; An International Perspective, p. 287 (Dekker, New York 1990).

6   Danna, R. P.; Rudnick, S. A.; Abels, R. I.: Erythropoietin therapy for anemic associated with AIDS and AIDS therapy and cancer; in Garnick, M. B., (ed.): Erythropoietin in Clinical Applications; An International Perspective, p. 301 (Dekker, New York 1990).

7   Fischl, M. A.; Richman, D. D.; Grieco, M. H., et al.: The efficacy of azidothymidine (AZT) in the treatment of patients with AIDS and AIDS-related complex: a double-blind, placebo-controlled trial. N. Engl. J. Med. 317: 185–191 (1987).

8   Richman, D. D.; Fischl, M. A.; Grieco, M. H., et al.: The toxicity of azidothymidine (AZT) in the treatment of patients with AIDS and AIDS-related complex: a double-blind, placebo-controlled trial. N. Engl. J. Med. 317: 192–197 (1987).

9   Henry, D. H.: Human recombinant erythropoietin in the treatment of severe anemia in patients with AIDS. Intern. Med. Specialist 10: 739–749 (1989).

10 Fischl, M. A.; Galpin, J. E.; Levine, J. D., et al.: Recombinant human erythropoietin for patients with AIDS treated with zidovudine. N. Engl. J. Med. 322: 1488–1493 (1990).

11 Kahan, B. D.: Effects of transfusion on recipient immune status: relationship to transplantation; in Dodd, R. Y.; Barker, L. F. (eds): Infection, Immunity, and Blood Transfusion. Prog. Clin. Biol. Res., vol. 182, pp. 345–374 (Liss, New York 1985).
12 Spivak, J. L.; Barnes, D. C.; Fuchs, E., et al.: Serum immunoreactive erythropoietin in HIV-infected patients. JAMA *261:* 3104–3107 (1989).
13 Johnson, M.; Caiazzo, T.; Molina, J. M., et al.: Inhibition of bone marrow myelopoiesis and erythropoiesis in vitro by antiretroviral nucleoside derivatives. Br. J. Haematol *70:* 137–141 (1988).

Marc B. Garnick, MD, Genetics Institute, Inc., 87 Cambridge Park Drive, Cambridge, MA 02140 (USA)

Gurland HJ, Moran J, Samtleben W, Scigalla P, Wieczorek L (eds): Erythropoietin in
Renal and Non-Renal Anemias. Contrib Nephrol. Basel, Karger, 1991, vol 88, pp 293–294

Discussion

to the Paper by M. B. Garnick et al.

Winearls (Oxford): At what stage of the trial design was an EPO concentration of
500 mIU/ml chosen as the cut-off between responders and non-responders? Was it before or
after the data was analysed?

Garnick: It was obtained during the course of the study evaluation, it was not prospectively determined.

Winearls: When were the levels of EPO measured? Was it before or after transfusion,
and were the hemoglobin concentrations comparable in the two groups at the time of sampling?

Garnick: It was at the time of study entry. The data I showed were in terms of the
baseline EPO levels as a function of hematocrit, performed at the time of study entry.

Winearls: Do you have any indication yet how those responsible for reimbursement of
the costs of EPO are going to respond to a cost of £25,000 per annum per patient to raise the
hematocrit to 30% and to allow some but not all to become transfusion independent? This is
relevant given the current difficulties in obtaining funding for the much smaller renal population, whose needs are more modest and in whom benefits are unequivocal.

Garnick: That's a point which has to be addressed nation by nation; we are wrestling
with that in the US right now.

Caro (Philadelphia): I wonder if you have any data on the platelet and white cell counts
in the two groups of patients. It seems that the difference in EPO levels reflects something
other than just production of EPO because your baseline transfusion requirements between
the two groups are significantly different. In the group with the lower EPO level you have
1.3 units of blood compared to 3.1 units in the group with the higher EPO level. It seems to me
that the bone marrow suppression in one group is different than in the other.

Garnick: We built into the study serial evaluations of count and differentials as well as
platelet counts. There was absolutely no difference in the treated versus the non-treated
population.

Essers (Aachen): What was the dose of AZT? Was it the same in all patients?

Garnick: The dose was 1,200 mg/day during the study. There was no substantial difference between the ability to deliver AZT in the placebo group compared to the EPO-treated
patients. There was actually a slight decrease in the total weekly dose of AZT administered in
the EPO group, but it was not statistically significantly different from the dose in the placebo
group.

Sobota (Rosemont): Was there any association between the level of EPO and any other factor such as the time of diagnosis of AIDS, the dose of AZT, the time on AZT and so forth?

Garnick: That data is unknown.

Klinkmann (Rostock): I was quite intrigued by your survival curve, and obviously there was no difference in opportunistic infections as well. Would you dare to speculate whether this is the last word, because then we may get into an argument about using EPO for these patients. If there is no difference in survival then the final decision depends on quality of life.

Garnick: Built into the study were quality of life assessments, energy level, and work capabilities. There was clearly a tendency towards an improvement in the quality of life.

Herrmann (Berlin): Did you look at the absolute number of T4 cells, and was there any difference?

Garnick: T4 cells were evaluated in the majority of patients but not in all.

Eschbach (Seattle): Is it possible that the high EPO level group represents a sicker group of patients than the lower EPO group? And if so, are they different? Are there other things that are different besides the EPO levels and the transfusion requirements? What I am getting at is: Did you look at separating out those patients that clearly responded to EPO and those that didn't, in other words those that had high EPO levels and those that didn't.

Garnick: That data is currently being analyzed.

Gurland HJ, Moran J, Samtleben W, Scigalla P, Wieczorek L (eds): Erythropoietin in
Renal and Non-Renal Anemias. Contrib Nephrol. Basel, Karger, 1991, vol 88, pp 295–303

Anemia of Chronic Inflammatory Arthritides: Treatment with Recombinant Human Erythropoietin

*Gunnar Birgegård[a], Björn Gudbjrönsson[a], Roger Hällgren[a],
Leif Wide[b, 1]*

Departments of [a]Internal Medicine and [b]Clinical Chemistry, University Hospital,
Uppsala, Sweden

Chronic inflammatory disease is often associated with a relatively moderate degree of anemia [12, 17]. The etiology is a matter of controversy. A shortened life span of the erythrocytes is accepted by most workers in the field, but this is quantitatively of minor importance [8]. A reduced production of erythrocytes is the most important cause, but there is no consensus concerning the reason for this. A block in the release of iron from the reticuloendothelial cells to the erythron has been advocated by some workers [7, 11] but recent studies have not been able to support this idea [4, 5]. Patients with anemia of chronic inflammation have elevated serum EPO (sEPO) levels. In spite of this, anemia is not corrected. Some studies have shown a blunted EPO response to anemia [2a, 10], others have shown appropriate EPO levels [3, 6, 13]. A previous report of response to treatment with recombinant human EPO (rhEPO) has been presented [14].

This is a preliminary report from an ongoing study of the efficacy of EPO treatment of the anemia of chronic inflammatory disease.

[1] Thanks are due to Mrs. Gudrun Lundgren, research nurse, for teaching the patients the injection techniques and to the staff at the Section of Rheumatology for thoroughly collecting blood samples and taking care of the patients.

Table 1. Clinical features of 6 patients with RA and 1 patient with ankylosing spondylitis undergoing 6 weeks' treatment with rhEPO

Patient No.	Sex	Age years	Disease duration years	Serology	X-ray[1]	Extra articular symptoms	Function class	Ritchie index	Antirheumatic medications
1 AE	F	69	31	RF+	Y	none	II	12	sulfasalazine[2]
2 KB	F	35	10	RF+	Y	none	II	16	p.o. gold
3 MP	F	76	39	RF+, ANA+	Y	amyloidosis renal insuff.	III	11	–[2]
4 GE	F	70	17	RF+, ANA+	Y	Sjögren's syndrome	II	20	azathioprine[2]
5 SO	F	56	22	RF+, ANA+	Y	rh. nodules cut. vasculitis	II	11	p.o. gold[2]
6 OE	M	42	10	neg	Y	none	III	14	i.m. gold salt[2]
7 RM[3]	M	47	18	neg	Psp	amyloidosis renal insuff.	III	–	NSAID

[1] X-ray: roentgenological erosions yes (Y) or no (N) and signs of ankylosing spondylitis (Psp).
[2] Patients taking corticosteroids.
[3] Patient with ankylosing spondylitis.

Patients and Methods

Patients

Seven patients, 5 women and 2 men, with inflammatory arthritides and with subjective symptoms of anemia (Hb < 105 g/l), were included in the study. Six patients, 5 women and 1 man, fulfilled the criteria of the American Rheumatism Association [1] for classical rheumatoid arthritis (RA) and one 47-year-old man had ankylosing spondylitis according to the New York criteria of the American Rheumatism Association [2b].

Mean age was 56 years, range 35–76 years, and the mean disease duration was 21 years, range 10–39 years. All patients, except 2 (cases 2 and 7), were taking nonsteroidal anti-inflammatory drugs (NSAID) or aspirin as well as a low dose of corticosteroids. Two patients were treated with peroral gold (Ridaura®; SK & F, Herts., UK) and 1 with parenteral gold salt (Myocrisin®; Rhône-Poulenc, Birkeröd, Denmark), respectively. Two additional patients were treated with disease-modifying antirheumatic drugs; 1 with sulfasalazine (Salazopyrin EN®; Pharmacia, Malmö, Sweden) and the other with azathioprine (Imurel®; Wellcome, London, UK), respectively.

Four patients had extra-articular manifestations; 1 patient had secondary Sjögren's syndrome and another patient had rheumatoid nodules and a history of cutaneous vasculitis. Further, 2 patients had secondary amyloidosis with moderate renal insufficiency (serum creatinine 350 and 280, respectively). Clinical data are presented in table 1.

Table 2. Laboratory features of 6 patients with RA and of 1 patient with ankylosing spondylitis before treatment with rhEPO

	Patients (n = 7)		Reference values
	mean ± SD	range	
Hb, g/l			
Female	94±8	82–103	113–134
Male	87±22	71–102	134–166
Hct, %			
Female	30±3.7	24–34	35–44
Male	28±5.3	24–32	40–49
MCV, μm^3	88±11	72–105	70–98
MCH, pg	28±5	20–6	28–35
MCHC, g/l	311±21	281–338	320–360
Reticulocytes, %	2.2±0.8	1.4–3.4	0.2–2.0
WBC, 10^9/l	8.6±3.0	4.9–13.1	4–9
Platelets, 10^9/l	502±268	224–758	150–400
ESR, mm/h	81±39	28–130	2–15
Haptoglobin, g/l	4.0±2.8	1.9–9.6	0.2–1.4
Serum iron, μmol/l	7.3±3.4	3.3–12.8	11–35
Serum transferrin, μmol/l	44.4±20.5	29–85	45–72
Serum ferritin, μmol/l	343±461	10–1353	10–240
sEPO	15.4±10.6	6.1–37.9	33.3–13.5

Treatment Schedule

All patients were studied as outpatients at the Department of Medicine, University Hospital, Uppsala. Informed consent was obtained and the study was approved by the Uppsala University Committee on Medical Ethics.

All patients received 50 IU/kg body weight of EPO subcutaneously 5 days/week, i.e., a weekly dose of 250 IU/kg. A maximum dose of 4,000 IU/day was not exceeded and patients who required a dose higher than 2,000 IU were given injections at two sites. EPO was provided as rhEPO manufactured and supplied by Boehringer Mannheim, Mannheim, FRG.

A treatment duration of 6 weeks was chosen in order to make it possible to avoid changes in the anti-inflammatory drug treatment during the study. Only patients with a relatively stable, although in some cases high, inflammatory activity, were accepted. No changes were made in the anti-inflammatory treatment. The treatment goal was an increase in Hb > 15 g/l in the individual patient. When this goal was reached, the rhEPO dose was reduced by 50% to 25 IU/kg 5 days/week.

Each patient underwent hematological evaluation, including serum iron, serum trans-ferrin, serum ferritin, tests for hemolysis and bone marrow aspiration with staining for iron to exclude other causes of anemia than the chronic inflammation (table 2). Patients with laboratory signs of increased hemolysis or without stainable bone marrow hemosiderin were not accepted in the study. If the ferritin value before the start of the rhEPO treatment was <250 µmol/l oral iron therapy (100 mg/day) was given (5 patients, all except cases 1 and 5).

Clinical and Laboratory Evaluation

Subjective symptoms (morning stiffness and joint pain during movements and at rest) were evaluated by interviews and graded with the use of a 10-grade visual analog scale. Objective signs of active arthritis were estimated by the Ritchie index [14] and the functional capacity was estimated according to Steinbrocker et al. [16]. This evaluation of disease activity was made before and after 6 weeks of treatment with rhEPO. During the treatment period the patients were interviewed and examined weekly. The blood pressure was also measured before each injection of EPO.

The following measurements were performed weekly; Hb, hematocrit (EVF), reticulocyte and white blood cell counts (WBC), platelets, serum creatinine, serum potassium, C-reactive protein (CRP), erythrocyte sedimentation rate (ESR) and haptoglobin, all measured according to standard clinical laboratory techniques. The same evaluation was made every other week during the 6 weeks after the treatment with rhEPO was discontinued.

sEPO was measured before the start of treatment, using a radioimmunoassay method previously published [18]. The lower detection limit is 0.5 IU/l, and the mean EPO level in a normal population is 6.7 IU/l, reference range 3.3–13.5 IU/l.

Results

All patients had signs of active inflammatory disease with elevated ESR, CRP and a high Ritchie index (table 3). The mean Hb for the whole group was 90.9 ± 9.5 g/l before treatment and 109.7 ± 11.0 g/l after 6 weeks (p = 0.01). The mean EVF increased from 29.3 ± 3.2 to $34.9 \pm 2.5\%$ (p = 0.01) (fig. 1). The highest Hb and EVF levels were reached after 5 weeks: 112.1 ± 8.9 g/l and $35.3 \pm 1.8\%$. Five of the 7 patients responded to therapy with an increase in Hb >15 g/l. The 2 patients with renal insufficiency both responded in spite of very active inflammation; Hb increased from 98 to 130 and 75 to 117 g/l, respectively (fig. 2). The individual Hb curves of the 5 patients with normal kidney function are shown in figure 3. Three of these patients responded with an increase in Hb >15 g/l, 2 showed no response. One of the nonresponders had an increase in reticulocyte count to 8% during the last week of treatment.

The 2 nonresponders differed from the other patients with regard to the inflammatory activity. Both had a very high CRP level, a high Ritchie index and clinically very active arthritis with more pain, redness and swelling than the others.

Not all patients have completed the 6 weeks of follow-up. Only 1 of the responders has maintained the Hb level so far, 3 have fallen, although not yet

Table 3. Laboratory features of 6 patients with RA and of 1 patient with ankylosing spondylitis on baseline and on follow-up after 6 weeks' treatment with rhEPO

Patient No.		Hb g/l (max)	Hct %	Retic. % (max)	WBC $10^9/l$ (max)	Platelets $10^9/l$	sEPO IU/l	SR mm/h	CRP mg/l	Ritchie index
1	baseline	81	24.0	2.8	5.7	306	11.9	28	19	12
	follow-up	108 (110)	34.0	0.5	5.8 (3.0)	196	–	12	48	–
2	baseline	98	31.5	2.2	7.8	289	12.5	40	36	16
	follow-up	110 (120)	34.0	2.2	8.9 (5.6)	375	–	40	57	11
3	baseline	98	29	1.4	11.9	318	8.1	120	62	11
	follow-up	130 (130)	40.0	1.4	10.3 (6.6)	334	–	60	25	8
4	baseline	98	34.0	1.4	13.1	519	37.9	62	114	20
	follow-up	98 (103)	32.0	4.2	10.0 (8.0)	565	–	19	122	11
5	baseline	89	29.0	1.4	8.3	559	15.3	90	97	10
	follow-up	100 (108)	34.0	2.8	8.9 (3.6)	448	–	42	56	8
6	baseline	97	30.0	1.8	8.4	841	16.9	94	174	14
	follow-up	105 (105)	34.8	2.0	8.5 (2.0)	718	–	73	198	14
7	baseline	75	27.0	3.4	4.9	227	6.1	71	130	–
	follow-up	117 (117)	35.4	1.0	8.1 (1.8)	258	–	117	80	–
p value		= 0.01	= 0.01	NS	NS	NS		NS	NS	NS

to pretreatment levels (fig. 1–3). Four weeks after cessation of treatment the mean Hb level was still significantly higher than before treatment (p = 0.01). No significant difference was observed in MCV, MCH, MCHC, serum iron, serum ferritin or serum transferrin before and after the study (data not shown). Mean sEPO before treatment was 15.4 ± 10.6 IU/l. Four patients had an sEPO within the reference range for normals, 2 just above this range. The patient with the highest sEPO (37.9 IU/l) did not respond to EPO therapy.

Neither the inflammatory activity, measured by ESR, CRP or the Ritchie index, nor the functional capacity according to Steinbrocker, were influenced by the rhEPO therapy (table 3). CRP increased in 4 patients, decreased in 3, ESR decreased in 5, increased in 1 and showed no change in 1 case. No adverse

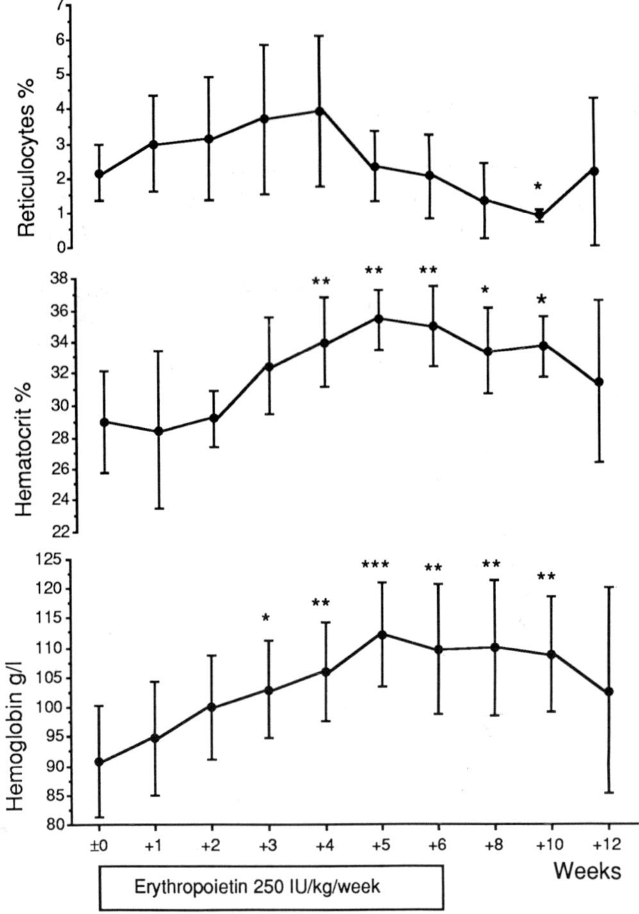

Fig. 1. Hb, Hct and reticulocytes from 6 patients with RA and from 1 patient with ankylosing spondylitis treated with rhEPO for 6 weeks. The data are presented as means ± SD.

effects could be attributed directly to the rhEPO therapy. One patient (case 2) had subjectively increased joint pain from the shoulders. Whether this was due to the rhEPO therapy or only joint pain associated to her RA is difficult to estimate. She did not require increased doses of analgesics. Two patients (cases 3 and 4) were taking antihypertensive medication when the study

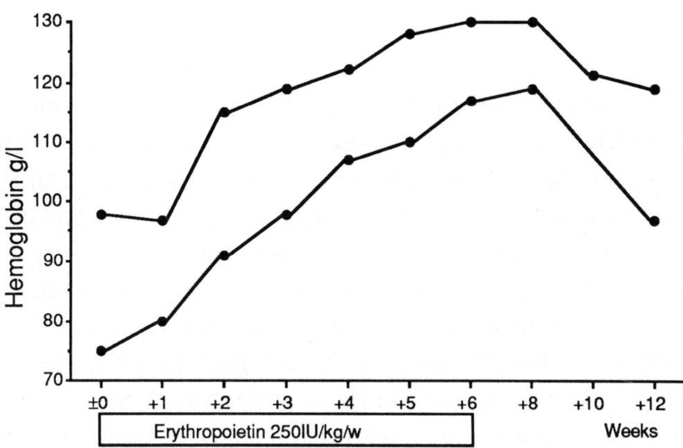

Fig. 2. Individual Hb curves for 2 patients with anemia of mixed etiology; ACI and renal insufficiency (amyloidosis) during treatment with rhEPO.

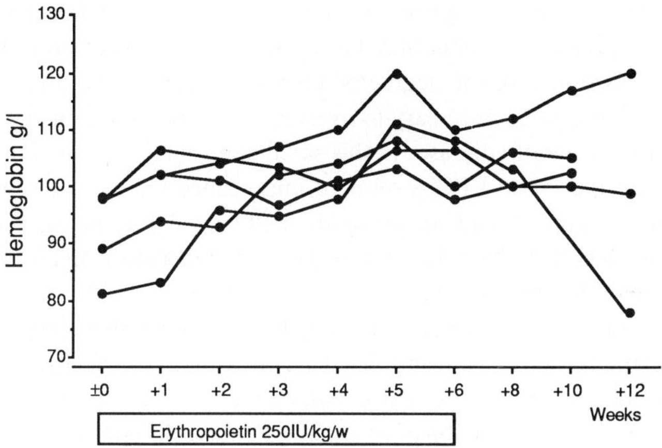

Fig. 3. Individual Hb curves for 5 patients with anemia of chronic inflammation during treatment with rhEPO.

began. Neither of these 2 patients required additional antihypertensive treatment during the study. Further, none of the normotensive patients had any signs of increased blood pressure during the study. The rhEPO injections were well tolerated and 5 of the patients learnt to handle the subcutaneous injections themselves after instruction from a nurse.

Discussion

The anemia of chronic inflammation (ACI) is generally of a moderate degree. It is often difficult to evaluate the role of the anemia for the well-being of the patient. The inflammatory disease itself gives general fatigue, and since many patients are limited in their functional capacity by joint pain and disfiguration, the cardiovascular system is not challenged by physical activities. Many clinicians, however, have noticed an improvement in general well-being when successful anemia treatment has been given, even when there has been no change in the activity of the inflammatory disease. Therefore it seems worthwhile to test the possibility of increasing Hb in patients with ACI.

rhEPO offers such a possibility. It has proven effective in overcoming the uremic inhibition of erythropoiesis [9], and spurious reports of response in other anemias have been presented lately. In the present study we have so far shown a response in the Hb level in 5/7 patients. Pincus et al. [13] have previously reported successful treatment of ACI with EPO.

The controversy concerning whether these patients have an adequate or blunted EPO response to anemia may be of minor importance; even if the EPO levels are adequate for the degree of anemia, a further elevation of the EPO concentration may be necessary to overcome the inhibition on erythropoiesis by the inflammatory disease. In this small material it is not possible to evaluate whether the initial EPO level is of importance for the response to treatment. Only 1 patient had an adequate EPO level for the degree of anemia. It is worth noticing that the 2 nonresponders had a more highly active inflammation than the responders.

The 2 patients with the combination of renal and inflammatory anemia had the most dramatic response, showing that EPO treatment is effective in this mixed type of anemia in spite of active inflammation. The duration of Hb response was limited after cessation of treatment. Four weeks after the last dose the mean Hb was still significantly higher (p = 0.01) than before treatment, but only 1 patient so far has maintained the Hb level for 6 weeks after treatment.

This study does not investigate whether there was any improvement in the quality of life. Five of the patients spontaneously expressed that they felt better when Hb was higher, and 3 wanted to restart EPO treatment after the study.

In conclusion, we have found that patients with ACI arthritides respond to treatment with moderate doses of subcutaneous rhEPO. The intensity of the inflammation may influence response. The study will be continued with collection of more patients and measurement of sEPO during and after the treatment.

References

1   Arnett FC, Edworthy SM, Bloch DA, et al: The American Rheumatism Association 1987. Revised criteria for the classification of rheumatoid arthritis. Arthritis Rheum 1988;31:315–324.

2a Baer AN, Dessypris EN, Goldwasser E, Krantz SB: Blunted erythropoietin response to anemia in rheumatoid arthritis. Br J Haematol 1987;66:559–564.

2b Bennet PH, Wood PHN: in Bennet PH, Wood PHN (eds): Population Studies of the Rheumatic Diseases. Amsterdam, Excerpta Medica Foundation, 1968, pp 456–457.

3   Birgegård G, Hällgren R, Caro J: Serum erythropoietin in rheumatoid arthritis and other inflammatory arthritides: relationship to anaemia and the effect of anti-inflammatory treatment. Br J Haematol 1987;65:479–483.

4   Bentley DP, Cavill I, Ricketts C, et al: A method for the investigation of reticuloendothelial iron kinetics in man. Br J Haematol 1979;43:619–624.

5   Bentley DP, Williams P: Serum ferritin concentrations as an index of iron stores in rheumatoid arthritis. J Clin Pathol 1974;27:786–790.

6   Erslev AJ, Caro J, Miller O, Silver R: Plasma erythropoietin in health and disease. Ann Clin Lab Sci 1980;10:250–259.

7   Cartwright GE: The anaemia of chronic disorders. Semin Hematol 1966;3:351–375.

8   Cavill I, Bentley DP: Erythropoiesis in the anemia of rheumatoid arthritis. Br J Haematol 1982;50:583–590.

9   Eschbach J, Egrie J, Downing M, Browne J, Adamson J: Correction of the anemia of end-stage renal disease with recombinant human erythropoietin. N Engl J Med 1987;316:73–78.

10 Hochberg MC, Arnold CM, Hogans BB, Spivak JL: Serum immunoreactive erythropoietin in rheumatoid arthritis: impaired response to anemia. Arthritis Rheum 1988;31:1318–1321.

11 Konijn AM, Hershko C: Ferritin synthesis in inflammation. I. Mechanism of impaired iron release. Br J Haematol 1977;37:7–15.

12 Miller RK, Altz-Smith M: Usefulness of serum ferritin in detecting iron deficiency in rheumatoid arthritis. Arthritis Rheum 1982;25(suppl):114.

13 Nielsen OJ, Andersen LS, Ludwigsen E, et al: Anaemia of rheumatoid arthritis. Ann Rheum Dis 1990;49:349–353.

14 Pincus T, Olsen NJ; Russell IJ, et al: Anemia in rheumatoid arthritis: correction using recombinant erythropoietin (abstract). Arthritis Rheum 1989;32(suppl 4):43.

15 Ritchie DM, Boyle JA, McInnes JM, et al: Clinical studies with an articular index for the assessment of joint tenderness in patients with rheumatoid arthritis. Q J Med 1968;37:393–406.

16 Steinbrocker O, Traeger CH, Batterman RC: Therapeutic criteria in rheumatoid arthritis. JAMA 1949;140:659–664.

17 Strandberg O: Anemia in rheumatoid arthritis. Acta Med Scand 1966; 180(suppl 454):7–153.

18 Wide L, Bengtsson C, Birgegård G: Circadian rhythm of erythropoietin in human serum. Br J Haematol 1989;72:85–90.

Gunnar Birgegård, MD, Department of Internal Medicine, University Hospital, S–75185 Uppsala (Sweden)

Gurland HJ, Moran J, Samtleben W, Scigalla P, Wieczorek L (eds): Erythropoietin in Renal and Non-Renal Anemias. Contrib Nephrol. Basel, Karger, 1991, vol 88, pp 304–305

Discussion

to the Paper by G. Birgegård et al.

Klinkmann (Rostock): I am going to invite Dr. Krantz to give a few comments.

Krantz (Nashville): Our results agree very closely. We had 17 patients with active rheumatoid arthritis, very similar to Dr. Birgegard's patients, who were placed in a double-blind, placebo-controlled, randomized study for the first 8 weeks. They received either placebo or 50, 100 or 150 U/kg i.v. 3 times a week. After 8 weeks they were allowed to go onto open maintenance treatment if they wished. There were 13 patients who received EPO in the first 8 weeks. One received 150 U/kg, six 100 U/kg, six 50 U/kg, and there were four placebo patients. We defined a response as an increase in hematocrit of 6%. There were 4 responders in the first 8 weeks of treatment: the one receiving 150 U/kg, 2 of the 6 receiving 100 U/kg and 1 of the 6 receiving 50 U/kg. None of the placebo group responded. Eight of the non-responders elected to go onto maintenance therapy, and all 8 responded when they were treated with EPO for a longer period and with increasing doses up to a maximum of 300 U/kg i.v. 3 times a week. All 3 of the placebo patients who entered the open phase responded to rhEPO. There were 4 patients who did not respond to EPO, and all received only 50 U/kg i.v. 3 times a week for 8 weeks. So it is possible that, had we been allowed to give the EPO for a longer period of time or in a higher dose, these 4 also would have responded. Nevertheless, 75% of the patients did respond, and of the 12 responders, 11 reached totally normal hematocrits.

So, I think that the majority of these patients are going to respond very well. We had no significant adverse effects which required stopping the drug or instituting any new form of treatment. We gave a quality-of-life questionnaire to these patients, a visual analogue pain scale, and found no change in the quality of life during the course of EPO administration. However, this was a very hard study for our patients. They had to come to the hospital 3 times a week, get out of the car, come into the hospital, get back in the car, something that rheumatoid arthritis patients don't like to do. So it's possible that if they were allowed to administer their EPO at home subcutaneously with less activity, then perhaps they would have some benefit.

I think the real use of EPO for these patients will be for hip prostheses or other surgery. We can get their hematocrits up to normal, so that they can donate autologous blood. EPO may also benefit patients who are very severely anemic. I don't think anybody is suggesting that we should go out and treat everybody who has rheumatoid arthritis with EPO.

O. Nielsen (Copenhagen): Could you speculate a little bit: your patients have hematocrits up to the high 40s, and one even higher. We try to keep our kidney patients between 35 and 40%. Did you see any adverse effects in your patients at 40–50?

Krantz: No, we didn't. I am not recommending that we should get that high. Our target was 35%. This was a multicenter study and some patients did get higher than we wanted, but we did not see any adverse effects. There was no effect on the white cell count or platelet count.

O. Nielsen: Do you think it's worthwhile putting our renal patients up to a hematocrit of 40%?

Krantz: No, I don't, I think that 33 or 35 would provide a maximum benefit to the patients with very little risk.

Scigalla: What is the incidence of the anemia in patients with RA, and is there a medical indication for treatment with EPO?

Birgegård: It varies a lot between different studies. The variation in incidence is as great as 30–70%, and it depends largely on where you draw the line for what you call anemia, severe, moderate or mild anemia. So there is no easy answer, but they very commonly have a moderate anemia at around 10.0–10.5 g/dl. It is uncommon for them to fall below 9.0 g/dl.

Bahlmann (Hannover): I wonder whether the response to EPO in your studies was influenced by the therapy necessary for the RA, especially the corticoid therapy?

Krantz: In our study the patients were not on any anti-rheumatoid drugs except the non-steroidal anti-inflammatory drugs. They were kept off corticoid drugs during the whole period and for at least 1 month beforehand.

Birgegård: In our study many patients were on a lot of cortisone and other therapy but we did not change any of the therapies during the study, so we do not have an answer to the question.

D'Andrea (Boston): Obviously, everyone who works with EPO is delighted by the fact that it is not immunogenic. That is, patients treated with rhEPO do not seem to develop antibodies. It is particularly interesting working with patients with RA or autoimmune diseases. Perhaps you should be aware of antibodies directed against EPO or even against the EPO receptor in these patients. One way we have generated monoclonal antibodies against EPO is by injecting autoimmune mice with the native hormone. I'm wondering if you are continuing to monitor the RA patients for the development of antibodies.

Krantz: We haven't seen any antibodies to EPO. I'm not sure that we are continuing to monitor that.

Birgegård: We are saving up the serum samples till the study is concluded, so we haven't analysed them yet.

Gurland HJ, Moran J, Samtleben W, Scigalla P, Wieczorek L (eds): Erythropoietin in Renal and Non-Renal Anemias. Contrib Nephrol. Basel, Karger, 1991, vol 88, pp 306–312

A Randomized, Placebo-Controlled Clinical Trial of Recombinant Human Erythropoietin in the Anemia of Prematurity[1]

William C. Mentzer[a], *Kevin M. Shannon*[a, b], *Robert I. Abels*[c], *Patricia Freeman*[a], *Nancy Newton*[a], *Dorothy Thompson*[c], *Roderic H. Phibbs*[a]

[a]Department of Pediatrics and Cardiovascular Research Institute, University of California, San Francisco, Calif.; [b]Department of Pediatrics, United States Naval Hospital, Oakland, Calif., and [c]Ortho Pharmaceutical Corporation, Raritan, N.J., USA

The normal postnatal decline in hematocrit is exaggerated in premature infants, sometimes to the extent that transfusions are required to treat symptoms of anemia. The anemia of prematurity, as this phenomenon is called, becomes apparent during the second month of life as the physiologic nadir in hemoglobin level is approached and is self-limited, disappearing as the rate of erythropoiesis increases during or after the third month of life [2]. Among the reasons for the anemia of prematurity are the lower hematocrit at birth found in premature infants, the remarkably rapid rate of somatic growth during the first few months of life requiring a concomitant expansion in red cell mass, diagnostic blood sampling necessary to manage frequent, complex, and often prolonged medical complications associated with prematurity, and a failure to produce enough erythropoietin (EPO) to stimulate erythropoiesis and arrest the decline of the hematocrit to subphysiological levels [9]. The recent availability of recombinant human EPO (rhEPO) has raised the possibility of correcting the relative EPO deficiency of premature infants in order to blunt or eliminate anemia and thus avoid exposure to red cell transfusions and their associated problems [7, 9, 14, 15]. Support for this therapeutic approach has come from in vitro studies that have demonstrated the presence of large

[1] Supported in part by grants from the R.W. Johnson Pharmaceutical Research Corporation and the National Institutes of Health (DK 32094).

numbers of the necessary erythroid progenitors in the blood and bone marrow of premature infants [10, 12]. These erythroid progenitors resemble those obtained from adults in their in vitro sensitivity to rhEPO [10, 12].

To evaluate its potential utility we conducted a randomized, placebo-controlled trial of rhEPO administration in a pilot group of small (BW < 1,200 g) premature infants [13]. The results of this trial, summarized briefly here and to be presented in full elsewhere [13], suggest that rhEPO may safely be administered to premature infants but that further investigation is needed to identify an optimal dosing strategy.

Materials and Methods

This study was reviewed and approved by the Human Experimentation Committee at the University of California San Francisco. Written consent was obtained from the parents of each infant who participated. We enrolled 10 extremely premature babies (BW < 900 g) and 10 slightly older and larger (BW 901–1250 g) infants; 5 members of each group received rhEPO and 5 the placebo. The mean birth weight was 896 g in babies who received rhEPO and 908 g in those who received the placebo (p = NS). Six of 10 infants in each group were female. Requirements for enrollment into the study in addition to a birth weight less than 1,250 g included a gestational age (at birth) ≤ 33 weeks, an age at enrollment between 10 and 35 days, and hematocrit $\leq 35\%$ on the first day of treatment. Study infants had to be on enteral feedings, have minimal requirements for respiratory support ($F_1O_2 < 0.3$, ventilator rate < 20 bpm, ventilator pressure $\leq 20/4$), and be free of seizures, congenital or acquired infections, intraventricular hemorrhage (grade I), and significant isoimmune hemolytic disease. Phlebotomy requirements for diagnostic testing could not exceed 7.5 ml/week.

rhEPO manufactured by Amgen (Thousand Oaks, Calif.) was provided to us by Ortho Pharmaceutical Co. (Raritan, N.J.). Vials of rhEPO or placebo were prepared and coded at Ortho; investigators and nursery personnel at the study site in San Francisco were unaware of the contents of vials utilized in the study until it was completed.

We gave 100 U/kg of rhEPO (or an equivalent volume of placebo) twice weekly by intravenous bolus injection for 6 weeks. An attempt was made to provide oral iron supplementation (3 mg/kg/day) to each infant; the actual amount received was often less than this due to feeding intolerance.

Blood was obtained for analyses at weekly intervals during the treatment phase and less frequently during the 6-month follow-up period. The volume of each phlebotomy was recorded. The total volume obtained for tests related to the study did not exceed 11.2 ml during the treatment phase and 11.2 ml thereafter. Complete blood counts were determined on an automated cell counter (Technicon H-1). Reticulocytes were estimated by flow cytometry [11], serum EPO by radioimmunoassay [3], and hemoglobin F either by densitometric scanning of cellulose acetate hemoglobin electrophoresis gels or by radial immunodiffusion using a commercially available system (Helena Labs). Red cell mass was estimated (using the reported average blood volume for premature infants of 76 ml/kg [8]) by multiplying body weight (kg) $\times$ hematocrit (%) $\times$ 76 (ml).

Table 1. Results of rhEPO administration during the 6-week treatment phase

	rhEPO infants	Placebo infants
Mean hematocrit, %	30.2	30.1
Mean reticulocyte count, %	170.6	156
Mean change in RBC mass, ml	+15.5	+16.8
Mean change in Hb F level, %	− 4.9	− 4.5
Mean phlebotomy, ml	22.5	20.7
Mean RBC phlebotomy, ml	6.9	6.5
Mean volume transfused, ml	23.5	26.6
Adjusted mean change in RBC mass, ml	− 0.12	+ 1.8
Mean platelet count, $\times 10^{-3}/\mu l$	401	435
Mean absolute neutrophil count, per μl	3,536	2,860

Results

Characteristics of the Population Studied

Mean values at study entry for rhEPO and placebo infants were not statistically different for weight (909 vs. 957 g), age (22.5 vs. 21.4 days), hematocrit (33.4 vs. 34.3%), reticulocyte count (84.8 vs. $87.7 \times 10^{-3}/\mu l$), serum EPO (7.7 vs. 4.4 U/ml), or hemoglobin F level (55.9 vs. 50.5%). The hemoglobin F level at entry ranged from 6.3 to 96.8% reflecting the differing prestudy transfusion history of the participants. Nineteen of 20 infants completed the treatment phase and were analyzed for the effects of the treatment regimen.

Effects of rhEPO on Erythropoiesis

Changes observed during the 6-week treatment phase are summarized in table 1. There was no difference (p = NS) between rhEPO and placebo infants in the mean hematocrit, reticulocyte count, red cell mass, or change in hemoglobin F percentage. The mean volume of blood or of red cells drawn for laboratory tests and the volume of blood transfused was comparable in the two groups, although a greater fraction (8/10) of placebo babies than of rhEPO infants received transfusions.

To evaluate the adequacy of red cell production, we corrected the raw change in red cell mass (from day 1 to day 42) for red cell losses as a result of diagnostic phlebotomy and red cell gains as a result of transfusions. The

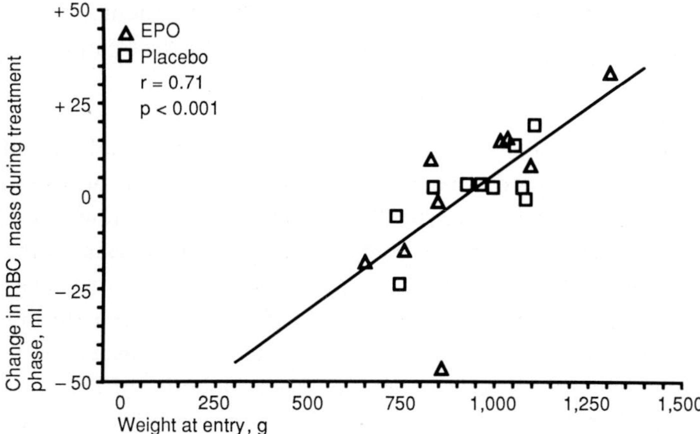

Fig. 1. Relationship between entry weight and change in RBC mass during the treatment phase.

results varied considerably depending on the entry weight of the infant (fig. 1). For each group as a whole there was virtually no change in the RBC mass and no difference between babies treated with rhEPO or placebo (table 1). However, in all babies whose entry weight was less than 800 g the red cell mass declined while in all but 1 whose entry weight was greater than 900 g it increased. A strong direct correlation was observed between entry weight and change in red cell mass (r = 0.71, p < 0.0005). There was a weaker correlation between entry weight and mean reticulocyte count (r = 0.51, p < 0.05) but the mean reticulocyte count did correlate strongly with the change in red cell mass (r = 0.71, p < 0.001). Taken together, these observations reflect a greater impairment of erythropoiesis in small premature babies, and consequently a greater need for transfusions. rhEPO had no clear influence on the change in red cell mass in either larger or small premature infants (fig. 1).

Serum EPO values rose in both rhEPO and placebo infants when remeasured at the end of the treatment period (21.4 vs. 15 U/ml, p = NS). Anti-EPO antibodies were absent at this time and subsequently during 6 further months of follow-up. Four infants received less than two-thirds of the prescribed daily doses of iron (3 rhEPO and 1 placebo). All had entry weights less than 900 g and together they comprised the entire group whose red cell masses declined by more than 6 ml during the treatment phase of the study (fig. 1). Two of 4 other infants with similar entry weights but more consistent iron supplementation were actually able to gain in RBC mass during the treatment phase.

Side Effects

No seizures or other major side effects clearly attributable to rhEPO administration were noted. One infant died of complications of necrotizing enterocolitis in the fifth week of rhEPO treatment and another, who received the placebo, developed meningitis complicated by brain abscesses at the end of the first week of the treatment phase. Mean platelet and neutrophil counts during the treatment phase did not vary significantly between rhEPO and placebo infants (table 1). An interesting direct correlation between the reticulocyte count and the platelet count was seen in both rhEPO ($r = 0.46$, $p < 0.001$) and in placebo ($r = 0.44$, $p < 0.001$) infants. Conversely, an inverse correlation between the absolute neutrophil count and the reticulocyte count was noted, again in both rhEPO ($r = 0.37$, $p < 0.01$) and placebo infants ($r = 0.46$, $p < 0.001$). Mean weight gain in rhEPO infants was 794 g and in placebo infants 913 g, reflecting an increase over day 0 weights of 85 and 95.1% respectively. When followed for a period of 6 months after the treatment phase, no differences in hematologic parameters, growth, or general well-being were noted between the rhEPO and placebo groups.

Discussion

In this initial pilot study we found that rhEPO could safely be given to very small premature infants but we failed to see any clear-cut stimulation of erythropoiesis. The dose of rhEPO was purposefully kept low to minimize potential toxicity but had been shown previously to elevate the hematocrit of adults with chronic renal failure [4].

Peak serum levels of rhEPO after intravenous injection are considerably lower in neonatal monkeys than in adults, reflecting developmental differences in pharmacokinetics [5]. If similar differences occur in humans, the dose we chose may not have reached the therapeutic range. An inadequate supply of iron may also have blunted the potential erythropoietic response. In another recently published evaluation of rhEPO therapy in larger premature infants (mean BW 1,394 g), Halperin et al. [6] found that serum iron and ferritin declined rapidly after initiation of treatment. Although we did not assess iron status directly, the 4 infants in our study who received the least iron supplementation were those with the greatest decline in red cell mass.

We believe that additional clinical trials of rhEPO in the anemia of prematurity are warranted and should explore the effect of higher doses and the relationship between the level of response and the adequacy of nutritional support with iron, vitamin E, and other nutrients. A concurrent, placebo-based control group is essential for interpretation of results since small premature infants may experience a variety of medical complications that may influence erythropoiesis independent of the effects of rhEPO. As in our initial pilot study, the focus of attention should be on infants whose gestational age is less than 30 weeks, since these infants are the most likely to require transfusion [1] and thus may benefit the most from an alternate form of treatment.

References

1   Brown, M.S.; Berman, E.R.; Luckey, D.: Prediction of the need for transfusion during anemia of prematurity. J. Pediatr. *116:* 773–778 (1990).
2   Dallmann, P.R.: Anemia of prematurity. Ann. Rev. Med. *32:* 143–160 (1981).
3   Egrie, J.C.; Cotes, P.M.; Lane, J.; Gaines Das, R.E.; Tan, R.C.; Development of radioimmunoassays for human erythropoietin using recombinant erythropoietin as tracer and immunogen. J. Immunol. Methods *99:* 235–241 (1987).
4   Eschbach, J.W.; Egrie, J.C.; Downing M.R.; Browne, J.K.; Adamson, J.W.: Correction of the anemia of end-stage renal disease with recombinant human erythropoietin. N. Engl. J. Med. *316:* 73–78 (1987).
5   George, J.W.; Bracco, C.; Shannon, K.; Phibbs, R.; Davis, J.; Smith, I.; Hendrickx, A.: Response of rhesus monkeys to recombinant human erythropoietin: comparison of adults and infants. Pediatr. Res. *25:* 269A (1989).
6   Halperin, D.S.; Wacker, P.; Lacourt, G.; Felix, M.; Babel, J.-F.; Aapro, M.; Wyss, M.: Effects of recombinant human erythropoietin in infants with anemia of prematurity: a pilot study. J. Pediatr. *116:* 779–786 (1990).
7   Mentzer, W.C.; Shannon, K.; Phibbs, R.H.: Prospects for the use of recombinant human erythropoietin in the anemia of prematurity; in Erslev, A.J.; Eschbach, J.W., Jr.; Winearls, C.G. (eds): Erythropoietin: Molecular, Cellular, and Clinical Biology (Johns Hopkins University Press, Baltimore, 1990)
8   Oski, F.A.: Normal blood values in the newborn period; in Oski, F.A.; Naiman J.L. (eds): Hematologic Problems of the Newborn; 3rd ed., pp.1–31 (Saunders, Philadelphia, 1982).
9   Phibbs, R.H.; Shannon, K.; Mentzer, W.C.: Rationale for using recombinant human erythropoietin to treat the anemia of prematurity; in Baldamus, C.A.; Scigalla, P.; Wieczorek, L.; Koch, K.M. (eds): Erythropoietin: From molecular structure to clinical application. Contrib. Nephrol., vol. 76, pp. 324–329 (Karger, Basel, 1989).
10 Rhondeau, S.M.; Christiansen, R.D.; Ross, M.P.; Rothstein, G.P.; Simmons, M.A.: Responsiveness to recombinant human erythropoietin of marrow erythroid progenitors from infants with the 'anemia of prematurity'. J. Pediatr. *112:* 935–940 (1988).

11   Sage, B.H.; O'Connell, J.P.; Mercolino, T.J.: A rapid, vital staining procedure for flow
     cytometric analysis of human reticulocytes. Cytometry *4:* 222–227 (1983).
12   Shannon, K.M.; Naylor, G.S.; Torkildson, J.C.; Clemons, G.K.; Schaffer, V.; Gold-
     man, S.L.; Lewis, K.; Phibbs, R.: Circulating erythroid progenitors in the anemia of
     prematurity. N. Engl. J. Med. *317:* 728–733 (1987).
13   Shannon, K.M.; Mentzer, W.C.; Abels, R.I.; Freeman, P.; Newton, N.; Thompson, D.;
     Sniderman, S.; Ballard, R.; Phibbs, R.H.: Recombinant human erythropoietin in the
     anemia of prematurity. Results of a placebo-controlled pilot study (submitted, 1990).
14   Shannon, K.M.: Anemia of prematurity: Progress and prospects. Am. J. Pediatr. He-
     matol. Oncol. *12:* 14–20 (1990).
15   Stockman, J.A., III: Erythropoietin: Off again, on again. J. Pediatr. *112:* 906–908 (1988).

William C. Mentzer, MD, Division of Pediatric Hematology, San Francisco General
Hospital 6J5, 1001 Potrero Avenue, San Francisco, CA 94110 (USA)

Gurland HJ, Moran J, Samtleben W, Scigalla P, Wieczorek L (eds): Erythropoietin in Renal and Non-Renal Anemias. Contrib Nephrol. Basel, Karger, 1991, vol 88, p 313

Discussion

to the Paper by W. C. Mentzer et al.

Caro (Philadelphia): I'd like to ask about the EPO levels. You showed very low EPO levels. At what level of hematocrit were those EPO levels measured? No-one found a correlation between hematocrit and EPO titers. We have measured EPO levels during gestation in humans. In babies with erythroblastosis fetalis there is a significant increase in EPO after 28 weeks of gestation. If the fetuses are under 28 weeks they don't respond to anemia; as long as they are at 28 or more weeks of gestation they have significant increases in EPO levels.

Mentzer: There is an increase in EPO levels in the first several months of life and both treated and control infants exhibited that expected general rise; EPO levels roughly tripled during the 6-week study period. There was no correlation between the serum EPO and hemoglobin levels in our small group of infants, possibly because the hemoglobin and hematocrit actually change rather quickly as a result of blood testing, as my colleagues have pointed out.

Halpérin (Geneva): We also found no correlation between the hematocrit and the EPO level.

Obladen (Berlin): You have to remember that the site of EPO production changes very dramatically during this period. EPO is no longer produced only in the liver since production slowly shifts to the kidney site.

Gurland HJ, Moran J, Samtleben W, Scigalla P, Wieczorek L (eds): Erythropoietin in
Renal and Non-Renal Anemias. Contrib Nephrol. Basel, Karger, 1991, vol 88, pp 314–326

Efficacy and Safety of Recombinant Human Erythropoietin to Prevent the Anaemias of Prematurity

European Randomized Multicenter Trial

*Michael Obladen[a], Rolf Maier[a], Hugo Segerer[a], E. Ludwig Grauel[b],
Barbara M. Holland[c], Graham Stewart[c], Gerhard Jorch[d], Heike Rabe[d],
Otwin Linderkamp[e], H. G. Hoffmann[e], Frieda Houghton[f],
Zuzana Herrmann[g], Paul Scigalla[g], Charles Wardrop[h]*

[a]Department of Neonatology, University Children's Hospital, Free University, Berlin,
FRG; [b]Department of Neonatology, Charité Children's Hospital, Humboldt
University, Berlin, GDR; [c]Department of Paediatrics, Queen Mother's Hospital,
University of Glasgow, UK; [d]University Children's Hospital, Münster, FRG;
[e]Department of Neonatology, University Children's Hospital, Heidelberg, FRG;
[f]Clinical Research Department, MCP Pharmaceuticals, Livingston, UK; [g]Boehringer
Mannheim GmbH, Mannheim, FRG; [h]Department of Haematology, University of
Wales, College of Medicine, Cardiff, UK

Anaemias are a common threat to very low birth weight infants and a
major problem in the intensive care of preterm infants. Contributing factors
include anaemia of prematurity and blood losses. The major cause of anaemia
of prematurity is an abrupt increase in oxygen availability after transition from
placental to pulmonary oxygenation with a consequent decrease in erythropoietin (EPO) production. As anaemia develops there is a diminished EPO
response to decreased oxygen availability. Additionally there is more rapid
destruction of fetal cells. Due to rapid growth between 30 and 40 weeks'
gestation there may also be haemodilution [1, 2]. Blood loss may be due to
spontaneous perinatal haemorrhage, but the most significant cause of anaemia in the first weeks of life is diagnostic sampling. The smallest preterm
infants requiring the highest level of intensive care may have their total blood
volume removed for sampling within the first 28 days of life [3]. The view has
become obsolete that anaemia is 'physiologic' in preterm infants [4]. It reduces
the amount of available oxygen [5] and contributes to apnoeic spells, mesen-
teric hypoperfusion [6], necrotizing enterocolitis, and failure to thrive [7].

Infants of less than 1,000 g birth weight requiring artificial ventilation will need frequent red cell transfusions. Therefore, they may be confronted with more than 8 donors within 28 days and thus the risk of acquiring viral infections is significant. 'Walking' donor systems, using a constant donor – preferably the infant's father – [8], do not exclude the risk of transfusion-acquired viral infections. Infants who are allowed to become anaemic may be symptomatic [9]. The best descriptors of this anaemia are red cell volume and haematocrit [10]. Infants with higher red cell volumes at birth require a shorter period of intensive care and have reduced morbidity and mortality.

Red cell volume can be manipulated by controlled placento-fetal transfusion at birth [11] or transfusion of adult red cells. Successful stimulation of the infant's own erythropoiesis will maintain red cell volume, i.e. the total amount of red cells in the circulation, thus reducing the need for red cell transfusion in the period of intensive care and prevent the anaemia of prematurity.

Recent studies have suggested that erythroid progenitors from preterm infants differentiate in response to recombinant human EPO (rhEPO) [12, 13]. rhEPO has been used successfully to stimulate erythropoiesis in more than 2,000 adults and children with anaemia due to renal failure [14, 15]. The aim of this study was to investigate whether treatment with rhEPO reduces the anaemias of prematurity and thus the need for transfusion by one third in preterm infants.

Patients, Materials and Methods

Ethical approval and informed consent was obtained by each participating centre. 171 preterm infants with gestational age of 28–32 completed weeks were admitted to the five study centres from April 1989 to February 1990. 47 infants were not eligible for study due to participation in other therapeutic trials (n = 28) or lack of parental consent (n = 19). 31 preterm infants were excluded prior to randomization for the following reasons: polycythaemia (venous haematocrit 55% or higher on 3rd day of life, regardless of cause), n = 10; congenital malformation, n = 8; haemolytic disease of the newborn, n = 3; exchange transfusion, n = 2; renal failure (urine output <30 ml/kg/24 h and/or serum creatinine >180 µmol/l on 3rd day of life), n = 2; other reasons (e.g. investigator absent), n = 6.

A total of 93 preterm infants were entered in the study. Details are shown in table 1. The study was of randomized open-controlled parallel-group design. Stratification was performed according to the need for ventilatory support on the 3rd day of life. Randomization was performed by prenumbered sealed envelopes.

EPO Treatment. rhEPO was supplied from Boehringer Mannheim GmbH in vials containing 500 U/ml in liquid preparation. A volume of 0.1 ml of the preparation was diluted with 0.9 ml 0.15 *M* NaCl and a dose of 30 U/kg was given by subcutaneous injection into the

Table 1. Randomized patients according to stratification, birth weight, and gestational age

	rhEPO n = 43	Control n = 50
Male/female, n	27/16	29/21
Birth weight, g (mean $\pm$ SD)	$1,380 \pm 324$	$1,295 \pm 323$
500– 999 g (n, vent/spont)	7/2	5/4
1,000–1,499 g (n, vent/spont)	9/11	10/17
$\geq 1,500$ g (n, vent/spont)	6/8	8/6
Gestational age, weeks (mean $\pm$ SD)	30 ± 1	30 ± 1
28 weeks, n	3	3
29 weeks, n	5	11
30 weeks, n	16	13
31 weeks, n	19	22
32 weeks, n	0	1

rhEPO = rhEPO-treated group; Control = control group; vent = artificial ventilation; spont = spontaneous breathing.

thigh every 3rd day from the 4th to the 25th day of life. Control infants were not given subcutaneous injections of placebo, but were otherwise managed identically. Iron treatment was started on day 14 with 2 mg Fe^{2+}/day orally, if there were no feeding or intestinal problems, and was given in the form of Fe(II)-chloride, Fe(II)-ascorbate or polysaccharide-iron complex.

Patient monitoring: Infants' heart rate, respiratory rate and blood pressure were recorded throughout the study. Monitoring for liver parenchymal damage and renal failure was performed on days 3, 13, and 25. Ultrasound brain scan for the detection of intraventricular haemorrhage and ophthalmoscopy for retinopathy of prematurity was carried out. During the study period, rhEPO treatment was withheld if the haematocrit rose to >50% or the haemoglobin to >17 g/dl. If these values were achieved by transfusions, and were maintained for at least 3 days after the last transfusion, rhEPO administration was discontinued until haemoglobin concentration had fallen below a value which was 3 g/dl above the level recommended as indication for transfusion (fig. 1). Moreover, the treatment was stopped if the platelet count was $>600 \times 10^9$/l, and if renal failure, hypertension or severe local reactions occurred. Patients were withdrawn from the study if they required an exchange transfusion, or medication with possible toxicity to bone marrow. Proven vertical infection and loss of parental consent were also indications for withdrawal.

Transfusion was strictly regulated as shown in figure 1. Volume of transfused red cells was determined by multiplying the total transfused volume by the haematocrit of the donor pack. Where the haematocrit of the transfused blood was unavailable the red cell volume transfused was calculated using a donor haematocrit of 70%. Transfused volume was divided

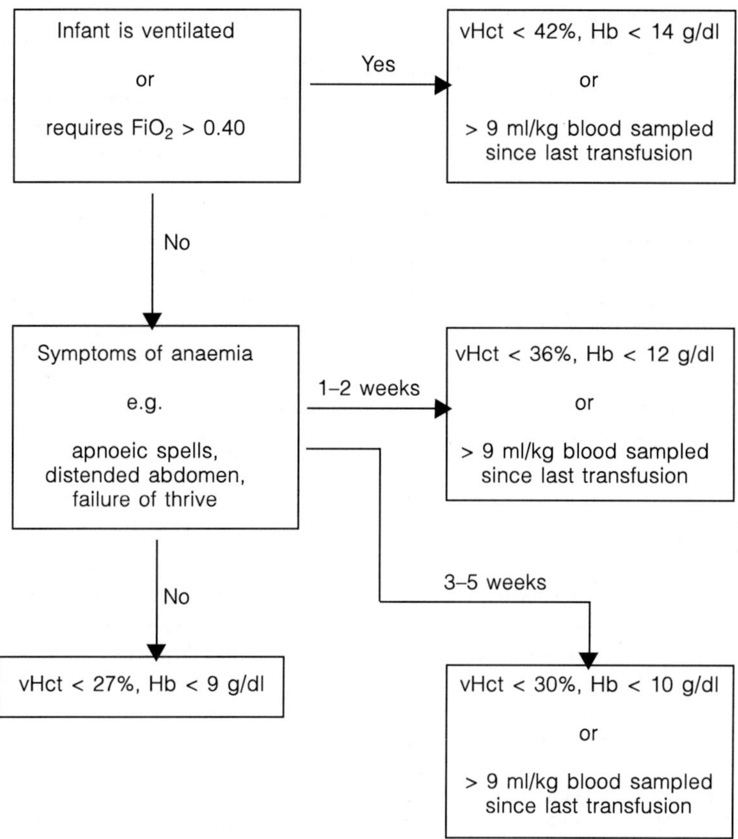

Fig. 1. Indication for transfusion of packed red cells.

by birth weight. The total volume of blood removed for diagnostic purposes during the study period was carefully recorded.

Haematological Studies. Venous haematocrit, haemoglobin and platelet counts were performed on days 3, 7, 10, 13, 19, and 25 prior to the administration of rhEPO. Reticulocyte count, serum ferritin, serum protein and serum EPO were checked on days 3, 13, and 25. The total volume of blood required for the study was 2,700 µl.

Statistical Methods. Mean values between groups were tested with the Mann-Whitney test. For categorical data the χ^2 test or Fisher's exact test were used respectively.

Table 2. Cumulated packed red cell volume transfused until day 25

	Red cells transfused, ml/kg				Number of infants with/ without transfusion	
	rhEPO		control		rhEPO	control
	mean	SD	mean	SD		
Spontaneous breathing	6.6	9.1	10.9	14.0	8/11	15/10
Artificial ventilation	21.2	21.1	22.3	25.8	15/4	14/6
All	14.1	17.8	16.5	20.8	23/15	29/16

rhEPO = rhEPO-treated group; control = control group.

Table 3. Haematologic values on day 25

	Spontaneous breathing				Artificial ventilation			
	rhEPO, n = 19		control, n = 25		rhEPO, n = 19		control, n = 20	
	mean	SD	mean	SD	mean	SD	mean	SD
Hct, %	36	8	38	5	41	6	39	7
Hb, g/dl	11.8	2.1	12.3	1.5	13.6	2.0	12.7	2.2
WBC, $\times 10^9$/l	10.2	2.0	10.3	3.3	10.6	3.8	11.2	3.1
Platelets, $\times 10^9$/l	390	149	381	165	318	179	336	162
Reticulocytes, %	5.0	6.2	3.7	4.8	7.7	14.9	2.5	2.1
Ferritin, ng/ml	163	74	170	78	252	171	201	90

rhEPO = rhEPO-treated group; control = control group.

Results

Efficacy

The cumulated volume of red cells transfused within the first 25 days is shown in table 2. A total of 31 infants (15 rhEPO, 16 control infants) did not require any transfusions. There was no significant difference between the two groups of infants. The effect of rhEPO treatment on haematological values is

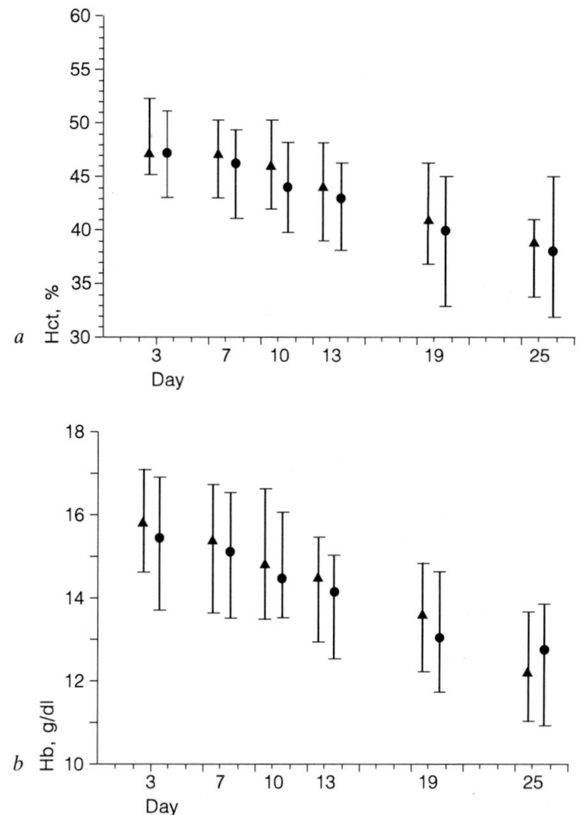

Fig. 2. Development of anaemia in preterm infants during the first 25 days of life. *a* Venous haematocrit. *b* Haemoglobin. Median ± quartiles. No difference can be observed between rhEPO-treated (●) and control infants (▲).

shown in table 3 and figures 2–4. There was no significant difference in any of the parameters among treated and nontreated, ventilated and nonventilated infants. Cumulated iron dose up to day 25 is shown in table 4. Although it was different in each centre, there were no signs of iron deficiency. Median ferritin levels on day 13 (before iron treatment was initiated) were 186 ng/ml in the rhEPO group and 189 ng/ml in the control group (NS). Ferritin levels of less than 100 ng/ml were never observed during the study period. The serum ferritin concentrations remained unchanged throughout the study (fig. 3). Total blood volume sampled for diagnostic purpose within 25 days is shown in

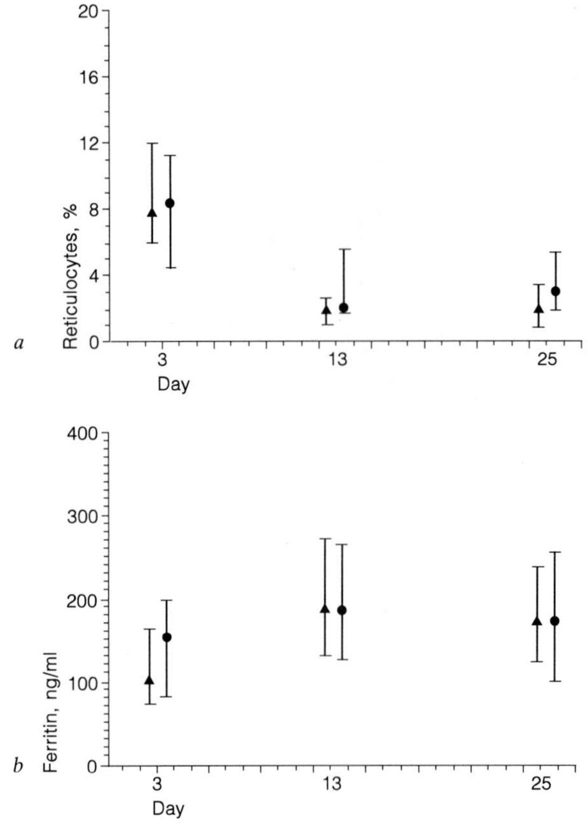

Fig. 3. Reticulocyte concentration *(a)* and serum ferritin levels *(b)* in preterm infants during the first 25 days of life. Median ± quartiles. No difference can be observed between rhEPO-treated (●) and control infants (▲).

figure 5. It is highest in the smallest infants and in each birth weight group is higher in infants requiring ventilatory support.

Safety

The study was discontinued in 10 infants as shown in table 5. No infant developed arterial hypertension (i.e. systolic blood pressure above 90 mm Hg) or suffered severe local reaction at the site of injection. The incidence of complications reported during the study is shown in table 6. No infant treated with rhEPO died. There were two deaths in the control group (one of a 610 g

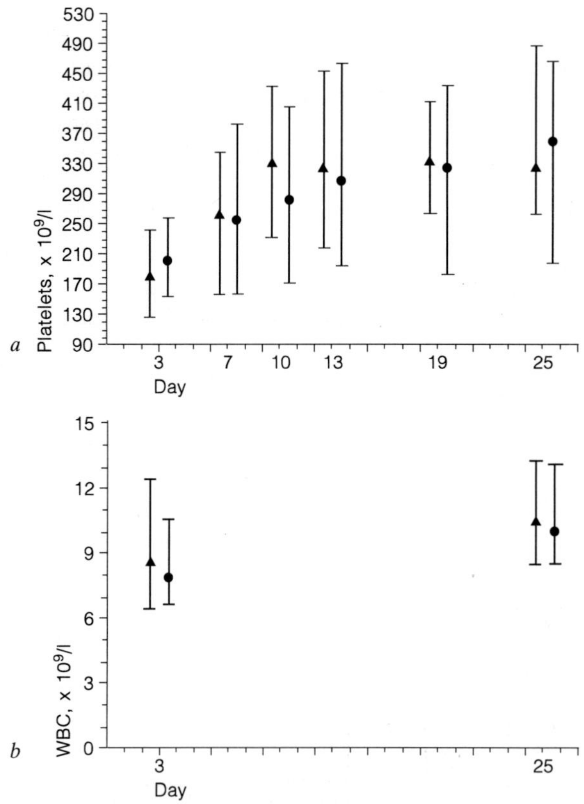

Fig. 4. a Typical rise of platelet count in preterm infants during the first 25 days of life.
b White blood cell count on days 3 and 25 in preterm infants. Median ± quartiles. No
difference can be observed between rhEPO-treated (●) and control infants (▲).

infant from necrotizing enterocolitis and one of a 1,380 g infant from hydro-
cephalus and brain atrophy).

Discussion

This study has shown that rhEPO at a subcutaneous dose of 70 U/kg/week
is safe in preterm infants. Treatment with this regimen did not affect haematocrit, haemoglobin or volume of red cells transfused per kilogram birth

Table 4. Iron administration up to day 25

	Infants without any iron, n	Infants treated with iron, n	Mean cumulated iron dose (mg) in iron-treated infants
Münster	1	18	25
Heidelberg	6	10	17
Glasgow	1	17	53
Berlin-Charité	4	6	31
Berlin-West	2	18	30
All	14	69	32

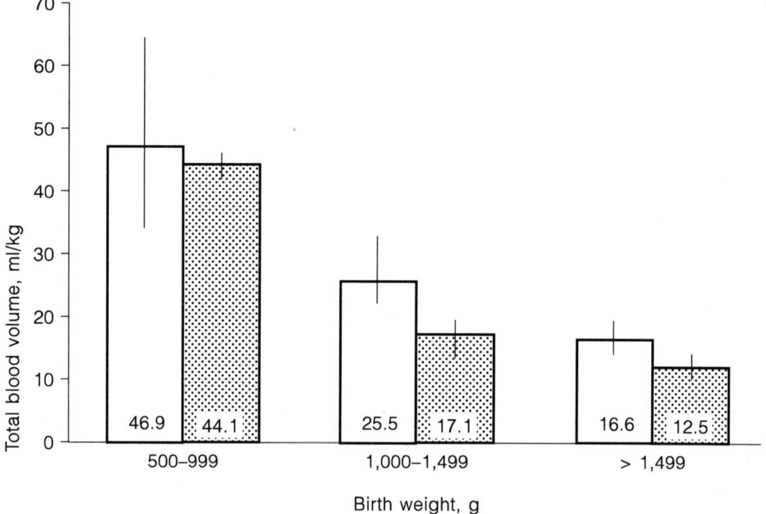

Fig. 5. Total blood volume sampled up to day 25 (ml/kg birth weight; median ± quartiles), according to birth weight and stratification. □ = Artificial ventilation; ▨ = spontaneous breathing.

weight. Although reticulocyte counts in infants receiving rhEPO were slightly higher than in the control infants at days 13 and 25, this failed to reach statistical significance. The expected fall in serum ferritin concentration did not occur, confirming that rhEPO given to preterm infants at this dose was not effective. Shannon et al. [16] in a double-blind placebo-controlled study administering 100 U/kg twice weekly to treat the anaemia of prematurity also

Table 5. Major reasons for discontinuation of the study in 10 infants, explaining the total number of 83 infants in tables 2–4 (only one reason is indicated per infant)

Stop rule	rhEPO	Control
Death	0	1
Hct >50%, Hb >17 g/dl	3	0
Platelets >600 × 10^3/l	1	0
Renal failure	0	1
Exchange transfusion	0	1
Consent withdrawal	1	1
Others (transfer)	0	1
All	5	5

rhEPO = rhEPO-treated group; control = control group.

Table 6. Incidence of complicating disorders of prematurity, independent of discontinuation of the trial

Complications	rhEPO (n = 43)	Control (n = 50)
Necrotizing enterocolitis	1	3
Patent ductus arteriosus	1	3
Intraventricular haemorrhage	5	5
Bronchopulmonary dysplasia	6	5
All complicating disorders	13	16

rhEPO = rhEPO-treated group; control = control group.

failed to show a response. This failure to demonstrate a haemopoietic response may be due to inadequate dosage, suboptimal nutrition including iron deficiency, inflammation, infection, or the requirement for other growth factors.

Premature infants may generally require larger doses of rhEPO than older children and adults: in an animal study using rhesus monkeys, George et al. [17] found that rhEPO doses of 100 or 250 U/kg, applied twice weekly, produced significant increases in haemoglobin in adults, but no change in newborn animals. Oster et al. [18] used doses of 300–600 U/kg/week to prevent chemotherapy-induced anaemia, Niemeyer [19] has used doses of up to 2,000 U/kg daily in an attempt to treat Blackfan-Diamond disease. EPO has been used in a dose of 1,200 U/kg/week to increase preoperative collection of autologous blood [20]. Halpérin et al. [21] in a recent uncontrolled pilot study reported an increase in reticulocytes and stabilization of haematocrit in preterm infants treated with higher doses (up to 300 U/kg/week) of EPO. However, since the EPO treatment was started after the 3rd week of life, the infants were slightly more mature; therefore, Halpérin's study was different from ours not only in terms of EPO dosage. It cannot be excluded that the positive response was due to a normal development of reticulocytes and haematocrit at this age.

Ohls et al. [22] studied the erythroid 'burst-promoting' activity in the serum of patients with the anaemia of prematurity. Burst-promoting activity was similar to that found in adult blood and cord sera. Their findings indicate that the anaemia of prematurity like the anaemia of end-stage renal disease is associated with a specific deficiency of EPO.

The erythropoietic potential of a fetus gaining weight from 1 to 3 kg is 90 ml red cells. If this potential is to be realized, maintenance of nutritional status, especially with regard to haematopoiesis, will be important. Achievement of optimal erythropoiesis should reduce the requirement for donor transfusion whilst maintaining blood volume for optimal oxygen delivery and tissue perfusion. Maintenance of this physiological state of the blood is also likely to minimize the complications of preterm delivery, especially those related to inadequate oxygenation and perfusion by the blood such as prolonged dependence on respiratory support [7]. For these reasons we believe that controlled studies with higher doses of rhEPO are now indicated in preterm infants.

References

1   Brown, M.S.; Garcia, J.F.; Phibbs, R.H.; Dallmann, P.R.: Decreased response of plasma immunoreactive erythropoietin to 'available oxygen' in anemia of prematurity. J. Pediatr. *105:* 793–798 (1984).
2   Dallmann, P.R.: Anemia of prematurity. Annu. Rev. Med. *32:* 143–160 (1981).
3   Obladen, M.; Sachsenweger, M.; Stahnke, M.: Blood sampling in very low birth weight infants receiving different levels of intensive care. Eur. J. Pediatr. *147:* 399–404 (1988).

4   Wardrop, C. A. J.; Holland, B. M.; Veale, K. E. A.; Jones, J. G.; Gray, O. P.: Nonphysi-ological anemia of prematurity. Arch. Dis. Child. *53:* 855–860 (1978).

5   Jones, J. G.; Holland, B. M.; Veale, R. E. A.; Wardrop, G. A. J.: 'Available oxygen', a realistic expression of the ability of the blood to supply oxygen to tissues. Scand. J. Haematol. *22:* 77–82 (1979).

6   Szabo, J. S.; Stonestreet, B.; Oh, W.: Effects of hypoxemia on gastrointestinal blood flow and gastric emptying in the newborn piglet. Pediatr. Res. *19:* 466–471 (1985).

7   Stockman, J. A.; Clark, D. A.; Levin, E. A.: Weight gain – response to transfusion in preterm infants. Pediatr. Res. *14:* 612 (1980).

8   Buchmann, S.; Kewitz, G.; Eckstein, R.; Obladen, M.: Blood donation from parents may limit risk of infection in preterm infants. Klin. Pädiatr. *2:* 148 (1988).

9   Stockman, J. A.: Anemia of prematurity. Current concepts in the issue of when to transfuse. Pediatr. Clin. North Am. *33:* 111–128 (1986).

10   Jones, J. G.; Holland, B. M.; Hudson, J. R. B.; Wardrop, C. A. J.: Total circulating red cells versus haematocrit as the primary descriptor of oxygen transport by the blood. Br. J. Haematol. (in press).

11   Kimmond, S.; Hudson, I. R. B.; Aitchison, T.; Holland, B. M.; Turner, T. L.; Jones, J. G.; Wardrop, C. A. J.: Placento-foetal transfusion in preterm infants. Early human development (in press).

12   Rhondeau, S. M.; Christensen, R. D.; Ross, M. P.; Rothstein, G.; Simmons, M. A.: Responsiveness to recombinant human erythropoietin of marrow erythroid progenitors from infants with 'anemia of prematurity'. J. Pediatr. *112:* 935–940 (1988).

13   Shannon, K. M.; Naylor, G. S.; Torkildson, J. C.; Clemons, G. K.; Schaffner, V.; Gold-man, S. L.; Lewis, K.; Bryant, P.; Phibbs, R.: Circulating erythroid progenitors in the anemia of prematurity. N. Engl. J. Med. *317:* 728–733 (1987).

14   Koch, K. M.; Kühn, K.; Nonnast-Daniel, B.; Scigalla, P. (eds): Treatment of Renal Anaemia with Recombinant Human Erythropoietin (Karger, Basel 1988).

15   Winearls, C. R.; Peppard, M. J.; Downing, M. R., et al.: Effect of human erythropoietin derived from recombinant DNA on the anemia of patients maintained by chronic haemodialysis. Lancet *ii:* 1175 (1986).

16   Shannon, K. M.; Mentzer, W. C.; Abels, R. I.; Freeman, P.; Newton, N.; Thompson, D.; Sniderman, S.; Ballard, R.; Phibbs, R. H.: Recombinant human erythropoietin (rhEPO) in anemia of prematurity (AOP): Preliminary results of a double-blind place-bo-controlled pilot study. Pediatr. Res. *27:* 269A (1990).

17   George, J. W.; Bracco, C.; Shannin, K.; Phibbs, R.; Davis, J.; Smith, J.; Hendrickx, A.: Response of rhesus monkeys to recombinant human erythropoietin. Comparison of adults and infants. Pediatr. Res. *25:* 269A (1989).

18   Oster, W.; Hermann, F.; Cicco, A.; Gamm, H.; Zeile, G.; Kolbe, K.; Lindemann, A.; Brune, T.; Schulz, G.; Mertelsmann, R.: Erythropoietin prevents chemotherapy-in-duced anaemia. Blut *59:* 341A (1989).

19   Niemeyer, C.: Blackfan-Diamond Disease. Third International Workshop on Treat-ment of Anemia with Recombinant Human Erythropoietin, Telfs, 1990.

20   Goodnough, L. T.; Rudnick, S.; Price, T. H.; Ballas, S. K.; Collins, M. L.; Crowley, J. P.; Kosmin, M.; Kruskall, M. S.; Lenes, B. A.; Menitove, J. E.; Silberstein, L. E.; Smith, K. J.; Wallas, C. H.; Abels, R.; Von Tress, M.: Increased preoperative collection of autologous blood with recombinant human erythropoietin therapy. N. Engl. Med. *321:* 1163–1168 (1989).

21 Halpérin, D. S.; Wacker, P.; Lacourt, G.; Felix, M.; Babel, J. F.; Aapro, M.; Wyss, M.: Effects of recombinant human erythropoietin in infants with the anaemia of prematurity: A pilot study. J. Pediatr. *116:* 779–786 (1990).

22 Ohls, R.; Liechty, K. W.; Turner, M. C.; Kimura, R. F.; Christensen, R. D.: Erythroid 'burst-promoting' activity in serum of patients with anaemia of prematurity. J. Pediatr. *116:* 786–789 (1990).

Prof. Dr. M. Obladen, University Children's Hospital, Free University, Department of Neonatology, Heubnerweg 4, D–1000 Berlin 19 (FRG)

Gurland HJ, Moran J, Samtleben W, Scigalla P, Wieczorek L (eds): Erythropoietin in Renal and Non-Renal Anemias. Contrib Nephrol. Basel, Karger, 1991, vol 88, pp 327–333

Increasing Autologous Blood Donation with Recombinant Human Erythropoietin

Edward A. Levine

Department of Surgery, Michael Reese Hospital and Medical Center,
Chicago, Ill., USA

The real and perceived risks of homologous blood administration have forced a reassessment of transfusion practice [1]. The screening of blood for infectious agents should make homologous transfusion safer [2]. However, it seems clear that the risk of infectious disease related to transfusion will never be nonexistent [3].

In patients undergoing surgical procedures, homologous red blood cell transfusions may be particularly hazardous. Blood transfusions have been shown to be immunosuppressive in a variety of laboratory [4, 5] and clinical settings [6, 7]. The immunosuppressive effects of transfusion have been shown, in retrospective analyses, to increase the incidence of perioperative septic complications [8, 9], burn sepsis [10], multisystem organ failure [11], as well as increased recurrence rates following resections of sarcomas [12] and carcinomas [13–15]. Therefore it is clear that avoidance of homologous blood exposure seems to be of particular importance to surgical patients.

The best alternative to homologous blood, with its attendant risks, is autologous blood [16]. Autologous blood for surgery can be made available by preoperative donation [17] or intraoperative salvage techniques [18]. Autologous blood can also be made available in the postoperative period by accelerated endogenous erythropoiesis [19, 20].

While accelerating erythropoiesis is not a new idea, it was not until recombinant human erythropoietin (rhEPO) became available in large quantities [21] that it became a serious possibility. Acceleration of erythropoiesis is an attractive alternative to the risks of homologous exposure. By accelerating erythropoiesis, rhEPO may make more autologous blood available. The purpose of this paper is to evaluate the utility of rhEPO in surgical patients who donate autologous blood preoperatively.

Discussion

Autologous blood donation prior to elective surgery has been widely endorsed as a safe and effective method of avoiding perioperative homologous blood exposure [16, 22, 23]. However, despite the advantages of perioperative autologous donation, these programs remain seriously underutilized [24]. Further, perioperative autologous blood donation programs require 2–5 weeks to complete and the average yield is only 2.2 units/patient [17]. This represents only 59% of the blood ordered by the referring surgeon and up to 34.5% of these patients still required homologous transfusion perioperatively [16, 25]. Increasing the autologous blood donor's erythropoietic rate with rhEPO could theoretically increase the yield and decrease the time required to complete preoperative blood donation.

The first study to evaluate the possible role of rhEPO in autologous blood donation appeared in *Surgery* in 1988 [26]. In that study, 12 baboons were randomized into two groups. The animals entered a model of an autologous blood donation program. Animals were studies thrice weekly for a 5-week period. If on any study day the hematocrit was >30%, a unit of blood (200 ml) was withdrawn. The animals then received either 750 units/kg of rhEPO or placebo on each study day. In addition, after each donation, iron dextran was given intravenously to replace 150% of shed iron.

The rhEPO group consistently donated more blood than the control group (fig. 1). The difference in the number of units donated became significant on day 11 (5.5 vs. 4.3 units, p<0.05) and remained significant thereafter. By the end of the 5-week protocol, the group given rhEPO had donated 3.5 units more than the control group (13.5 vs. 10.0 units). The percent increase in donation for the rhEPO group remained similar (28–35%) from weeks 2 to 5.

The hematocrit values of both groups fell during the first week of the protocol (3% per unit drawn) (fig. 2). The rhEPO group tended to have higher hematocrit values than the control group. The rhEPO group had a higher mean hematocrit on 13 of 15 study days (p = 0.007, sign test).

The results of this study show that rhEPO increased the yield of an aggressive autologous blood program by 35%. The substantial yield of blood by the control group suggests that an aggressive schedule of autologous blood donation should increase yields over present programs. The American Association of Blood Banks recommends a minimum hematocrit value of 34% for autologous donations which are commonly scheduled 7 days apart [27]. This necessitates delaying surgical procedures up to 5 weeks to meet the expected

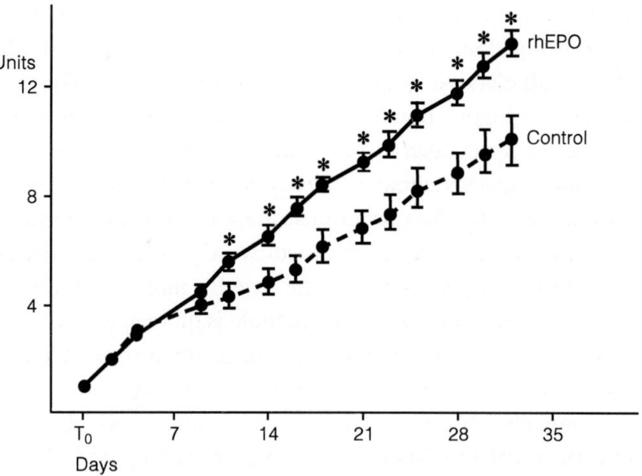

Fig. 1. Total number of donations, in units ± SEM, versus study day. Asterisks, difference between groups significant at $p < 0.05$ level.

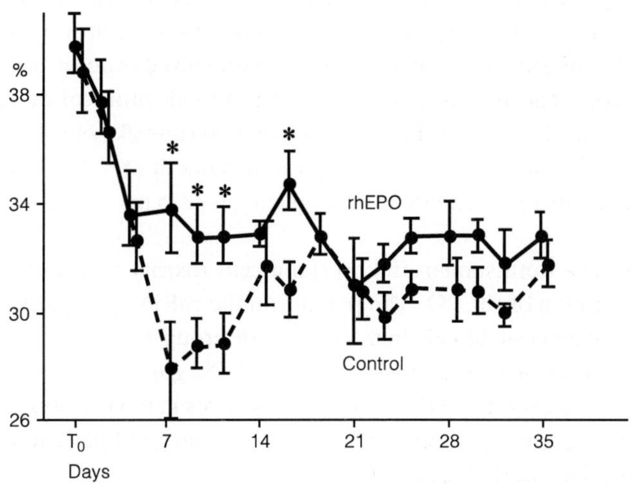

Fig. 2. Hematocrit % ± SEM versus study day. The rhEPO group had a higher hematocrit than the control group on 13 of 15 study days ($p = 0.007$). Asterisks, difference between groups significant at $p < 0.05$ level.

operative requirements for autologous blood. During the first 14 days of this trial, the rhEPO group donated an average of 6.5 units of blood which is sufficient for nearly all elective surgical elective surgical cases. This suggests than an aggressive autologous donation schedule with supplemental rhEPO could minimize the delay necessary to fill autologous blood orders.

While this study suggests clinical efficacy for rhEPO as an adjuvant in preoperative autologous donation programs, there are several questions that must be raised. First, animals in this protocol were healthy, unstressed and given iron parenterally which may not be the case for most autologous blood donors. Further, the autologous donation schedule is quite aggressive by most standards. Therefore, while this animal study suggested possible clinical efficacy, it remained for clinical trials to truly evaluate efficacy.

A small uncontrolled trial was recently published, in which 5 patients received 6,000 units of rhEPO thrice weekly and were compared to a control group of 7 patients [28]. These patients received oral iron supplementation during a 17-day autologous blood donation protocol. This study showed that after the third donation the hemoglobin was significantly higher in the rhEPO-treated patients (12.7 vs. 10.6 g/dl, $p<0.001$). This small study suggests that significant increases in preoperative hematocrit may be attainable with the administration of small doses of rhEPO during autologous donation.

A multicenter, prospective, randomized, placebo-controlled trial of rhEPO in autologous blood donors was published in the *New England Journal of Medicine* in October 1989 [29]. In this study, 47 otherwise healthy patients, scheduled for elective orthopedic surgery, were randomized to receive either rhEPO or placebo. The patients then entered a 3-week protocol of twice weekly donations at which time they received either 600 units/kg of rhEPO or placebo. Donation of blood was excluded for a hematocrit of $<34\%$ on any study day. All patients received oral iron supplements (325 mg of iron sulfate thrice daily).

The two groups were similar and no significant toxicity was associated with the administration of rhEPO. The patients in the rhEPO group donated significantly more units of blood than the control group (5.4 vs. 4.1 units, $p<0.05$). Further, only 1 of the 23 patients in the rhEPO groups was unable to donate at least 4 units as compared to 7 of the 24 patients in the placebo group (table 1). Perioperatively, 2 patients in the placebo group and 1 patient in the rhEPO group received homologous transfusions.

The hematocrits of patients in the rhEPO group were significantly higher after the third visit and remained so for the duration of the study. The control group had a larger decline in hematocrit from baseline (-8.8 vs. -5.5%,

Table 1. Total number of units donated by patients receiving rhEPO or placebo [28]

Group	Units donated					
	1	2	3	4	5	6
Placebo	0	1	6	9	5	3
rhEPO	0	0	1	3	4	15

$p < 0.05$) which correlated with a lower admitting hematocrit (35.2 vs. 38.6%, $p < 0.05$).

This study clearly shows that the increased erythropoiesis stimulated by rhEPO increased the ability of healthy patients to donate autologous blood. Further, this study corroborates the amelioration of anemia associated with preoperative donation [28], and parallelled the findings in the primate study [26].

The goal of preoperative donation is the avoidance of perioperative homologous exposure, not simply the amelioration of anemia. This study did not show a significant difference in homologous blood exposure. The most obvious reason is the average of 4.1 units of blood donated by the control group. This yield of autologous blood is clearly better than that commonly achieved [17, 24]. While intuitively, the greater the amount of autologous blood deposited, the less likely homologous exposure should be, proving it on a statistical basis would require the randomization of many more patients.

Summary and Conclusion

The ability of rhEPO to stimulate endogenous erythropoiesis makes it an attractive alternative to the risks of homologous exposure. The ability of rhEPO to increase the yields of preoperative autologous blood donation programs is clear. However, the amount of autologous blood that can be donated by otherwise healthy surgical patients makes the increase in donations achievable with rhEPO relatively small. This suggests that administration of rhEPO to autologous donors should be limited to selected indications. Patients who will need large amounts of blood (>3 units), have a limited time available for donation preoperatively, or who are anemic preoperatively, are most likely to benefit from rhEPO administration during preoperative donation. The addition of rhEPO to autologous donation programs may decrease the need for homologous transfusion in patients that would otherwise be poor candidates for these programs.

References

1   Zuck TF: Transfusion-transmitted AIDS reassessed. N Engl J Med 1988;318:511–512.

2   Bove JR: Transfusion-associated hepatitis and AIDS. N Engl J Med 1987;317:242–245.

3   Ward JW, Holmsberg SD, Allen JR, et al: Transmission of human immunodeficiency virus (HIV) by blood transfusions screened as negative for HIV antibody. N Engl J Med 1988;310:473–478.

4   Waymack JP, Chance WT: Effect of blood transfusions on immune function. IV. Effect on tumor growth. J Surg Oncol 1988;39:159–164.

5   Waymack JP, Yurt RW: The effect of blood transfusions on immune function. J Surg Res 1990;48:147–153.

6   Blumberg N, Heal JM: Transfusion and recipient immune functions. Arch Pathol Lab Med 1989;113:246–253.

7   Opelz G, Terasaki PI: Improvement in kidney graft survival with increased numbers of blood transfusions. N Engl J Med 1978;299:799–803.

8   Tartter PI, Quintero S, Barron DM: Perioperative blood transfusion associated with infectious complications after colorectal cancer operations. Am J Surg 1986;152: 479–482.

9   Tartter PI, Driefuss RM, Malon AM, et al: Relationship of postoperative septic complications and blood transfusions in patients with Crohn's disease. Am J Surg 1988;155:43–48.

10 Graves TA, Cioffi WG, Mason AD, et al: Relationship of transfusion and infection in a burn population. J Trauma 1989;29:948–954.

11 Maetani S, Nishikawa T, Hirakawa A, Tobe T: Role of blood transfusion in organ system failure following major abdominal surgery. Ann Surg 1986;203:275–281.

12 Rosenberg SA, Seipp CA, White DE, Wesley R: Perioperative blood transfusions are associated with increased rates of recurrence and decreased survival in patients with high grade soft tissue sarcomas of the extremities. J Clin Oncol 1985;3:693–709.

13 Blumberg N, Heal J, Chuang C, et al: Further evidence supporting a cause-and-effect relationship between blood transfusion and earlier cancer recurrence. Ann Surg 1988;207:410–415.

14 Stephenson KR, Steinberg SM, Hughes KS, et al: Perioperative blood transfusions are associated with decreased time to recurrence and decreased survival after resection of colorectal liver metastases. Ann Surg 1988;208:679–687.

15 Crowe JP, Gordon NH, Fry DE, et al: Breast cancer survival and perioperative blood transfusion. Surgery 1989;106:836–841.

16 Surgenor DM: The patient's own blood is the safest blood. N Engl J Med 1987;316: 542–544.

17 Toy PTCY, Straus RG, Stehling LC, et al: Predeposited autologous blood for elective surgery. N Engl J Med 1987;316:517–520.

18 Popovsky MA, Devine PA, Taswell HF: Intraoperative autologous transfusion. Mayo Clin Proc 1985;60:125–134.
19 Dudrick SJ, O'Donnell JJ, Matheny RG, et al: Stimulation of hematopoiesis as an alternative to transfusion. South Med J 1986;79:669–673.
20 Levine EA, Gould SA, Rosen AR, et al: Perioperative recombinant human erythro-poietin. Surgery 1989;106:932–938.
21 Lin F, Suggs S, Lin C, et al: Cloning and expression of the human erythropoietin gene. Proc Natl Acad Sci USA 1985;82:7580–7584.
22 Mintz PD: Autologous transfusion endorsed. JAMA 1985;254:507–508.
23 Perioperative red blood cell transfusion. JAMA 1988;260:2700–2703.
24 Toy PT, Stehling LC, Strauss RG, et al: Underutilization of autologous blood donation eligible elective surgical patients. Am J Surg 1986;152:483–486.
25 Kruskall MS, Glazer EE, Leonhard SS, et al: Utilization and effectiveness of a hospital autologous preoperative blood donor program. Transfusion 1986;26:335–340.
26 Levine EA, Rosen AL, Gould SA, et al: Recombinant human erythropoietin and autologous blood donation. Surgery 1988;104:365–369.
27 Council on Scientific Affairs. JAMA 1988;256:2378–2380.
28 Maeda H, Hitomi Y, Hirata R, et al: Erythropoietin and autologous blood donation. Lancet 1989;334:284.
29 Goodnough LT, Rudnick S, Price TH, et al: Increased preoperative collection of autologous blood with recombinant human erythropoietin therapy. N Engl J Med 1989;321:163–168.

Edward A. Levine, MD, Department of Surgery, Michael Reese Hospital and Medical Center, Lake Shore Drive at 31st Street, Chicago, IL 60616 (USA)

Gurland HJ, Moran J, Samtleben W, Scigalla P, Wieczorek L (eds): Erythropoietin in
Renal and Non-Renal Anemias. Contrib Nephrol. Basel, Karger, 1991, vol 88, pp 334–348

The Role of Recombinant Human Erythropoietin in Homologous Transfusion Avoidance

Joseph T. Sobota[1]

Chugai-Upjohn, Inc., Rosemont, Ill., and Northwestern University Medical School,
Chicago, Ill., USA

Transfusion of red blood cells, by itself, is not a curative therapy but does replace red cells lost by disease mechanisms, trauma, surgery or coagulation disorders. An increasing number of surgical procedures and a medical and public perception of transfusions as safe and unavoidably necessary resulted in an upward trend in the number of transfusions documented by progressively increased requirements placed on transfusion services throughout the world [1]. The lethal nature of AIDS transmission via red cell transfusions has generated a complete rethinking of homologous transfusion benefits and risks. There is no documented improvement of wound healing, accelerated convalescence or infection defense derived from red cell transfusions. Evidence continues to mount that transfusions of homologous blood can induce immunosuppression which impairs host resistance in patients [2, 3]. Despite the heightened sensitivity to the risks of red blood cell transfusions, the procedure remains a life-saving measure and homologous transfusions will continue to permit surgical procedures that otherwise would be impossible for many patients who may need them because of a variety of reasons. The challenge to surgeons, anesthesiologists, blood bank professionals and public health authorities is to devise safe and effective strategies, procedures and therapies which minimize the necessity and therefore the risk of a homologous transfusion.

[1] I wish to thank S. Bosi for her expert transcription, slide preparation and corrections to the manuscript, B. Solomon for the reference research, and S. Shroads and K. Andow for assistance in the preparation of the figures.

Table 1. Present alternatives to homologous transfusions

Method	Capacity	Contraindications
Preoperative donations	3–4 units	bacteremia, anemia, angina, aortic stenosis
Acute hemodilution	1–2 units	vasovagal reactions, intolerance to rapid blood withdrawal
Intraoperative blood salvage	dependent on blood loss at surgery	infection, tumor, dilutional coagulopathy, DIC, renal failure

A number of alternatives to homologous blood transfusions have been explored in the past several years and are based on the precept that the patient's own blood is the safest for transfusion [4]. These strategies include: (1) predeposit autologous blood transfusion; (2) hemodilution, and (3) cell salvage. Predeposit autologous transfusion is the presurgical collection and perioperative reinfusion of the patient's own blood. Preoperative hemodilution and autotransfusion is a procedure usually done immediately before or after the induction of anesthesia with a simultaneous infusion of a crystalloid or colloid solution in order to maintain normovolemia [5]. Perioperative blood salvage is the collection and reinfusion of blood shed from a wound or body cavity during and after surgery. Blood is collected from the patient and then reinfused directly as whole blood or infused as washed red blood cells. Table 1 notes the contraindications and general capacity in units of each method except intraoperative blood salvage which depends on actual blood loss.

Recombinant human erythropoietin (rhEPO) has been shown to increase erythropoiesis [6, 7]. A short supply of the hormone was the major obstacle to the conduct of clinical studies of rhEPO effectiveness in a number of medical and surgical indications. With the purification of the human EPO from urine by Miyake et al. [8] in 1977 and the cloning of the complementary DNA EPO in 1985 by Jacobs et al. [9], it was possible to engineer active glycosylated rhEPO in sufficient quantities for clinical trials. rhEPO preparations have regulatory approval for the treatment of anemia secondary to chronic renal failure (dialysis) in Western Europe, Japan and the United States with a number of other indications being explored including its potential role in homologous transfusion avoidance.

Background and Rationale for rhEPO Use in
Homologous Transfusion Avoidance

rhEPO accelerates endogenous erythropoiesis to increase red cell recovery following acute blood loss. It is generally recognized that EPO is the primary regulator of red cell formation and its major source in adults is the kidneys. EPO of renal origin has been characterized as a glycoprotein containing 165 amino acids with a molecular weight of approximately 30,000 daltons. A large portion (about 40%) of the molecule consists of carbohydrate. The main action of EPO is to stimulate the differentiation of erythroid progenitor cells in the bone marrow into functional erythroblasts. The subsequent maturation requires 5–9 days under normal physiologic conditions.

One of the first reports on the clinical use of rhEPO was in patients with anemia, due to end-stage renal disease [10]. This report demonstrated that intravenous doses of rhEPO between 15 and 500 IU/kg resulted in an increase in hematocrit during periods of therapy of up to 20 weeks. Increases in hematocrits of 30% above the patient's baseline were associated with the development of iron deficiency as a result of increased erythrocyte production, an increase in azotemia and increased risk of hyperkalemia. Iron deficiency is the most consistent side effect of rhEPO treatment irrespective of condition treated.

Over 2,500 North American and Japanese patients have been studied on rhEPO anemia secondary to chronic renal failure investigational protocols [11]. The commercial availability of rhEPO has placed the compound in the hands of practitioners and in the service of thousands of additional patients. rhEPO produces a dose-dependent stimulation of erythropoiesis. Single doses have been given up to 3,600 IU/kg in Japan and up to 1,000 IU/kg in the United States. Doses of rhEPO of 150 IU/kg or higher induced a dose-related increase in the group mean reticulocyte count when compared to baseline values 2–3 days postdose [Chugai-Upjohn, Inc., data on file].

Kickler and Spivak [12] explored the effect of repeated whole blood donations on serum-immunoreactive EPO levels in 69 autologous blood donors. At the time of the initial phlebotomy, 33% of the men and 6% of the women were anemic as defined by a hematocrit of less than 41% for men and 36% for women. In the course of the blood donations, anemia developed in an additional 71% of men and 45% of women. Although there was an increase in the level of serum-immunoreactive EPO with successive phlebotomies, the increase was not substantially out of the normal range. Since iron deficiency was ruled out, the authors concluded that within the hematocrit range recommended for autologous blood donation, the degree of anemia experienced is insufficient to initiate an adequate increase in EPO production. Mild anemia develops in autologous blood donors in the majority of circumstances and in many instances the volume of blood that can be donated is inadequate to meet their operative needs.

Since rhEPO was active in baboons [13], additional baboon studies were begun to determine the effects of rhEPO on an aggressive autologous donation program. Levine et al. [14] studied 12 adult male baboons which were randomized into two groups of 6 and studied 3 times per week for 5 weeks. A unit of blood was donated by the animals when on any study day the hematocrit was greater than 30%. One group of animals received 750 IU/kg of rhEPO and the other group received placebo on each study day. Iron dextran was given intravenously to replace 150% of shed iron. The rhEPO-treated animal group had an earlier onset of reticulocytosis (2.7 vs. 5.5 days) and donated 35% more blood (13.5% vs. 10.0 units) than the control group. No adverse reactions to rhEPO were observed.

To evaluate the effect of rhEPO on acute postoperative anemia [15], 11 adult male baboons were randomized into two groups, all of which underwent a laparotomy and an exchange transfusion with 6% hetastarch to a hematocrit of 15%. Six of the animals received 1,000 IU/kg of rhEPO each day for the first 14 postoperative days. The second group of animals received an equivalent volume of placebo. While hematocrits were similar between groups at the baseline and after exchange transfusion, the maximal rate of erythropoiesis was significantly faster in the rhEPO group (2.1 vs. 1.3%/day) and the time required to return to hematocrits of 30% was 9.9 days for the rhEPO group versus 17.4 days for the placebo-treated control (table 2, Study 1).

In an extension of that experiment, in addition to postoperative doses of rhEPO, another group of animals received five daily preoperative doses of 1,000 IU/kg rhEPO [16]. The time and days required to recover to hematocrits of 20% was significantly shorter in the pre- and postoperatively treated groups when compared to that of controls (3.3 vs. 5.7 days). Thus, in the baboon model, both perioperative and postoperative use of rhEPO significantly accelerates postoperative erythropoiesis (table 2, Study 2). The availability of rhEPO, the insufficient EPO response levels in humans donating autologous transfusions and the animal study results indicating an increased ability to supply additional predeposit units and accelerate erythropoiesis pre- and postoperatively set the stage for human studies using rhEPO in an effort to avoid homologous transfusions and their attendant risks.

Table 2. Recovery time to specific hematocrits: baboon animal studies

	Hematocrits			
	20%	25%	30%	baseline
Study 1[a]				
rhEPO (1,000 IU/kg × 14 postop. days)	5.7	7.7	9.9	11.9
Control	5.7	8.9	17.4	32.1
p	–	<0.08	<0.001	<0.01
Study 2[b]				
rhEPO (1,000 IU/kg × 5 pre-op. days)	3.3[c]	7.6	12.4	25.7
rhEPO (1,000 IU/kg × 5 pre-op. and				
14 postop. days)	3.2[c]	5.8	8.0[c]	12.6[c]
Control	5.7	8.8	17.7	28.2

[a] Data from Levine et al. [15].
[b] Data from Levine et al. [16].
[c] Recovery time significantly shorter than control (p<0.01).

Human Use of rhEPO in the Preoperative Collection of Autologous Blood

Phase I rhEPO safety studies indicated that doses of 1,000 IU/kg were well tolerated while renal anemia studies showed the effective erythropoiesis stimulation by rhEPO in humans [11]. These studies gave impetus to investigations to determine if rhEPO would enhance elective presurgical patient's donation of autologous blood.

A two-center, double-blind, parallel-group study was done in which 39 healthy male subjects were randomized equally to receive either 250, 500 or 1,000 IU/kg of rhEPO or placebo on study days 1, 4 and 7. The subjects were phlebotomized of 450 ml whole blood before dosing on days 1 and 4. Results of that study reported by Vlasses et al. [17] show that the three doses of rhEPO increased the reticulocyte count in an apparent dose-response relationship. Serial mean hemoglobin values determined as the change from baseline are seen in table 3. The median number of days required for hemoglobin to return to 95% of baseline values were approximately 50, 22, 36 and 8 days for the placebo, 250, 500 and 1,000 IU/kg treatment groups, respectively (table 4).

Table 3. Mean hemoglobin (g/dl) changes: baseline after 450 ml phlebotomy on days 1 and 4

Dose	n	Day 8	Day 15	Day 22	Recovery days[a]
Placebo	11	−2.84	−2.05	−1.58	50
250 IU/kg	9	−2.24	−1.36	−1.30	22
500 IU/kg	9	−2.34	−1.51	−1.05	36
1,000 IU/kg	10	−1.43	−0.30	−0.21	8

[a] Median days for hemoglobin to return to 95% of baseline.

Table 4. Days for various percentages of hemoglobin recovery

Hb recovery, %	Dose groups, IU/kg			
	placebo	250	500	1,000
85	8.0	8.0	8.5	1.0
90	15.0	11.5	15.0	2.0
95	50.0	22.0	36.0	8.0

The rhEPO was well tolerated and associated with a dose-related ($p < 0.05$ bilinear regression analysis over time) hematopoietic recovery after phlebotomy. No serious adverse experiences were reported during this trial period.

In a subsequent double-blind, parallel-group study conducted at three sites, 92 healthy male subjects were hospitalized for 26 days and randomized equally to receive either 250, 500 or 1,000 IU/kg of rhEPO or placebo 3 times weekly. A total of twelve doses were administered to each patient. On each day of dosing, beginning with day 3, subjects were phlebotomized to remove 450 ml of whole blood, provided their hemoglobin was ≥12.0 g/dl. Subjects could donate a maximum of 11 units during the study. The results of this trial shown in table 5 indicated that subjects treated with rhEPO were able to donate an average of 1.78, 2.22 and 2.36 units more than the placebo group at doses of rhEPO of 250, 500 and 1,000 IU/kg, respectively. Also, subjects given 500 or 1,000 IU/kg of rhEPO were more likely to maintain hemoglobin values above 12.0 g/dl even though they were phlebotomized more frequently than

Table 5. Number and percent of subjects by total number of phlebotomies at double-blind endpoint[a]

Total number of phlebotomies performed	Placebo (n = 23)		250 IU/kg (n = 23)		500 IU/kg (n = 19)		1,000 IU/kg (n = 22)	
	n	%	n	%	n	%	n	%
3	1	4	0	0	0	0	0	0
4	1	4	0	0	0	0	0	0
5	4	17	1	4	0	0	1	5
6	6	26	3	13	1	5	2	9
7	4	17	2	9	3	16	5	23
8	5	22	5	22	5	26	1	5
9	2	9	6	26	3	16	1	5
10	0	0	5	22	5	26	9	41
11	0	0	1	4	2	11	3	14
Total units	149		192		166		192	
n	23		23		19		22	
Adjusted mean[b]	6.32		8.10		8.53		8.68	
SE	0.228		0.230		0.251		0.236	

[a] Subjects who did not complete the double-blind period were excluded.
[b] Mean adjusted by analysis of covariance.

subjects treated with 250 IU/kg of rhEPO or placebo. Figure 1 charts the mean hemoglobin values while figure 2 depicts the mean reticulocyte counts in the double-blind study period. No serious adverse experiences were reported during this trial; however, patients did complain of fatigue, nausea, asthenia, rhinitis, pharyngitis and myalgia [Chugai-Upjohn, Inc., data on file].

Maeda et al. [18] report the use of rhEPO in a Japanese population prior to orthopedic surgery. Patients donated 400 ml of blood 17, 10 and 3 days prior to surgery. Seven patients received oral iron therapy only beginning 2 weeks prior to the first donation and 5 patients received 6,000 IU of rhEPO 3 times a week, beginning 1 week prior to the first donation. Hemoglobin levels were measured at each donation and remained above 11.0 g/dl. The average hemoglobin after the third donation was significantly higher in rhEPO-treated patients compared to nontreated patients (12.7 vs. 10.7 g/dl). Two patients who

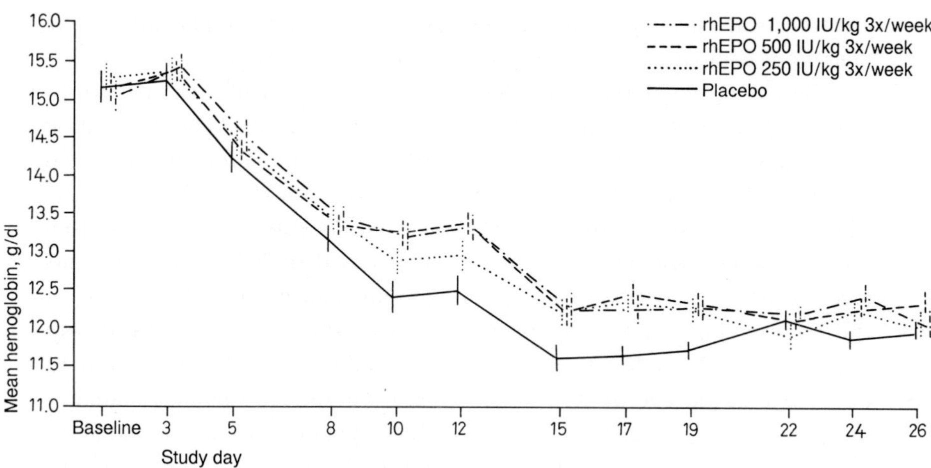

Fig. 1. Mean hemoglobin values of patients phlebotomized every third day if their hemoglobin value was ≥12 g/dl and treated with placebo or 250, 500 or 1,000 IU/kg or rhEPO 3 times weekly for a total of twelve doses. Error bars represent 1 SEM.

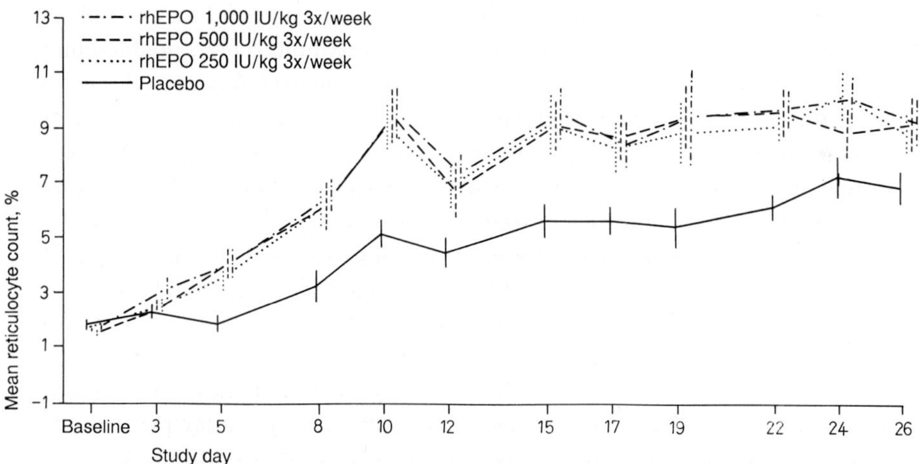

Fig. 2. Mean reticulocyte counts of patients described in figure 1 showing a higher and consistent increase in erythropoiesis evident on day 5 and persistent to day 26 in all rhEPO-treated groups compared to the placebo group. Error bars represent 1 SEM.

received iron only required homologous blood (1 and 2 units) after their operations compared to none of those who received rhEPO.

Goodnough et al. [19] confirmed the results of the Maeda et al. [18] study. This group conducted a randomized, controlled trial of rhEPO administration in 47 adults scheduled for elective orthopedic procedures. Patients received rhEPO at 600 IU/kg or placebo intravenously twice weekly for 21 days during which time up to 6 units of blood was collected. Patients were excluded from donation when their hematocrit values were less than 34% and all patients received iron sulfate at a dose of 325 mg orally 3 times daily. The dosing of rhEPO was done whether or not blood was donated. Patients treated with rhEPO were able to donate an average of 5.4 units of blood compared to 4.1 units from the placebo-treated patients. The mean red cell volume donated by the patients who received rhEPO was 41% greater than that donated by patients who received placebo (961 vs. 683 ml, $p < 0.05$). Seven of the 24 patients who received placebo were unable to donate ≥ 4 units of blood while only 1 of the 23 patients treated with rhEPO was unable to donate that volume. The frequency of adverse affects was comparable in the rhEPO and placebo groups.

Pre- and Postoperative Use of rhEPO

Animal studies have shown that pre- and postoperative use of rhEPO can be effective in accelerating the time of recovery to normal baseline red cell values in comparison to control [16]. A phase II multicenter, double-blind, parallel, randomized study was initiated to evaluate the safety and tolerability of rhEPO when administered daily in patients undergoing elective or semi-emergency surgery. The goals of the study included the exploration of safety and tolerability and the ability of rhEPO, when administered daily, to accelerate human erythropoiesis in the postoperative period. The ability of rhEPO to reduce homologous transfusions in the perioperative and postoperative periods was the most important goal. Patients eligible for the study required an operative procedure which usually resulted in blood loss which required replacement of 2 to a maximum of 6 units of red blood cells. Patients were to be randomized to receive either 250, 500 or 1,000 IU/kg of rhEPO or placebo. Medication is administered intravenously daily during a 5-day preoperative period, including the day of surgery and for up to 5 days during the postoperative period. All patients must receive a minimum of four doses of rhEPO or placebo prior to the surgery in order to continue in the study unless their hemoglobin is ≥ 16 g/dl.

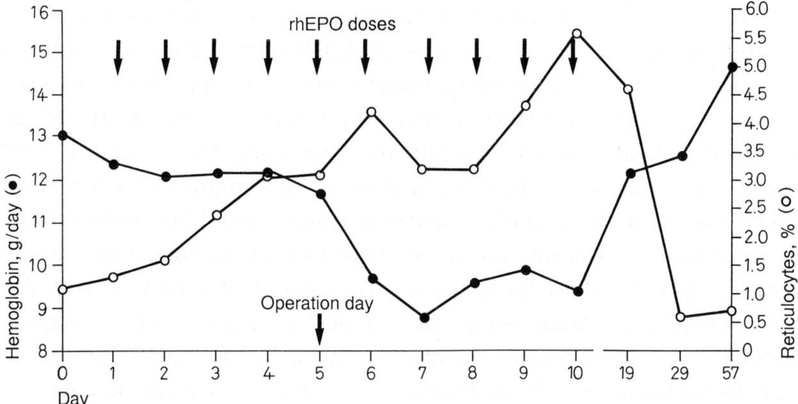

Fig. 3. Hemoglobin and reticulocyte values of an elective surgical patient treated with rhEPO 5 days pre- and postoperatively.

The decision to transfuse packed red blood cells was standardized. In this protocol, patients are considered eligible for transfusion if the hemoglobin is ≤8g/dl or their hematocrit is ≤25% or if clinical symptoms demand such an intervention. Intraoperative cell salvage and reinfusion is permitted along with predeposit autologous reinfusions. Any patient who is diagnosed with postoperative bleeding necessitating a return to the operating room for control of the bleeding is disqualified from the study.

A small number of patients have been entered into this study and since it is blinded, no dose-related patient data is available at this time. Data on 1 patient, who we believe to be on rhEPO because of the high reticulocyte count, is shown in figure 3. The preoperative hemoglobin was 13.1g/dl with the nadir at 9.6g/dl on day 6 (1 day postoperatively) and a level of 12.2 and 12.6g/dl on days 19 and 29, respectively. This example suggests that rhEPO pre- and postoperative therapy can achieve results seen in animal studies.

Discussion

Despite the efforts of a few enthusiasts, the implementation of autologous blood donation programs has been very slow to develop with considerable underutilization of those programs in eligible elective surgical patients [20]. The public's fear of AIDS transmission from homologous donors has not been quieted by the continuing advances in AIDS testing programs, which still remain imperfect. Patients facing major surgery, at which time they may be exposed to blood from a large number of homologous donors, are not eager to run the risk of surviving the procedure but contracting AIDS, hepatitis or other blood-borne infections. There now appears to be a confluence of forces which provide momentum for a major expansion of autologous blood collection methods, including preoperative predeposit, hemodilution techniques and intraoperative cell salvage. These forces include: (1.) a rising demand for blood, driven by population increases and greater surgical capabilities; (2.) a decreasing supply of donors secondary to more stringent requirements for donation; (3.) the application of new technology based on longer preservation of refrigerated red blood cells, and (4.) the availability of rhEPO to increase predeposit autologous donations and stimulate postoperative erythropoiesis.

In the most comprehensive study of predeposited autologous blood for elective surgery, Toy et al. [20] showed that only 5% of the eligible patients actually predeposited blood, indicating that predonation is not widely used. Of those who predeposited, only 13% subsequently received homologous blood, as compared with 36% of those who did not predeposit. Predonation could have avoided 68% of homologous transfusions. If all eligible patients predeposited autologous blood, they could have supplied as much as 72% of their own transfused cells.

Wasman and Goodnough [21] reported the effect on physician transfusion behavior when autologous blood donors undergoing elective surgical procedures were compared with matched controls without predeposit. Physicians tolerated significantly lower admission hematocrits (37.2 vs. 43.7%) and discharge hematocrits (32.6 vs. 35.8%) in patients with autologous predeposits compared with matched controls. Ten of 17 patients could have avoided homologous blood if 4 units of autologous blood had been donated and stored. With preoperative blood donation, patients are making two statements to their physicians. First, they agree that the likelihood of acquiring a blood transfusion during elective surgical hospitalization is significant; and second, they want to avoid, if possible, any exposure to homologous blood.

This patient signal has changed physician transfusion practice and has fueled discussion of a lower 'transfusion trigger'. Levine et al. [22] explored the optimal threshold for the initiation of transfusion therapy to a level of 15% hematocrit in unanesthetized animals. The adult baboons studied underwent an exchange transfusion with 6% hetastarch to a final hematocrit of 15%. The animals were followed for 2 months during which there was no morbidity or significant change in oxygen consumption. The animals adapted well to severe anemia. A perioperative red blood cell transfusion consensus conference also addressed the transfusion trigger in humans [23]. The conferees concluded that available evidence does not support the use of a single criteria for transfusion such as a hemoglobin concentration of $\leq 10\,g/dl$ or a hematocrit of 30%. Also, there was no evidence that mild to moderate anemia contributes to perioperative morbidity and that cardiac output does not increase dramatically in healthy humans until the hemoglobin value decreases to approximately 7.0 g/dl.

With the advent of the availability of rhEPO, the knowledge that autologous predeposits cannot generate sufficient EPO to overcome 'phlebotomy' anemia and that a significant percent of individuals can avoid homologous transfusions with just an additional predeposit of 1 or 2 units pharmacologic stimulation of erythropoiesis may help an enormous number of people avoid homologous transfusion. Studies described in this paper show that with treatment of rhEPO, 2–3 times in successive days prior to operation will increase the number of predeposit units from 1 to 2 over the usually tolerated donations by patients. There still remains a considerable amount of research required on the exact dosage schedule and dosage level. The animal and human data are, however, substantially similar.

The data supporting rhEPO treatment postoperatively is incomplete. A number of studies are underway but none have been analyzed or fully reported. The future use of rhEPO in combination with autologous blood collection methods will have to be based, as is usual in the practice of medicine, on individual circumstances. It seems that patients with infections cannot benefit from the techniques we have discussed. Artificial blood may be of eventual help in such cases. Individuals requiring immediate surgery from traumatic events will benefit from intraoperative salvage, but not from predeposit or hemodilution. Acute hemodilution also suffers from operational problems including unmonitored storage in the operating room while cell salvage may lead to air embolism and reinfusion of body fluids, fragments and irrigants and topical agents.

More patients seem to desire a zero exposure to homologous transfusions in elective surgery. It is very possible that a lower transfusion trigger and the use of rhEPO can combine to altogether avoid homologous transfusions in circumstances where 1–2 units of blood were previously administered. This is no small benefit since it is estimated that there are 6.2 million units of blood ordered (but not necessarily transfused) in procedures which require 2 or less pints of blood [Chugai-Upjohn, Inc., data on file].

There will be adverse reactions related to the use of rhEPO but none from the studies described thus far seem significant. Studies done on thousands on individuals with rhEPO given to treat anemia of chronic renal disease show rhEPO dose-related adverse events connected with AV grafts, headaches and nausea. Compared to control groups, hypertension has also been associated with rhEPO treatment as is a higher incidence of seizures in seizure-prone individuals [11]. The advent of rhEPO treatment in the practice of surgery to increase predeposit autologous transfusions and a lower transfusion trigger may be clearly beneficial to thousands of patients who wish to avoid homologous transfusions. Every transfusion that is not given has potential for lowering costs for compatibility testing, transfusion complications and increasing the general supply of blood for emergency circumstances.

Conclusions

A number of strategies are available to avoid homologous transfusions. They include preoperative donations of autologous blood of up to 3–4 units of blood in the 3–4 weeks prior to surgery. Hemodilution is another technique where 1–2 units of blood can be collected in the operating room just prior to surgery. Intraoperative cell salvage provides a means of reusing the patient's cells after being washed or filtered in circumstances where massive bleeding occurs secondary to surgery. In many circumstances, these techniques are underutilized and their use should be encouraged in the face of increasing demand for blood, secondary to greater surgical capabilities and population increases along with a decreasing supply of donors with more stringent requirements for donation. The fear of AIDS and other blood-borne diseases which can be transmitted through blood transfusions made patients extremely sensitive to the receipt of homologous transfusions. Changes in technology based on longer preservability of refrigerated blood cells and the availability of rhEPO to increase erythropoiesis are promising technological advances which will help avoid homologous transfusion exposure.

Animal studies have demonstrated that, when compared to controls, rhEPO can accelerate erythropoietic recovery as measured by hematocrit when administered in doses up to 1,000 IU/kg for 14 days postoperatively. Animal studies have also shown that increased amounts of blood can be donated with the use of rhEPO doses of 1,000 IU/kg given 5 days preoperatively and 14 days postoperatively.

Human studies of rhEPO at doses of 250, 500, 600 and 1,000 IU/kg confirmed the potential of the pharmacological erythropoietic effect to increase the ability of individuals to donate an additional 1 or 2 units of whole blood prior to elective operative procedures. Studies using rhEPO pre- and postoperatively are ongoing and preliminary results are encouraging. The use of rhEPO in combination with other autologous donation techniques already in use by surgeons, anesthesiologists and blood-bank physicians offer the potential to significantly decrease the exposure of patients to homologous transfusions and subsequently decrease transfusion reactions, lower costs and increase the blood supply in emergency circumstances.

References

1 Beal, R.; Isbister, J.: Blood component therapy in clinical practice. Oxford Scientific, Oxford 1985.

2 Fielding, L.; Red for danger: Blood transfusion and colorectal cancer (editorial). Br. Med. J. *291:* 841–842 (1985).

3 Kessler, C.; Schulob, R.; Goldstein, A.: Abnormal T-lymphocyte subpopulations associated with transfusion of blood-derived products. Lancet *i:* 991 (1983).

4 Surgenor, D.: The patient's own blood is the safest blood. N. Engl. J. Med. *316:* 542–544 (1987).

5 Council on Scientific Affairs: Autologous blood transfusions. JAMA *256:* 2378–2380 (1986).

6 Erslev, A.: Humoral regulations of red blood cell production. Blood *8:* 349–387 (1953).

7 McGonigle, R.; Wallin, J.; Shadduck, R.; Fisher, J.: Erythropoietin deficiency and inhibition of erythropoiesis in renal insufficiency. Kidney Int. *35:* 437–444 (1984).

8 Miyake, T.; Kung, C.; Goldwasser, E.: Purification of human erythropoietin. J. Biol. Chem. *252:* 5558–5564 (1977).

9 Jacobs, K.; Shoemaker, C.; Rudersdorf, R.; Neill, S.; Kaufman, R.; Mufson, A.; Seehra, J.; Jones, S.; Hewick, R; Fritsch, E.; Kawakita, M.; Shimizu, T.; Miyake, T.: Isolation and characterization of genomic and cDNA clones of human erythropoietin. Nature *313:* 806–810 (1985).

10 Eschbach, J.; Egrie, J.; Downing, M.; Browne, J.; Adamson, J.: Correction of the anemia of end-stage renal disease with recombinant human erythropoietin. N. Engl. J. Med. *316:* 73–78 (1987).

11 Sobota, J.: Erythropoietin treatment of end-stage renal disease: North American and Japanese experiences; in Garnick (ed.): Erythropoietin in Clinical Applications: An International Perspective; 1st ed. (Dekker, New York 1990).

12 Kickler, T.; Spivak, J.: Effect of repeated whole blood donations on serum immunoreactive erythropoietin levels in autologous donors. JAMA *260:* 65–67 (1988).

13 Al-Khatti, A.; Veith, R.; Papayannopoulou, T. et al.: Stimulation of fetal hemoglobin synthesis by erythropoietin in baboons. N. Engl. J. Med. *317:* 415–420 (1987).

14 Levine, E.; Rosen, A.; Gould, S.; Sehgal, L.; Egrie, J.; Browne, J.; Sehgal, H.; Moss,

G.: Recombinant human erythropoietin and autologous blood donation. Surgery. *104:* 365–369 (1988).

15 Levine, E.; Rosen, A.; Sehgal, L.; Gould, S.; Egrie, J.; Sehgal, H.; Moss, G.: Treatment of acute postoperative anemia with recombinant human erythropoietin. J. Trauma *29:* 1134–1139 (1989).

16 Levine, E.; Gould, S.; Rosen, A.; Sehgal, L.; Egrie, J.; Sehgal, H.; Levine, H.; Moss, G.: Perioperative recombinant human erythropoietin. Surgery *106:* 432–438 (1989).

17 Vlasses, P.; Flamenbaum, W.; Whalen, J.; Bennett, D.; Bjornsson, T.; Erslev, A.: Initial evalution of hematopoietic effects of recombinant human erythropoietin in healthy subjects undergoing phlebotomy (abstract). Clin. Pharmacol. Ther. *45:* 136 (1989).

18 Madea, H.; Hitomi, Y.; Hirata, R.; Tohyama, H.; Suwata, J.; Tsuzuki, N.; Shindo, H.: Erythropoietin and autologous blood donation. Lancet *i:* 284 (1989).

19 Goodnough, L.; Rudnick, S.; Price, T.; Ballas, S.; Collins, M.;Crowley, J.; Kosmin, M.; Kruskall, M.; Lenes, B.; Menitove, J.; Silberstein, L.; Smith, K.; Wallas, C.; Abels, R.; Von Tress, M.: Increased preoperative collection of autologous blood with recombinant human erythropoietin therapy. N. Engl. J. Med. *321:* 1163–1168 (1989).

20 Toy, P.; Strauss, R.; Stehling, L.; Sears, R.; Price, T.; Rossi, E.; Collins, M.; Crowley, J.; Eisenstaedt, R.; Goodnough, T.; Greenwalt, T.; Johnston, M.; Kennedy, M.; Lenes, B.; Lusher, J.; Mintz, P.; Patten, E.; Simon, T.; Westphal, R.: Predeposited autologous blood for elective surgery. N. Engl. J. Med. *316:* 517–520 (1987).

21 Wasman, J.; Goodnough, L.: Autologous blood donation for elective surgery. JAMA *258:* 3135–3137 (1987).

22 Levine, E.; Rosen, A.; Sehgal, L.; Gould, S.; Moss, G.: Physiologic effects of acute anemia: implications for a reduced transfusion trigger. Transfusion *30:*11–14 (1990).

23 National Institutes of Health, Red Blood Cell Transfusion Consensus Conference: Perioperative red blood cell transfusion. JAMA *260:* 2700–2703 (1988).

Joseph T. Sobota, MD, Executive Vice President and Chief Operating Officer, Chugai-Upjohn, Inc., 6133 North River Road, Suite 800, Rosemont, IL 60018 (USA)

Gurland HJ, Moran J, Samtleben W, Scigalla P, Wieczorek L (eds): Erythropoietin in
Renal and Non-Renal Anemias. Contrib Nephrol. Basel, Karger, 1991, vol 88, pp 349–350

Discussion

to the Papers by E. A. Levine and J. T. Sobota

Birgegård (Uppsala): Dr. Levine, you set the criterion for the use of EPO at a need for a
3 unit transfusion at operation. Now I want to ask what makes it so difficult to obtain 4 units
from a patient before operation. You said that you had a mean donation of less than 3 units
and I don't understand the reason for that. We have published a study on hip joint surgery in
an elderly population where it was very easy to take 4 U within 11 days. We then let them rest
for 3 weeks. They had not come back to the original hemoglobin level at the time of
operation, but still it was quite feasible to do it in that way. So I think that if you are going to
give EPO to every patient who needs 3 units of blood a lot of patients will be treated
unnecessarily.

Levine: When you talk about autologous donation there are a number of variables that
come into play. One is, as I suggested, many patients who might need them are unable to
donate 3 units very easily. Even in a group of elderly patients there are a number of things that
can be done to avoid homologous exposure. I don't think there is anything magic about the
figure of 3 units, and I don't mean to imply that there should be an iron-clad guideline. On the
other hand, if you have a patient whom you expect to require more than 3 units of blood, I
think you should probably do something more than preoperative autologous donation, because the majority of patients, perhaps unlike your group, will be unable to donate the amount
of blood you hope to have available when you operate.

Wardrop (Cardiff): Sometimes inflammatory and infective complications occur after
surgery. Have you evidence that, when they occurred in your patients, the response to
perioperative EPO was depressed?

Sobota: We have not analysed that data.

Levine: I don't think it is known what will happen to someone who develops a septic
complication in the perioperative period. All patients who undergo an operative procedure
are going to have some element of inflammation, by the nature of surgery, and it is difficult to
predict what a patient's erythropoietic response would be, as you suggest. One advantage of
giving the patients rhEPO preoperatively as part of an autologous blood donation program is
that this may avoid that sort of problem in the perioperative period.

Eschbach (Seattle): I look forward to seeing the results of your data, Dr. Sobota,
because I hope that patients will respond at the large doses you are giving. However, I am a
little sceptical, based upon some experience in our dialysis population. We published in the

Quarterly Journal of Medicine in December 1989 a graph of 4 patients who had elective hip surgery. They had stable hematocrits prior to surgery on doses of rhEPO of about 75–150 U/kg 3 times a week. Several of the patients self-donated their own blood. In 3 of the 4 patients, despite transfusion, the hematocrits dropped to 18%. They stayed at this level for 5 weeks despite continuing the same dose of rhEPO. After this time they started to respond again. The serum iron, percent transferrin saturation and the ferritin levels changed markedly, indicative of an inflammatory disorder. So I think hip surgery represents a fairly severe type of surgical inflammation which temporarily blocks the response to rhEPO.

Levine: The Goodnough study was done exclusively on orthopedic surgical patients. Those patients were followed for longer than the time I actually discussed here and they didn't have the sort of problems you described. Whether those problems are unique to the dialysis population I cannot say.

Jacobs (Cardiff): Can I ask Dr. Sobota about his perioperative EPO. You refer to patients who might need 1 or 2 U of blood and sometimes of course they don't in fact need transfusion. If you have given them perioperative EPO, might you not end up with an increase in hemoglobin more than you actually want with a consequent increased risk of post-operative thrombosis?

Sobota: Such side effects are possible, but in the normal practice of medicine if you have no blood loss during surgery, and therefore no perioperative transfusion, no perioperative or postoperative rhEPO should be given. Preoperative treatment with multiple doses of 1,000 U/kg are recommended only when autologous predeposits of blood are made by the patient.

Essers (Aachen): I wonder about Dr. Levine's sampling time. You need 6 weeks to get the blood. If you store the blood for 6 weeks, you cannot store it at 4°C but must freeze it.

Levine: I didn't mean to suggest that you should store the blood for 6 weeks. CPDA-1 bags are only good for 5 weeks, according to the American Association of Blood Banks standards. My experimental protocol lasted 5 weeks, and this was for the purposes of the study. This length of time is not suggested for clinical practice.

Gurland HJ, Moran J, Samtleben W, Scigalla P, Wieczorek L (eds): Erythropoietin in
Renal and Non-Renal Anemias. Contrib Nephrol. Basel, Karger, 1991, vol 88, pp 351–357

Concluding Remarks

by *E. Goldwasser* and *J.W. Eschbach*

E. Goldwasser: I hope I can be permitted the luxury of rambling a bit
because I didn't realize until this afternoon that I had to replace half of David
Golde (unfortunately prevented from attending the Workshop [The Eds]). So
that the rambling won't be too bad, I will try to restrict my comments to those
aspects of this meeting which involve something I know a little bit about, and
that is the basic science of EPO. As far as the clinical matters go, my ignorance
is so profound that I'm very glad to have Joe Eschbach sitting next to me to
handle that aspect of the meeting.

Those of us who have been in the EPO field for a long time, and I can spot
them in the audience, must all feel a sense of great gratification, that meetings
like this have developed from rather obscure beginnings; from a field which
nobody took very seriously except those of us working in it, and even then,
sometimes, we didn't take it too seriously. It is an astonishing turn of events,
for me at any rate, that here is a room full of people interested in EPO. Not too
long ago, I doubt if we could have filled two tables with people interested in
EPO. So the gratification is quite significant.

Along with the gratification we also get, I confess, problems. One of the
problems that came immediately to mind, listening to today's and yesterday's
presentations, is the question of what happened to the simple biology that we
all knew about with regard to EPO. It used to be a very simple subject. If you
are anemic you make EPO and it corrected, the anemia, that was about it. I'm
completely baffled by so many things that have been said in the last couple of
days that I can't even begin to approach an understanding of them.

Let me briefly summarize what I considered the features of the basic
science part of the program: We jointly discussed the control of the expression
of the EPO gene both at the transcriptional and at the translational level and I

think we all are in fairly reasonable agreement that the control is not a simple one, there are several factors involving control of the EPO gene: they can include those factors that are involved in transcription, those involving the stability of the transcript and factors involving translation and a lot of other things that weren't spoken about, remembering that EPO is a secreted product. It must get to the outside of the cell and there may well be control mechanisms on how the package of this glycoprotein gets delivered to the circulation. The question of what are the kidney cells that make and secrete EPO is still one that excites a lot of passion and a determination to do more experiments. I think we need a lot more experimental work to resolve the problems and get some critical data. The mechanism by which the cell, whatever it may be, recognizes hypoxia is beginning to be understood. And I have a lot of confidence that that problem may be solved before there's another meeting similar to this one.

There are two problems related to that, which don't seem immediately on the verge of solution. Assuming, for the moment, that the mechanism by which Mark Goldberg and Frank Bunn have explained the mechanism of response to hypoxia, involving a hemeprotein is correct the next step must be studied. How does the chromosome know what happened to that hypoxia sensor? It is still not at all clear, nor is the experimental approach to it clear.

On the other side of the EPO: target cell axis, we heard a great deal about receptors. There are still many problems involving the EPO receptors and how EPO does what it does. I have to confess, parenthetically, that after about 35 years in the EPO field, I still feel that it's absolutely remarkable that there is a very ordinary glycoprotein that can tell cells that their progeny are going to be red cells. This, to me, is a remarkable biological phenomenon. The chemistry of the receptors, as with the chemistry of EPO, is still far from being understood. We don't yet have a clear idea, whether the receptors are monomers, multimers, heterodimers, or homodimers. Nor do we have a clue yet about the meaning of the two classes of receptors, or about the great mystery that Alan D'Andrea has talked about – the gp 55 interacting with the receptor. The follow-up steps of what happens after the ligand-receptor interaction occurs are not known. What is the signal transduction mechanism? How do the genes in the target cells know that this interaction has happened and tell the cell to become a red cell? We don't have a clear understanding of that yet, in spite of a lot of work in a lot of laboratories. So what we need, in addition to more work, is some good ideas.

The question that we discussed at great length this morning about a possible down-regulation of EPO secretion permitted Stanley Shaldon to describe me (I'm paraphrasing a bit) as an aging dogmatist. I've always thought of myself as a youthful iconoclast, but I agree with Stanley that it's very easy to be dogmatic about other peoples' experiments and so I'll continue to do that. I can't do anything about the aging. The speculation that came out of the discussion, I think, is a good thing, it's good to shake things up every now and then, to focus our attention on the fact that there is a lot we don't understand. We can fill days and days full of slides with all sorts of data but there's lot of biology that needs to be understood.

Some of the material that was presented in this meeting points up some of the problems that we have to come to grips with. For instance, what happens to EPO after it is administered? That seems to be a big mystery. Where does it go, how does it get broken down? It must get broken down; it does disappear, but we don't know a thing about it. The question was raised informally, that maybe we're facing this kind of problem because recombinant EPO and natural EPO may be not identical. I don't think that is the case. All the structural information that is available to date, including really remarkable details on carbohydrate structure, has revealed essentially no significant difference between urinary or natural and recombinant EPO. I don't think we can blame it on the fact that material is expressed by Chinese hamster ovary cells with an amplified human gene. I think we better design experimental approaches to the problem and not try and explain it away. The other problem can be expressed as: what is happening in human beings with very large EPO concentrations who don't seem to respond to all of that endogenous EPO and then after receiving a modest amount more do respond? I don't understand it and I hope that someone who does can explain it to me. For instance, the circulating level of EPO in normal human beings is about 20 mU/ml. That value, (perhaps with some disagreement by a factor of 2 or 3) permits or drives the synthesis of about 2.5 million red cells per second for all of our lives. It is fairly easy to get that rate of synthesis up to 17–20 million red cells per second at an EPO titer which won't be much greater than 1,000 mU/ml, if that high. What is the meaning then, of seeing titers much higher than that, where there doesn't seem to be much response and then, finding a response when exogenous material is administered on top of the endogenous amount, I just don't understand it. In that context, I can add, perhaps, a note of caution which I alluded to earlier today. Much of what we are doing now is dependent on interpreting radioimmunoassays and as Mary Cotes can testify, because she has done some of the more definitive studies, there are lots of ways that the RIA can fool us. Remember that the radioimmunoassay is a competitive assay, that the fewer counts you get at the end, the more EPO you had in what was competing. There are lots of ways of getting few counts without having any EPO in there, proteolytic action on the labeled material is one way. So I think we have to be very careful about interpreting these results and to be somewhat hesitant about accepting titers as reflecting something of great importance biologically until we can verify that what we measure is biologically active. There is clearly a great need for better assays. We need an assay which is more specific biologically, more convenient than the bioassay, more sensitive than the bioassay; and which will be able to discriminate between intact EPO and pieces of EPO which might have immunologic epitopes.

I can finish my rambling comments by quoting what I have heard attributed to Albert Einstein. He is reported to have said that biology was too complicated for biologists. Unfortunately we biologists are the only ones doing biology so we have to face up to the variety of problems. If they are too complicated for us, we may have to shatter them into less complicated bits so we can work on them.

I would like to end by saying that meetings like this are very useful, not so much for the data which can always be published and we can all read, but for the fact that we talk to each other as well as sit here and think our thoughts while other people are talking. Those thoughts frequently include things we would like to do, experiments we would like to be able to do to answer questions raised by other people. Now I'll turn the microphone over to Dr. Eschbach who can explain all these complicated things to me.

J.W. Eschbach: Thank you, Dr. Goldwasser. I want to thank Prof. Gurland and Boehringer Mannheim for this meeting. As we look back to the first meeting two and a half years ago, there has certainly been a lot of progress. I think that we now know that rhEPO is as remarkably safe and effective hormone in renal failure and now we are learning about its use in other conditions. What I would like to do is summarize very briefly what I have heard these last 2 days and then end with 6 or 7 issues that I would like to present to you for our future consideration. Dr. Keown, in talking about quality of life for dialysis patients treated with rhEPO in Canada, showed a slight, but not significant, improvement in some aspects of quality of life when the hemoglobin was 11.5–13 g vs. 9.5–11 g. One of the issues is what should the target hematocrit be for dialysis patients? We need more data like that. Dr. Bahlmann showed there was no change in the mortality with erythropoietin therapy and Dr. Samtleben showed that patients' survival was 94% at 2 years vs. 81% of non-treated EPO patients in Europe, but we have to realize that the EPO-treated patients were a selected group of patients and it really does not indicate a true improvement in survival. Many of us would like to hope that survival is improved, but we need more data to determine that. Dr. Koch showed that one of the risk factors for the hypertension that develops in some patients receiving recombinant human erythropoietin that have renal failure may be an inability of the elevated cardiac output to decrease as the anemia is improved. That whole area needs further investigation. Four different centers looked at the issue of subcutaneous administration: Dr. Bommer, Dr. Granolleras, Dr. Mion, and Dr. Bergström. And all of them have shown that subcutaneous administration, at least in small groups of patients, seems to be far more effective than intravenous therapy especially when given daily. So it appears that around 70 U/kg per week when given daily subcutaneously may be enough to increase the hematocrit up to the target range, both for CAPD patients and hemodialysis patients. Dr. Macdougall indicated that the site of subcutaneous injection based upon studies in normal volunteers, would be best in the thigh, the absorption is about twice as much in the thigh versus the abdomen or upper arm and that the bioavailability is increased from that site. Dr. Brown showed that viscosity, which increases as the hematocrit increases, does not seem to be deleterious to the patient with diabetes mellitus who we know has increased vascular problems, and doesn't seem to interfere with renal function. And this was confirmed by Dr. Koene who showed in predialysis patients that renal dysfunction is not accelerated with improvement in the hematocrit. In children, the data so far show that growth is not enhanced when the hematocrit is increased to 28–31 and hopefully with earlier treatment and higher hematocrits there may be improvement in growth. Of the other anemias unrelated to renal disease, we've heard that anemias of tumors seem to respond to rhEPO, whether they are solid or hematologic tumors, although there is some variability depending upon the erythropoietin levels of these patients. Dr. Herrmann, Dr. Miller, Dr. Jacobs, and Dr. Hirashima all presented very fascinating reports to us. And, finally, this afternoon, we've heard about the response to rhEPO in anemias of AIDS patients treated with AZT, and patients with rheumatoid arthritis which are very promising. Hopefully, the anemia of prematurity will respond to larger doses of EPO. The role of rhEPO in pre- and postoperative autologous blood donations? There is no question it works preoperatively, but, postoperatively, it remains to be determined. I think one of the issues is whether it will be cost effective.

Let me close by mentioning 7 issues of biologic and practical concern. Dr. Goldwasser has already mentioned my first concern: Why do patients with high endogenous erythropoietin levels respond when their EPO levels increase only modestly with subcutaneous rhEPO injections? A second issue is why is erythropoietin production inappropriately decreased in some anemias with normal exocrine renal function? In the past, we have only discussed renal function in relation to exocrine function. I think we need to think in terms of both endocrine and exocrine function of the kidney since there may be a dichotomy between the two. There may be rises in serum creatinine that imply that there is some exocrine dysfunction, but that doesn't necessarily tell us whether there is abnormal renal endocrine function and there may be normal exocrine functions with inappropriate endocrine function. So I wonder whether we are going to have to define renal function in different ways than we have in the past. A third issue is whether the receptor response is different in different diseases? I look forward to more information on that. In terms of the use of rhEPO for patients with renal disease I see three other major issues: (1) What should be the target hematocrit or hemoglobin? Our clinical trials have set different levels, yet we have no good yardstick to say what it should be. It's basically empiric, but we need some kind of objective, quantitative test that would help us in this regard. I suspect there are some patients that clearly need higher levels, those patients that are probably anephric with hypotension and, patients with chronic obstructive pulmonary disease who require more oxygen-carrying capacity. We need to be careful that we don't fix ourselves at a specific target hematocrit or hemoglobin just because patients start to feel better. We need some objective criteria that tells us what is the best level for patients. (2) The second issue in terms of practice is what should our route of administration be and what should be the frequency? We've heard today that daily subcutaneous injections appear to be the best and yet, there is some controversy on that. I think Dr. Bommer showed us that there was only about a 15–20% reduction from i.v. to s.c. in the requirements of EPO in a larger center study. He was able to achieve a much greater reduction in EPO dosage with subcutaneous versus intravenous than this other center. If these early results hold up, then I certainly would favor that all dialysis and predialysis patients be treated daily with subcutaneous erythropoietin just as any other hormone deficiency is treated, i.e. like diabetes mellitus. We are dealing with a hormonal deficiency state and we might as well forget about treating it in relationship to dialysis and treat it in relation to the hormone deficiency. Why not teach everybody to inject themselves daily? I think it can be done, but it's going to be hard for some patients that are on hemodialysis that are used to having everything injected intravenously. But I think it may probably make more physiologic sense to do it that way. (3) The third point on practice is : Will the adverse effects really be decreased with subcutaneous injections? I think we need more experience to answer this. I suspect that iron deficiency will be less because we are not going to be driving the marrow quite as hard with lower doses subcutaneously. And, whether there will be less hypertension remains to be determined. We have heard from Dr. Mion that many of his patients became more hypertensive with daily subcutaneous injections, whereas Dr. Bergström's patients didn't become more hypertensive.

My seventh and closing comment has to do with the abuse of erythropoietin. I am very concerned about this and I hope the rest of you are as well. I think all of us – physicians, as well as industry – need to do our best to make sure that this drug remains the wonder-drug that it is, and that it does not get tainted, as did androgens, by its abuse by athletes. We all know it will be difficult to monitor the use of rhEPO in athletes. Athletes, assuming that they use rhEPO illicitly, will have the tendency to think that, if a little makes a difference, a lot more rhEPO will even be better. It will be tragic if young athletes die from hyperviscosity problems. I personally think it's going to take a lot of education on our part to speak to athletes, trainees in high schools and colleges, and professional athletic organizations to try to minimize the abuse of rhEPO, because it will only hurt our profession, the biotechnology industry, and our patients in the long run. Thank you.

Subject Index